Core Curriculum for Nephrology Nursing

Sixth Edition

Editor: Caroline S. Counts, MSN, RN, CNN

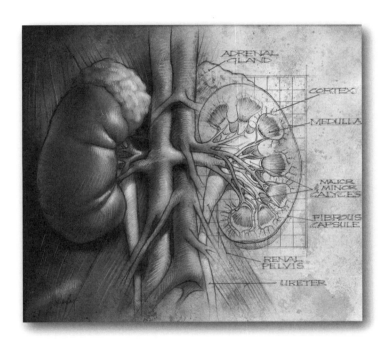

MODULE 4

Acute Kidney Injury

ANNA American Nephrology Nurses' Association
www.annanurse.org

Core Curriculum for Nephrology Nursing, 6th Edition

Editor and Project Director
Caroline S. Counts, MSN, RN, CNN

MODULE 4 • Acute Kidney Injury
Module Editor: Helen F. Williams

Publication Management
Anthony J. Jannetti, Inc.
East Holly Avenue/Box 56
Pitman, New Jersey 08071-0056

Managing Editor: Claudia Cuddy
Editorial Coordinator: Joseph Tonzelli
Layout Design and Production: Claudia Cuddy
Layout Assistants: Kaytlyn Mroz, Katerina DeFelice, Casey Shea, Courtney Klauber
Design Consultants: Darin Peters, Jack M. Bryant
Proofreaders: Joseph Tonzelli, Evelyn Haney, Alex Grover, Nicole Ward
Cover Design: Darin Peters
Cover Illustration: Scott M. Holladay © 2006
Photography: Kim Counts and Marty Morganello (*unless otherwise credited*)

ANNA National Office Staff
Executive Director: Michael Cunningham
Director of Membership Services: Lou Ann Leary
Membership/Marketing Services Coordinator: Lauren McKeown
Manager, Chapter Services: Janet Betts
Education Services Coordinator: Kristen Kellenyi
Executive Assistant & Marketing Manager, Advertising: Susan Iannelli
Co-Directors of Education Services: Hazel A. Dennison and Sally Russell
Program Manager, Special Projects: Celess Tyrell
Director, Jannetti Publications, Inc.: Kenneth J. Thomas
Managing Editor, *Nephrology Nursing Journal*: Carol Ford
Editorial Coordinator, *Nephrology Nursing Journal:* Joseph Tonzelli
Subscription Manager, *Nephrology Nursing Journal*: Rob McIlvaine
Managing Editor, *ANNA Update*, *ANNA E-News*, & Web Editor: Kathleen Thomas
Director of Creative Design & Production: Jack M. Bryant
Layout and Design Specialist: Darin Peters
Creative Designer: Bob Taylor
Director of Public Relations and Association Marketing Services: Janet D'Alesandro
Public Relations Specialist: Rosaria Mineo
Vice President, Fulfillment and Information Services: Rae Ann Cummings
Director, Internet Services: Todd Lockhart
Director of Corporate Marketing: Tom Greene
Exhibit Coordinator: Miriam Martin
Conference Manager: Jeri Hendrie
Comptroller: Patti Fortney

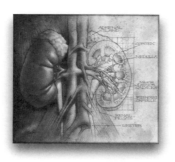

Foreword

The American Nephrology Nurses' Association has had a long-standing commitment to providing the tools and resources needed for individuals to be successful in their professional nephrology roles. With that commitment, we proudly present the sixth edition of the *Core Curriculum for Nephrology Nursing*.

This edition has a new concept and look that we hope you find valuable. Offered in six separate modules, each one will focus on a different component of our specialty and provide essential, updated, high-quality information. Since our last publication of the *Core Curriculum* in 2008, our practice has evolved, and our publication has been transformed to keep pace with those changes.

Under the expert guidance of Editor and Project Director Caroline S. Counts, MSN, RN, CNN (who was also the editor for the 2008 *Core Curriculum!*), this sixth edition continues to build on our fundamental principles and standards of practice. From the basics of each modality to our roles in advocacy, patient engagement, evidence-based practice, and more, you will find crucial information to facilitate the important work you do on a daily basis.

The ANNA Board of Directors and I extend our sincerest gratitude to Caroline and commend her for the stellar work that she and all of the section editors, authors, and reviewers have put forth in developing this new edition of the *Core Curriculum for Nephrology Nursing*. These individuals have spent many hours working to provide you with this important nephrology nursing publication. We hope you enjoy this exemplary professional resource.

Sharon Longton, BSN, RN, CNN, CCTC
ANNA President, 2014-2015

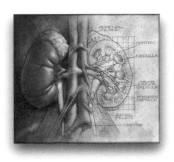

What's new in the sixth edition?

The 2015 edition of the *Core Curriculum for Nephrology Nursing* reflects several changes in format and content. These changes have been made to make life easier for the reader and to improve the scientific value of the *Core*.

1. The *Core Curriculum* is divided into six separate modules that can be purchased as a set or as individual texts. Keep in mind there is likely additional relevant information in more than one module. For example, in Module 2 there is a specific chapter for nutrition, but the topic of nutrition is also addressed in several chapters in other modules.

2. The *Core* is available in both print and electronic formats. The electronic format contains links to other websites with additional helpful information that can be reached with a simple click. With this useful feature comes a potential issue: when an organization changes its website and reroutes its links, the URLs that are provided may not connect. When at the organization's website, use their search feature to easily find your topic. The links in the *Core* were updated as of March 2015.

3. As with the last edition of the *Core*, the pictures on chapter covers depict actual nephrology staff members and patients with kidney disease. Their willingness to participate is greatly appreciated.

4. Self-assessment questions are included at the end of each module for self-testing. Completion of these exercises is not required to obtain CNE. CNE credit can be obtained by accessing the Evaluation Forms on the ANNA website.

5. References are cited in the text and listed at the end of each chapter.

6. We've provided examples of references in APA format at the beginning of each chapter, as well as on the last page of this front matter, to help the readers know how to properly format references if they use citations from the *Core*. The guesswork has been eliminated!

7. The information contained in the *Core* has been expanded, and new topics have been included. For example, there is information on leadership and management, material on caring for Veterans, more emphasis on patient and staff safety, and more.

8. Many individuals assisted in making the *Core* come to fruition; they brought with them their own experience, knowledge, and literature search. As a result, a topic can be addressed from different perspectives, which in turn gives the reader a more global view of nephrology nursing.

9. This edition employs usage of the latest terminology in nephrology patterned after the National Kidney Foundation.

10. The *Core Curriculum for Nephrology Nursing*, 6th edition contains 233 figures, 234 tables, and 29 appendices. These add valuable tools in delivering the contents of the text.

Thanks to B. Braun Medical Inc. for its grant in support of ANNA's *Core Curriculum*.

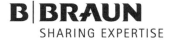

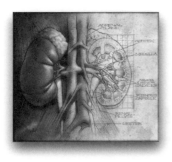

Preface

The sixth edition of the *Core Curriculum for Nephrology Nursing* has been written and published due to the efforts of many individuals. Thank you to the editors, authors, reviewers, and everyone who helped pull the *Core* together to make it the publication it became. A special thank you to Claudia Cuddy and Joe Tonzelli, who were involved from the beginning to the end — I could not have done my job without them!

The overall achievement is the result of the unselfish contributions of each and every individual team member. At times it was a daunting, challenging task, but the work is done, and all members of the "Core-team" should feel proud of the end product.

Now, the work is turned over to you — the reader and learner. I hope you learn at least half as much as I did as pieces of the *Core* were submitted, edited, and refined. Considering the changes that have taken place since the first edition of the *Core* in 1987 (322 pages!), one could say it is a whole new world! Even since the fifth edition in 2008, many changes in nephrology have transpired. This, the 2015 edition, is filled with the latest information regarding kidney disease, its treatment, and the nursing care involved.

But, buyer, beware! Evolution continues, and what is said today can be better said tomorrow. Information continues to change and did so even as the chapters were being written; yet, change reflects progress. Our collective challenge is to learn from the *Core*, be flexible, keep an open mind, and question what could be different or how nephrology nursing practice could be improved.

Nephrology nursing will always be stimulating, learning will never end, and progress will continue! So, the *Core* not only represents what we know now, but also serves as a springboard for what the learner can become and what nephrology nursing can be. A Chinese proverb says this: "Learning is like rowing upstream; not to advance is to drop back."

A final thank-you to the Core-team and a very special note of appreciation to those I love the most. (Those I love the most have also grown since the last edition!) For their love, support, and encouragement, I especially thank my husband, Henry, who thought I had retired; my son and daughter-in law, Chris and Christina, and our two amazing grandchildren, Cate and Olin; and my son-in-law, Marty Morganello, and our daughter, Kim, who provided many of the photographs used in this version of the *Core*. It has been a family project!

Last, but certainly not least, I thank the readers and learners. It is your charge to use the *Core* to grow your minds. Minds can grow as long as we live — don't drop back!

Caroline S. Counts
Editor, Sixth Edition

Module 4

Acute is described on MedicineNet.com as an illness with an abrupt onset that is often of short duration, rapidly progressive, and in need of urgent care. Once the symptoms appear, they can change or worsen swiftly. Synonyms of acute include severe, critical, drastic, dire, dreadful, terrible, awful, grave, bad, serious, desperate, and dangerous. The nurses who work with patients with acute kidney injury (AKI) know these descriptions are accurate. They also know that there is enough information to warrant a separate module devoted to AKI. The work of Helen Williams, who served as the module's editor, is greatly appreciated.

This module offers information on managing an acute care program, causes of AKI, and the nutritional needs of the patient. Hemodialysis, water treatment, peritoneal dialysis, continuous renal replacement therapy (CRRT), slow low-efficiency daily dialysis (SLEDD), and therapeutic apheresis are all topics addressed in this module. There is also a new chapter that nurses in the chronic setting will find useful; it addresses the patient who has a ventricular assist device (VAD). More patients with VADs are requiring dialysis, yet there has been little published on this subject.

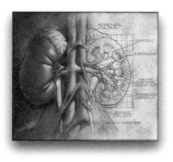

Chapter Editors and Authors

Lisa Ales, MSN, NP-C, FNP-BC, CNN
Clinical Educator, Renal
Baxter Healthcare Corporation
Deerfield, IL
Author: Module 3, Chapter 4

Kim Alleman, MS, APRN, FNP-BC, CNN-NP
Nurse Practitioner
Hartford Hospital Transplant Program
Hartford, CT
Editor: Module 6

Billie Axley, MSN, RN, CNN
Director, Innovations Group
FMS Medical Office
Franklin, TN
Author: Module 4, Chapter 3

Donna Bednarski, MSN, RN, ANP-BC, CNN, CNP
Nurse Practitioner, Dialysis Access Center
Harper University Hospital
Detroit, MI
Editor & Author: Module 1, Chapter 3
Editor & Author: Module 2, Chapter 3
Author: Module 6, Chapter 3

Brandy Begin, BSN, RN, CNN
Pediatric Dialysis Coordinator
Lucile Packard Children's Hospital at Stanford
Palo Alto, CA
Author: Module 5, Chapter 1

Deborah Brommage, MS, RDN, CSR, CDN
Program Director
National Kidney Foundation
New York, NY
Editor & Author: Module 2, Chapter 4
Editor: Module 4, Chapter 3

Deborah H. Brooks, MSN, ANP-BC, CNN, CNN-NP
Nurse Practitioner
Medical University of South Carolina
Charleston, SC
Author: Module 6, Chapter 1

Colleen M. Brown, MSN, APRN, ANP-BC
Transplant Nurse Practitioner
Hartford Hospital
Hartford, CT
Author: Module 6, Chapter 3

Loretta Jackson Brown, PhD, RN, CNN
Health Communication Specialist
Centers for Disease Control and Prevention
Atlanta, GA
Author: Module 2, Chapter 3

Molly Cahill, MSN, RN, APRN, BC, ANP-C, CNN
Nurse Practitioner
KC Kidney Consultants
Kansas City, MO
Author: Module 2, Chapter 3

Sally F. Campoy, DNP, ANP-BC, CNN-NP
Nurse Practitioner, Renal Section
Department of Veterans Affairs
Eastern Colorado Health System
Denver VA Medical Center, Denver, CO
Author: Module 6, Chapter 2

Laurie Carlson, MSN, RN
Transplant Coordinator
University of California –
   San Francisco Medical Center
San Francisco, CA
Author: Module 3, Chapter 1

Deb Castner, MSN, APRN, ACNP, CNN
Nurse Practitioner
Jersey Coast Nephrology & Hypertension
   Associates
Brick, NJ
Author: Module 2, Chapter 3
Author: Module 3, Chapter 2

Louise Clement, MS, RDN, CSR, LD
Renal Dietitian
Fresenius Medical Care
Lubbock, TX
Author: Module 2, Chapter 4

Jean Colaneri, ACNP-BC, CNN
Clinical Nurse Specialist and Nurse
   Practitioner, Dialysis Apheresis
Albany Medical Center Hospital, Albany, NY
Editor & Author: Module 3, Chapter 1

Ann Beemer Cotton, MS, RDN, CNSC
Clinical Dietitian Specialist in Critical Care
IV Health/Methodist Campus
Indianapolis, IN
Author: Module 2, Chapter 4
Author: Module 4, Chapter 2

Caroline S. Counts, MSN, RN, CNN
Research Coordinator, Retired
Division of Nephrology
Medical Unversity of South Carolina
Charleston, SC
Editor: Core Curriculum for Nephrology Nursing
Author: Module 1, Chapter 2
Author: Module 2, Chapter 6
Author: Module 3, Chapter 3

Helen Currier, BSN, RN, CNN, CENP
Director, Renal Services, Dialysis/Pheresis,
   Vascular Access/Wound, Ostomy,
   Continence, & Palliative Care Services
Texas Children's Hospital, Houston, TX
Author: Module 6, Chapter 5

Kim Deaver, MSN, RN, CNN
Program Manager
University of Virginia
Charlottesville, VA
Editor & Author: Module 3, Chapter 3

Anne Diroll, MA, BSN, BS, RN, CNN
Consultant
Volume Management
Rocklin, CA
Author: Module 5, Chapter 1

Daniel Diroll, MA, BSN, BS, RN
Education Coordinator
Fresenius Medical Care North America
Rocklin, CA
Author: Module 2, Chapter 3

Sheila J. Doss-McQuitty, MBA, BSN, RN, CNN, CCRA
Director, Clinical Programs and Research
Satellite Healthcare, Inc., San Jose, CA
Author: Module 2, Chapter 1

Paula Dutka, MSN, RN, CNN
Director, Education and Research
Nephrology Network
Winthrop University Hospital, Mineola, NY
Author: Module 2, Chapter 1

Andrea Easom, MA, MNSc, APRN, FNP-BC, CNN-NP
Instructor, College of Medicine
Nephrology Division
University of Arkansas for Medical Sciences
Little Rock, AR
Author: Module 6, Chapter 2

Rowena W. Elliott, PhD, RN, CNN, CNE, AGNP-C, FAAN
Associate Professor and Chairperson
Department of Advanced Practice
College of Nursing
University of Southern Mississippi
Hattiesburg, MS
Editor & Author: Module 5, Chapter 2

Susan Fallone, MS, RN, CNN
Clinical Nurse Specialist, Retired
Adult and Pediatric Dialysis
Albany Medical Center, Albany, NY
Author: Module 4, Chapter 2

Jessica J. Geer, MSN, C-PNP, CNN-NP
Pediatric Nurse Practitioner
Texas Children's Hospital, Houston, TX
Instructor, Renal Services, Dept. of Pediatrics
Baylor College of Medicine, Houston, TX
Author: Module 6, Chapter 5

Silvia German, RN, CNN
Clinical Writer, CE Coordinator
Manager, DaVita HealthCare Partners Inc.
Denver, CO
Author: Module 2, Chapter 6

Elaine Go, MSN, NP, CNN-NP
Nurse Practitioner
St. Joseph Hospital Renal Center
Orange, CA
Author: Module 6, Chapter 3

Norma Gomez, MSN, MBA, RN, CNN
Nephrology Nurse Consultant
Russellville, TN
Editor & Author: Module 1, Chapter 4

Janelle Gonyea, RDN, LD
Clinical Dietitian
Mayo Clinic
Rochester, MN
Author: Module 2, Chapter 4

Karen Greco, PhD, RN, ANP-BC, FAAN
Nurse Practitioner
Independent Contractor/Consultant
West Linn, OR
Author: Module 2, Chapter 1

Bonnie Bacon Greenspan, MBA, BSN, RN
Consultant, BBG Consulting, LLC
Alexandria, VA
Author: Module 1, Chapter 1

Cheryl L. Groenhoff, MSN, MBA, RN, CNN
Clinical Educator, Baxter Healthcare
Plantation, FL
Author: Module 2, Chapter 3
Author: Module 3, Chapter 4

Debra J. Hain, PhD, ARNP, ANP-BC, GNP-BC, FAANP
Assistant Professor/Lead AGNP Faculty
Florida Atlantic University
Christine E. Lynn College of Nursing
Boca Raton, FL
Nurse Practitioner, Cleveland Clinic Florida
Department of Nephrology, Weston, FL
Editor & Author: Module 2, Chapter 2

Lisa Hall, MSSW, LICSW
Patient Services Director
Northwest Renal Network (ESRD Network 16)
Seattle, WA
Author: Module 2, Chapter 3

Mary S. Haras, PhD, MS, MBA, APN, NP-C, CNN
Assistant Professor and Interim Associate
 Dean of Graduate Nursing
Saint Xavier University School of Nursing
Chicago, IL
Author: Module 2, Chapter 2

Carol Motes Headley, DNSc, ACNP-BC, RN, CNN
Nephrology Nurse Practitioner
Veterans Affairs Medical Center
Memphis, TN
Editor & Author: Module 2, Chapter 1

Mary Kay Hensley, MS, RDN, CSR
Chair/Immediate Past Chair
Renal Dietitians Dietetic Practice Group
Renal Dietitian, Retired
DaVita HealthCare Partners Inc.
Gary, IN
Author: Module 2, Chapter 4

Kerri Holloway, RN, CNN
Clinical Quality Manager
Corporate Infection Control Specialist
Fresenius Medical Services, Waltham, MA
Author: Module 2, Chapter 6

Alicia M. Horkan, MSN, RN, CNN
Assistant Director, Dialysis Services
Dialysis Center at Colquitt Regional
 Medical Center
Moultrie, GA
Author: Module 1, Chapter 2

Katherine Houle, MSN, APRN, CFNP, CNN-NP
Nephrology Nurse Practitioner
Marquette General Hospital
Marquette, MI
Editor: Module 6
Author: Module 6, Chapter 3

Liz Howard, RN, CNN
Director
DaVita HealthCare Partners Inc.
Oldsmar, FL
Author: Module 2, Chapter 6

Darlene Jalbert, BSN, RN, CNN
HHD Education Manager
DaVita University School of Clinical
 Education Wisdom Team
DaVita HealthCare Partners Inc., Denver, CO
Author: Module 3, Chapter 2

Judy Kauffman, MSN, RN, CNN
Manager, Acute Dialysis and Apheresis Unit
University of Virginia Health Systems
Charlottesville, VA
Author: Module 3, Chapter 2

Tamara Kear, PhD, RN, CNS, CNN
Assistant Professor of Nursing
Villanova University, Villanova, PA
Nephrology Nurse, Fresenius Medical Care
Philadelphia, PA
Editor & Author: Module 1, Chapter 2

Lois Kelley, MSW, LSW, ACSW, NSW-C
Master Social Worker
DaVita HealthCare Partners Inc.
Harrisonburg Dialysis
Harrisonburg, VA
Author: Module 2, Chapter 3

Pamela S. Kent, MS, RDN, CSR, LD
Patient Education Coordinator
Centers for Dialysis Care
Cleveland, OH
Author: Module 2, Chapter 4

Carol L. Kinzner, MSN, ARNP, GNP-BC, CNN-NP
Nurse Practitioner
Pacific Nephrology Associates
Tacoma, WA
Author: Module 6, Chapter 3

Kim Lambertson, MSN, RN, CNN
Clinical Educator
Baxter Healthcare
Deerfield, IL
Author: Module 3, Chapter 4

Sharon Longton, BSN, RN, CNN, CCTC
Transplant Coordinator/Educator
Harper University Hospital
Detroit, MI
Author: Module 2, Chapter 3

Maria Luongo, MSN, RN
CAPD Nurse Manager
Massachusetts General Hospital
Boston, MA
Author: Module 3, Chapter 5

Suzanne M. Mahon, DNSc, RN, AOCN, APNG
Professor, Internal Medicine
Division of Hematology/Oncology
Professor, Adult Nursing, School of Nursing
St. Louis University, St. Louis, MO
Author: Module 2, Chapter 1

Nancy McAfee, MN, RN, CNN
CNS – Pediatric Dialysis and Vascular Access
Seattle Children's Hospital
Seattle, WA
Editor & Author: Module 5, Chapter 1

Maureen P. McCarthy, MPH, RDN, CSR, LD
Assistant Professor/Transplant Dietitian
Oregon Health & Science University
Portland, OR
Author: Module 2, Chapter 4

M. Sue McManus, PhD, APRN, FNP-BC, CNN
Nephrology Nurse Practitioner
Kidney Transplant Nurse Practitioner
Richard L. Roudebush VA Medical Center
Indianapolis, IN
Author: Module 1, Chapter 2

Lisa Micklos, BSN, RN
Clinical Educator
NxStage Medical, Inc.
Los Angeles, CA
Author: Module 1, Chapter 2

Michele Mills, MS, RN, CPNP
Pediatric Nurse Practitioner
Pediatric Nephrology
University of Michigan
C.S. Mott Children's Hospital, Ann Arbor, MI
Author: Module 5, Chapter 1

Geraldine F. Morrison, BSHSA, RN
Clinical Director, Home Programs & CKD
Northwest Kidney Center
Seattle, WA
Author: Module 3, Chapter 5

Theresa Mottes, RN, CDN
Pediatric Research Nurse
Cincinnati Children's Hospital & Medical Center
Center for Acute Care Nephrology
Cincinnati, OH
Author: Module 5, Chapter 1

Linda L. Myers, BS, RN, CNN, HP
RN Administrative Coordinator, Retired
Home Dialysis Therapies
University of Virginia Health System
Charlottesville, VA
Author: Module 4, Chapter 5

Clara Neyhart, BSN, RN, CNN
Nephrology Nurse Clinician
UNC Chapel Hill
Chapel Hill, NC
Editor & Author: Module 3, Chapter 1

Mary Alice Norton, BSN, FNP-C
Senior Heart Failure/LVAD/Transplant
 Coordinator
Albany Medical Center Hospital
Albany, NY
Author: Module 4, Chapter 6

Jessie M. Pavlinac, MS, RDN, CSR, LD
Director, Clinical Nutrition
Oregon Health and Science University
Portland, OR
Author: Module 2, Chapter 4

Glenda M. Payne, MS, RN, CNN
Director of Clinical Services
Nephrology Clinical Solutions
Duncanville, TX
Editor & Author: Module 1, Chapter 1
Author: Module 3, Chapter 2
Author: Module 4, Chapter 4

**Eileen J. Peacock, MSN, RN, CNN,
 CIC, CPHQ, CLNC**
Infection Control and Surveillance
 Management Specialist
DaVita HealthCare Partners Inc.
Maple Glen, PA
Editor & Author: Module 2, Chapter 6

Mary Perrecone, MS, RN, CNN, CCRN
Clinical Manager
Fresenius Medical Care
Charleston, SC
Author: Module 4, Chapter 1

Susan A. Pfettscher, PhD, RN
California State University Bakersfield
 Department of Nursing, Retired
Satellite Health Care, San Jose, CA, Retired
Bakersfield, CA
Author: Module 1, Chapter 1

Nancy B. Pierce, BSN, RN, CNN
Dialysis Director
St. Peter's Hospital
Helena, MT
Author: Module 1, Chapter 1

Leonor P. Ponferrada, BSN, RN, CNN
Education Coordinator
University of Missouri School of Medicine –
 Columbia
Columbia, MO
Author: Module 3, Chapter 4

Lillian A. Pryor, MSN, RN, CNN
Clinical Manager
FMC Loganville, LLC
Loganville, GA
Author: Module 1, Chapter 1

Timothy Ray, DNP, CNP, CNN-NP
Nurse Practitioner
Cleveland Kidney & Hypertension Consultants
Euclid, OH
Author: Module 6, Chapter 4

Cindy Richards, BSN, RN, CNN
Transplant Coordinator
Children's of Alabama
Birmingham, AL
Author: Module 5, Chapter 1

Karen C. Robbins, MS, RN, CNN
Nephrology Nurse Consultant
Associate Editor, *Nephrology Nursing Journal*
Past President, American Nephrology Nurses'
 Association
West Hartford, CT
Editor: Module 3, Chapter 2

Regina Rohe, BS, RN, HP(ASCP)
Regional Vice President, Inpatient Services
Fresenius Medical Care, North America
San Francisco, CA
Author: Module 4, Chapter 8

Francine D. Salinitri, PharmD
Associate (Clinical) Professor of
 Pharmacy Practice
Wayne State University, Applebaum College of
 Pharmacy and Health Sciences, Detroit, MI
Clinical Pharmacy Specialist, Nephrology
Oakwood Hospital and Medical Center
Dearborn, MI
Author: Module 2, Chapter 5

Karen E. Schardin, BSN, RN, CNN
Clinical Director, National Accounts
NxStage Medical, Inc.
Lawrence, MA
Editor & Author: Module 3, Chapter 5

Mary Schira, PhD, RN, ACNP-BC
Associate Professor
Univ. of Texas at Arlington – College of Nursing
Arlington, TX
Author: Module 6, Chapter 1

Deidra Schmidt, PharmD
Clinical Pharmacy Specialist
Pediatric Renal Transplantation
Children's of Alabama
Birmingham, AL
Author: Module 5, Chapter 1

Joan E. Speranza-Reid, BSHM, RN, CNN
Clinic Manager
ARA/Miami Regional Dialysis Center
North Miami Beach, FL
Author: Module 3, Chapter 2

Jean Stover, RDN, CSR, LDN
Renal Dietitian
DaVita HealthCare Partners Inc.
Philadelphia, PA
Author: Module 2, Chapter 4

Charlotte Szromba, MSN, APRN, CNNe
Nurse Consultant, Retired
Department Editor, Nephrology Nursing
 Journal
Naperville, IL
Author: Module 2, Chapter 1

Kirsten L. Thompson, MPH, RDN, CSR
Clinical Dietitian
Seattle Children's Hospital, Seattle, WA
Author: Module 5, Chapter 1

Lucy B. Todd, MSN, ACNP-BC, CNN
Medical Science Liaison
Baxter Healthcare
Asheville, NC
Editor & Author: Module 3, Chapter 4

Susan C. Vogel, MHA, RN, CNN
Clinical Manager, National Accounts
NxStage Medical, Inc.
Los Angeles, CA
Author: Module 3, Chapter 5

Joni Walton, PhD, RN, ACNS-BC, NPc
Family Nurse Practitioner
Marias HealthCare
Shelby, MT
Author: Module 2, Chapter 1

Gail S. Wick, MHSA, BSN, RN, CNNe
Consultant
Atlanta, GA
Author: Module 1, Chapter 2

Helen F. Williams, MSN, BSN, RN, CNN
Special Projects – Acute Dialysis Team
Fresenius Medical Care
Denver, CO
Editor: Module 4
Editor & Author: Module 4, Chapter 7

Elizabeth Wilpula, PharmD, BCPS
Clinical Pharmacy Specialist
Nephrology/Transplant
Harper University Hospital, Detroit, MI
Editor & Author: Module 2, Chapter 5

Karen Wiseman, MSN, RN, CNN
Manager, Regulatory Affairs
Fresenius Medical Services
Waltham, MA
Author: Module 2, Chapter 6

Linda S. Wright, DrNP, RN, CNN, CCTC
Lead Kidney and Pancreas Transplant
  Coordinator
Thomas Jefferson University Hospital
Philadelphia, PA
Author: Module 1, Chapter 2

Mary M. Zorzanello, MSN, APRN
Nurse Practitioner, Section of Nephrology
Yale University School of Medicine
New Haven, CT
Author: Module 6, Chapter 3

STATEMENTS OF DISCLOSURE

Editors

Carol Motes Headley DNSc, ACNP-BC, RN, CNN, is a consultant and/or member of the Corporate Speakers Bureau for Sanofi Renal, and a member of the Advisory Board for Amgen.

Karen E. Schardin, BSN, RN, CNN, is an employee of NxStage Medical, Inc.

Lucy B. Todd, MSN, ACNP-BC, CNN, is an employee of Baxter Healthcare Corporation.

Authors

Lisa Ales, MSN, NP-C, FNP-BC, CNN, is an employee of Baxter Healthcare Corporation.

Billie Axley, MSN, RN, CNN, is an employee of Fresenius Medical Care.

Brandy Begin, BSN, RN, CNN, is a consultant for CHA-SCOPE Collaborative Faculty and has prior received financial support as an injection-training nurse for nutropin from Genentech.

Molly Cahill, MSN, RN, APRN, BC, ANP-C, CNN, is a member of the advisory board for the National Kidney Foundation and Otsuka America Pharmaceutical, Inc., and has received financial support from DaVita HealthCare Partners Inc. [Author states none of this pertains to the material present in her chapter.]

Ann Diroll, MA, BSN, BS, RN, CNN, is a previous employee of Hema Metrics LLC/Fresenius Medical Care (through March 2013).

Sheila J. Doss-McQuitty, MBA, BSN, RN, CNN, CCRA, is a member of the consultant presenter bureau and the advisory board for Takeda Pharmaceuticals U.S.A., Inc., and Affymax, Inc.

Paula Dutka, MSN, RN, CNN, is a coordinator of Clinical Trials for the following sponsors: Amgen, Rockwell Medical Technologies, Inc.; Keryx Biopharmaceuticals, Inc.; Akebia Therapeutics; and Dynavax Technologies.

Elaine Go, MSN, NP, CNN-NP, is on the Speakers Bureau for Sanofi Renal.

Bonnie B. Greenspan, MSN, MBA, RN, has a spouse who works as a medical director of a DaVita HealthCare Partners Inc. dialysis facility.

Mary Kay Hensley, MS, RDN, CSR, is a member of the Academy of Nutrition & Dietitians Renal Practitioners advisory board.

Tamara M. Kear, PhD, RN, CNS, CNN, is a Fresenius Medical Care employee and freelance editor for Lippincott Williams & Wilkins and Elsevier publishing companies.

Kim Lambertson, MSN, RN, CNN, is an employee of Baxter Healthcare Corporation.

Regina Rhoe, BS, RN, HP(ASCP), is an employee of Fresenius Medical Care.

Francine D. Salinitri, Pharm D, received financial support from Otsuka America Pharmaceutical, Inc., through August 2013.

Susan Vogel, MHA, RN, CNN, is an employee of NxStage Medical, Inc.

Reviewers

Jacke L. Corbett, DNP, FNP-BC, CCTC, was on the Novartis Speakers Bureau in 2013.

Deborah Glidden, MSN, ARNP, BC, CNN, is a consultant or member of Corporate Speakers Bureau for Amgen, Pentec Health, and Sanofi-Aventis, and she has received financial support from Amgen.

David Grubbs, RN, CDN, Paramedic, ACLS, PALS, BCLS, TNCC, NIH, has familial relations employed by GlaxoSmithKline (GSK).

Diana Hlebovy, BSN, RN, CHN, CNN, was a clinical support specialist for Fresenius Medical Care RTG in 2013.

Kristin Larson, RN, ANP, GNP, CNN, is an employee of NxStage Medical, Inc.

All other contributors to the *Core Curriculum for Nephrology Nursing* (6th ed.) reported no actual or potential conflict of interest in relation to this continuing nursing education activity.

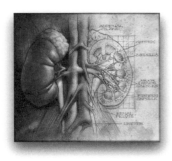

Reviewers

The Blind Review Process

The contents of the *Core Curriculum* underwent a "blind" review process by qualified individuals. One or more chapters were sent to chosen people for critical evaluation. The reviewer did not know the author's identity at the time of the review.

The work could be accepted (1) as originally submitted without revisions, (2) with minor revisons, or (3) with major revisions. The reviewers offered tremendous insight and suggestions; some even submitted additional references they thought might be useful. The results of the review were then sent back to the chapter/module editors to incorporate the suggestions and make revisions.

The reviewers will discover who the authors are now that the *Core* is published. However, while there is this published list of reviewers, no one will know who reviewed which part of the *Core*. That part of the process remains blind.

Because of the efforts of individuals listed below, value was added to the sixth edition. Their hard work is greatly appreciated.

Caroline S. Counts, Editor

Marilyn R. Bartucci, MSN, RN, ACNS-BC, CCTC
Case Manager
Kidney Foundation of Ohio
Cleveland, OH

Christina M. Beale, RN, CNN
Director, Outreach and Education
Lifeline Vascular Access
Vernon Hills, IL

Jenny Bell, BSN, RN, CNN
Clinical Transplant Coordinator
Banner Good Samaritan Transplant Center
Phoenix, AZ

M. Geraldine Biddle, RN, CNN, CPHQ
President, Nephrology Nurse Consultants
Pittsford, NY

Randee Breiterman White, MS, RN
Nurse Case Manager Nephrology
Vanderbilt University Hospital
Nashville, TN

Jerrilynn D. Burrowes, PhD, RDN, CDN
Professor and Chair
Director, Graduate Programs in Nutrition
Department of Nutrition
Long Island University (LIU) Post
Brookville, NY

Sally Burrows-Hudson, MSN, RN, CNN
Deceased 2014
Director, Nephrology Clinical Solutions
Lisle, IL

LaVonne Burrows, APRN, BC, CNN
Advanced Practice Registered Nurse
Springfield Nephrology Associates
Springfield, MO

Karen T. Burwell, BSN, RN, CNN
Acute Dialysis Nurse
DaVita HealthCare Partners Inc.
Phoenix, AZ

Laura D. Byham-Gray, PhD, RDN
Associate Professor and Director
Graduate Programs in Clinical Nutrition
Department of Nutritional Sciences
School of Health Related Professions
Rutgers University
Stratford, NJ

Theresa J. Campbell, DNP, APRN, FNP-BC
Doctor of Nursing Practice
Family Nurse Practitioner
Carolina Kidney Care
Adjunct Professor of Nursing
University of North Caroline at Pembroke
Fayetteville, NC

Monet Carnahan, BSN, RN, CDN
Renal Care Coordinator Program Manager
Fresenius Medical Care
Nashville, TN

Jacke L. Corbett, DNP, FNP-BC, CCTC
Nurse Practitioner
Kidney/Pancreas Transplant Program
University of Utah Health Care
Salt Lake City, UT

Christine Corbett, MSN, APRN, FNP-BC, CNN-NP
Nephrology Nurse Practitioner
Truman Medical Centers
Kansas City, MO

Sandra Corrigan, FNP-BC, CNN
Nurse Practitioner
California Kidney Medical Group
Thousand Oaks, CA

Maureen Craig, MSN, RN, CNN
Clinical Nurse Specialist – Nephrology
University of California Davis Medical Center
Sacramento, CA

Diane M. Derkowski, MA, RN, CNN, CCTC
Kidney Transplant Coordinator
Carolinas Medical Center
Charlotte, NC

Linda Duval, BSN, RN
Executive Director, FMQAI: ESRD Network 13
ESRD Network
Oklahoma City, OK

Damian Eker, DNP, GNP-C
ARNP, Geriatrics & Adult Health
Adult & Geriatric Health Center
Ft. Lauderdale, FL

Elizabeth Evans, DNP
Nephrology Nurse Practitioner
Renal Medicine Associates
Albuquerque, NM

Susan Fallone, MS, RN, CNN
Clinical Nurse Specialist, Retired
Adult and Pediatric Dialysis
Albany Medical Center
Albany, NY

Karen Joann Gaietto, MSN, BSN, RN, CNN
Acute Clinical Service Specialist
DaVita HealthCare Partners Inc.
Tiffin, OH

Deborah Glidden, MSN, ARNP, BC, CNN
Nurse Practitioner
Nephrology Associates of Central Florida
Orlando, FL

David Jeremiah Grubbs, RN, CDN, Paramedic, ACLS, PALS, BCLS, TNCC, NIH
Clinical Nurse Manager
Crestwood, KY

Debra J. Hain, PhD, ARNP, ANP-BC, GNP-BC, FAANP
Associate Professor/Lead Faculty AGNP Track
Florida Atlantic University
Christine E. Lynn College of Nursing
Boca Raton, FL
Nurse Practitioner, Cleveland Clinic Florida
Department of Nephrology
Weston, FL

Brenda C. Halstead, MSN, RN, AcNP, CNN
Nurse Practitioner
Mid-Atlantic Kidney Center
Richmond and Petersburg, VA

Emel Hamilton, RN, CNN
Director of Clinical Technology
Fresenius Medical Care
Waltham, MA

Mary S. Haras, PhD, MBA, APN, NP-C, CNN
Associate Dean, Graduate Nursing Programs
Saint Xavier University School of Nursing
Chicago, IL

Malinda C. Harrington, MSN, RN, FNP-BC, ANCC
Pediatric Nephrology Nurse Practitioner
Vidant Medical Center
Greenville, NC

Diana Hlebovy, BSN, RN, CHN, CNN
Nephrology Nurse Consultant
Elyria, OH

Sara K. Kennedy, BSN, RN, CNN
UAB Medicine, Kirklin Clinic
Diabetes Care Coordinator
Birmingham, AL

Nadine "Niki" Kobes, BSN, RN
Manager Staff Education/Quality
Fresenius Medical Care – Alaska JV Clinics
Anchorage, AK

Deuzimar Kulawik, MSN, RN
Director of Clinical Quality
DaVita HealthCare Partners Inc.
Westlake Village, CA

Kristin Larson, RN, ANP, GNP, CNN
Clinical Instructor
College of Nursing
Family Nurse Practitioner Program
University of North Dakota
Grand Forks, ND

Deborah Leggett, BSN, RN, CNN
Director, Acute Dialysis
Jackson Madison County General Hospital
Jackson, TN

Charla Litton, MSN, APRN, FNP-BC, CNN
Nurse Practitioner
UHG/Optum
East Texas, TX

Greg Lopez, BSN, RN, CNN
IMPAQ Business Process Manager
Fresenius Medical Care
New Orleans, LA

Terri (Theresa) Luckino, BSN, RN, CCRN
President, Acute Services
RPNT Acute Services, Inc.
Irving, TX

Alice Luehr, BA, RN, CNN
Home Therapy RN
St. Peter's Hospital
Helena, MT

Maryam W. Lyon, MSN, RN, CNN
Education Coordinator
Fresenius Medical Care
Dayton, OH

Christine Mudge, MS, RN, PNP/CNS, CNN, FAAN
Mill Valley, CA

Mary Lee Neuberger, MSN, APRN, RN, CNN
Pediatric Nephrology
University of Iowa Children's Hospital
Iowa City, IA

Jennifer Payton, MHCA, BSN, RN, CNN
Clinical Support Specialist
HealthStar CES
Goose Creek, SC

April Peters, MSN, RN, CNN
Clinical Informatics Specialist
Brookhaven Memorial Hospital Medical Center
Patchogue, NY

David J. Quan, PharmD, BCPS
Health Sciences Clinical Professor of Pharmacy
Clinical Pharmacist, Liver Transplant Services
UCSF Medical Center
San Francisco, CA

Kristi Robertson, CFNP
Nephrology Nurse Practitioner
Nephrology Associates
Columbus, MS

E. James Ryan, BSN, RN, CDN
Hemodialysis Clinical Services Coordinator
Lakeland Regional Medical Center
Lakeland, FL

June Shi, BSN, RN
Vascular Access Coordinator
Transplant Surgery
Medical University of South Carolina
Charleston, SC

Elizabeth St. John, MSN, RN, CNN
Education Coordinator, UMW Region
Fresenius Medical Care
Milwaukee, WI

Sharon Swofford, MA, RN, CNN, CCTC
Transplant Case Manager
OptumHealth
The Villages, FL

Beth Ulrich, EdD, RN, FACHE, FAAN
Senior Partner, Innovative Health Resources
Editor, *Nephrology Nursing Journal*
Pearland, TX

David F. Walz, MBA, BSN, RN, CNN
Program Director
CentraCare Kidney Program
St. Cloud, MN

Gail S. Wick, MHSA, BSN, RN, CNNe
Consultant
Atlanta, GA

Phyllis D. Wille, MS, RN, FNP-C, CNN, CNE
Nursing Faculty
Danville Area Community College
Danville, Il

Donna L. Willingham, RN, CPNP
Pediatric Nephrology Nurse Practitioner
Washington University St. Louis
St. Louis, MO

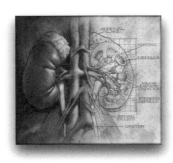

Contents at a Glance

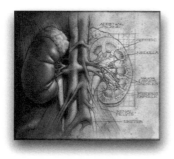

Expanded Contents

The table of contents contains chapters and sections with editors and authors for all six modules. The contents section of this specific module is highlighted in a blue background.

Module 1　Foundations for Practice in Nephrology Nursing

Module 2   Physiologic and Psychosocial Basis for Nephrology Nursing Practice

Module 3 Treatment Options for Patients with Chronic Kidney Failure

Module 5   Kidney Disease in Patient Populations Across the Life Span

Module 6   The APRN's Approaches to Care in Nephrology

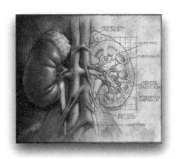

Examples of APA-formatted references

A guide for citing material from Module 4 of the *Core Curriculum for Nephrology Nursing, 6th edition.*

All examples for Module 4 are similar in that each chapter has only one or two authors.

Interpreted: Chapter author(s). (Date). Title of chapter. In …

For citation in text: (Author, 2015)

Module 4, Chapter 1

Perrecone, M. (2015). Program management in the acute care setting. In C.S. Counts (Ed.), *Core curriculum for nephrology nursing: Module 4. Acute kidney injury* (6th ed., pp. 1-18). Pitman, NJ: American Nephrology Nurses' Association.

Module 4, Chapter 2

Fallone, S., & Cotton, A.B. (2015). Acute kidney injury. In C.S. Counts (Ed.), *Core curriculum for nephrology nursing: Module 4. Acute kidney injury* (6th ed., pp. 19-54). Pitman, NJ: American Nephrology Nurses' Association.

Module 4, Chapter 3

Axley, B. (2015). Hemodialysis in the acute setting. In C.S. Counts (Ed.), *Core curriculum for nephrology nursing: Module 4. Acute kidney injury* (6th ed., pp. 55-106). Pitman, NJ: American Nephrology Nurses' Association.

Module 4, Chapter 4

Payne, G. . (2015). Water treatment in the acute care setting. In C.S. Counts (Ed.), *Core curriculum for nephrology nursing: Module 4. Acute kidney injury* (6th ed., pp. 107-118). Pitman, NJ: American Nephrology Nurses' Association.

Module 4, Chapter 5

Myers, L.L. (2015). Peritoneal dialysis in the acute care setting. In C.S. Counts (Ed.), *Core curriculum for nephrology nursing: Module 4. Acute kidney injury* (6th ed., pp. 119-142). Pitman, NJ: American Nephrology Nurses' Association.

Module 4, Chapter 6

Norton, M.A. (2015). The patient with a ventricular assist device. In C.S. Counts (Ed.), *Core curriculum for nephrology nursing: Module 4. Acute kidney injury* (6th ed., pp. 143-160). Pitman, NJ: American Nephrology Nurses' Association.

Module 4, Chapter 7

Williams, H.F. (2015). Continuous renal replacement therapies. In C.S. Counts (Ed.), *Core curriculum for nephrology nursing: Module 4. Acute kidney injury* (6th ed., pp. 161-210). Pitman, NJ: American Nephrology Nurses' Association.

Module 4, Chapter 8

Rohe, R. (2015). Therapeutic apheresis. In C.S. Counts (Ed.), *Core curriculum for nephrology nursing: Module 4. Acute kidney injury* (6th ed., pp. 211-234). Pitman, NJ: American Nephrology Nurses' Association.

CHAPTER 1

Program Management in the Acute Care Setting

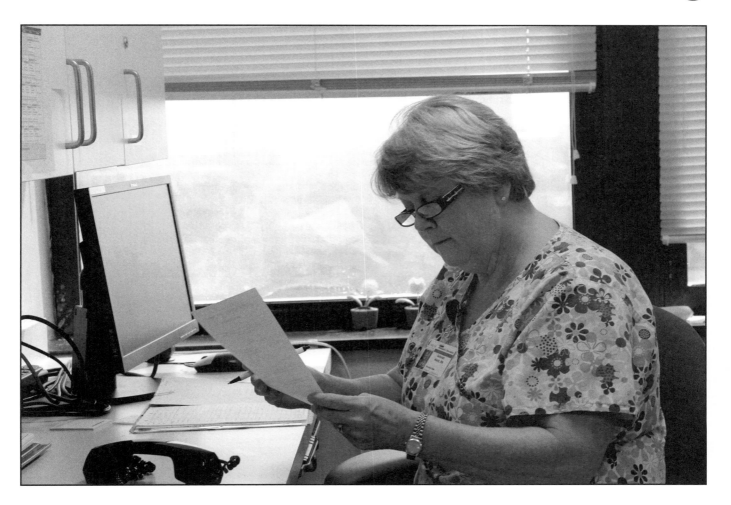

Chapter Editor
Helen F. Williams, MSN, BSN, RN, CNN

Author
Mary Perrecone, MS, RN, CNN, CCRN

CHAPTER **1**

Program Management in the Acute Care Setting

This offering for **1.2 contact hours** is provided by the American Nephrology Nurses' Association (ANNA).

American Nephrology Nurses' Association is accredited as a provider of continuing nursing education by the American Nurses Credentialing Center Commission on Accreditation.

ANNA is a provider approved by the California Board of Registered Nursing, provider number CEP 00910.

This CNE offering meets the continuing nursing education requirements for certification and recertification by the Nephrology Nursing Certification Commission (NNCC).

To be awarded contact hours for this activity, read this chapter in its entirety. Then complete the CNE evaluation found at **www.annanurse.org/corecne** and submit it; or print it, complete it, and mail it in. Contact hours are not awarded until the evaluation for the activity is complete.

Example of reference for Chapter 1 in APA format. One author for entire chapter.

Perrecone, M. (2015). Program management in the acute care setting. In C.S. Counts (Ed.), *Core curriculum for nephrology nursing: Module 4. Acute kidney injury* (6th ed., pp. 1-18). Pitman, NJ: American Nephrology Nurses' Association.

Interpreted: Chapter author. (Date). Title of chapter. In ...

Cover photo by Counts/Morganello.

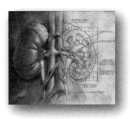

CHAPTER 1

Program Management in the Acute Care Setting

Purpose

The purpose of this chapter is to consider the variety of services, roles, and issues that are a part of providing nephrology nursing care in the acute care setting.

Objectives

Upon completion of this chapter, the learner will be able to:
1. Describe three settings and three services common to acute care nephrology.
2. Discuss the nephrology nurse's role in acute care program management.
3. Identify three challenges that the acute care nephrology nurse encounters.

I. **Acute care nephrology services are provided in various types of facilities.**

A. Facilities, locations, and treatment options.
   1. Large teaching hospitals with multiple treatment sites on multiple campuses providing a full array of treatment options.
   2. Large teaching hospitals with multiple intensive care units (ICU) on one campus providing a full array of nephrology treatment options.
   3. Private hospitals with multiple ICUs on one campus providing a full array of nephrology treatment options.
   4. Medium-sized hospitals with one or two ICUs and a dedicated dialysis treatment room (two to four beds) providing hemodialysis, continuous renal replacement therapy (CRRT), and peritoneal dialysis (PD) coverage.
   5. Small hospitals with a dedicated dialysis room (two beds) providing only hemodialysis treatments.
   6. Small hospitals with a dedicated dialysis storage area providing all hemodialysis treatments at the patient's bedside.
   7. Acute care hospitals accepting patients on long-term ventilator management, complex wounds, and acute nursing needs with hemodialysis and peritoneal dialysis therapies.
   8. Rehabilitation hospitals accepting patients with a need for chronic hemodialysis and/or peritoneal dialysis.
   9. Multiple hospitals of various sizes contracting for a variety of levels of dialysis support with one provider.
   10. Medium or larger hospitals using their own employees for dialysis services, floating dialysis employees to other units in the hospital when census dictates.
   11. Correctional institutions contracting for chronic hemodialysis services for inmates with an acute dialysis provider.
   12. Correctional institutions that hire their own staff to provide hemodialysis services.

B. Departments within institutions where acute nephrology nursing services are provided.
   1. Dialysis/pheresis treatment room or unit.
   2. Patient bedside.
   3. ICU.
      a. Dialytic therapy postoperatively for fluid and electrolyte management.
      b. Maintenance dialytic therapy for the critically ill patient.
   4. Emergency department (ED).
      a. Hemodialysis treatment for patient with hyperkalemia or fluid overload with impending intubation when no beds are available in the ICU or telemetry unit.
      b. Fistula needle removal from a patient who has arrived via ambulance from an in-center dialysis unit with needles left in place to expedite the patients' rapid transfer to emergency care.

c. Vascular access assessment and care for a patient with bleeding at the fistula needle site.

d. Dialysis catheter care to repair disconnected or severed dialysis catheter port/s or to refer the patient to interventional radiology (IR).

e. A peritoneal dialysis exchange performed to obtain a sample of effluent to send to the laboratory to rule out peritonitis.

f. Assessing the PD catheter exit site and tunnel for signs and symptoms of infection.

5. The cardiac catheterization lab.

a. CRRT or intermittent hemodialysis (IHD) may be started or maintained on a patient sensitive to volume and electrolyte shifts during or shortly after a cardiac catheterization procedure.

b. Hemodialysis treatments during or immediately following contrast exposure to minimize contrast nephropathy for patients with residual kidney function.

6. The operating room (OR).

a. During open hearts, transplants, or other major vascular procedures, hemodialysis or CRRT may be started to assist with electrolyte and fluid management.

b. During transplant surgery to maintain homeostasis.

II. The nephrology multidisciplinary team.

Staff in the acute care setting can range from a small to a large team depending on the program needs. Positions may be filled by hospital employees, contracted dialysis employees, vendor-provided employees under contract, or a combination of these options.

A. Hospital care providers.

B. Nurse manager.

C. Administrative assistant.

D. Nephrology nurses.

E. Dialysis technicians or patient care technicians working under the direct supervision of the nephrology nurse.

F. Facility technician responsible for machine disinfection and culturing.

G. Biomed technician responsible for preventive maintenance and repairs on equipment.

H. Inventory technician responsible for supplies: ordering, receiving, delivering to sites, and ensuring supply availability where and when needed.

I. Social worker.

J. Dietitian.

K. Home training nurse.

L. Transplant coordinators.

M. Case managers/discharge planners.

N. Vascular access (VA) center coordinator.

III. Nephrology nurse roles and responsibilities in the acute care setting.

A. Provide direct patient care using a variety of modalities of treatment.

B. Communicate with hospital care providers before, during, and after the dialysis treatment to ensure continuity of care.

C. Provide direct supervision of unlicensed dialysis personnel.

D. Provide dialysis coverage 24 hours a day, 7 days a week.

E. Educate hospital staff regarding care of the nephrology patient.

F. Educate hospital staff regarding treatment modalities used to treat acute kidney injury (AKI) and chronic kidney disease (CKD) stage 5.

G. Coordinate schedule for dialytic procedures with hospital staff and departments.

H. Communicate patient care needs to physicians and other hospital care providers.

I. Educate patients and families regarding their diagnosis, the plan of care, and treatment options. (Refer to Appendix 1.1. Patient Education Pamphlet at the end of this chapter.)

J. Provide predialysis modality education for in-patients with CKD stage 4, approaching the need for dialysis treatments.

K. Use research to build evidence-based practice and to participate in personal education to improve the services provided.

L. Participate in Quality Assurance and Performance Improvement (QAPI) activities.

M. Participate in orientation and training of new employees, developing a mentoring relationship to strengthen the nephrology specialty.

N. Report equipment and supply issues to management to ensure a safe working environment.

O. Collaborate with the patient's chronic dialysis unit care providers prior to discharge from acute care regarding the hospitalization, procedures performed, medication changes, vascular access issues, and other changes in the patient's condition as a result of his/her hospital visit.

P. As a member of the nephrology service, ensure positive interactions with the staff of every facility or unit.

Q. Assist emergency department (ED) personnel in caring for patients with nephrology issues.

R. Coordinate with insurance providers for outpatient procedures, such as therapeutic plasma exchange (TPE) or hemodialysis.

S. Collaborate with the social worker/discharge planner to coordinate care for the patient who is uninsured or underinsured.

T. Support discharge planners and utilization review managers when they intervene with the Immigration and Naturalization Service (INS) or other government agencies (such as Centers for Medicare and Medicaid [CMS] or Social Security).

U. Coordinate insurance coverage and scheduling of treatments for acute kidney injury patients pending return of kidney function as well as CKD stage 5 patients new to dialysis.

V. Provide weekly dialysis access catheter care, including site care, aspirating, flushing, and recapping the catheter, for patients discharged from the hospital who are not being cared for by a chronic outpatient unit.

IV. Patients encountered in the acute care setting encompass a wide range of needs and interventions.

A. CKD stage 5 patients admitted for non-nephrology issues needing dialytic support during the acute care stay.

B. Newly diagnosed CKD stage 5 patients.
  1. Patients living in areas where the chronic dialysis units are saturated and there is a waiting list for new patient placement.
  2. Patients who are without a funding source, either undocumented or uninsured, that report to the ED or come to the hospital on a regularly scheduled basis for routine, urgent, or emergent dialysis care.

C. CKD stage 5 patients with urgent dialysis or vascular access needs.
  1. Outpatients who have had an access revision or catheter placement and missed their outpatient appointment time may be dialyzed in the acute setting.

a. In some states, these treatments may be billed under a special Medicare billing code specific for this situation.
b. The patient's treatment may be performed by the acute nephrology nurse in the ED, the dialysis unit, an Infusion Center, or an assigned patient room, depending on the facility and the situation.
  2. Outpatients having dialytic needs for fluid overload or electrolyte disturbances not adequately managed by their regularly scheduled chronic dialysis unit treatments.

D. CKD stage 5 patients without chronic dialysis unit affiliation.
  1. Patients who have been dismissed from their chronic dialysis center because of nonadherence to the treatment plan. These patients will come to the ED for treatment until another chronic dialysis center can be established.
  2. Patients who have been dismissed because of aggressive or violent behaviors against staff or patients at a chronic dialysis unit.
    a. These patients will come to the ED for treatment and will benefit from the help of the ESRD network to reestablish a chronic dialysis center, usually under a signed behavioral contract.
    b. Patients with behavioral issues may not be able to reestablish with a chronic dialysis center.

E. Conservatively managed patients with CKD stage 4 to 5 admitted for conservative management of uremic symptoms and palliative care.

F. AKI patients.
  1. Acutely ill patient with AKI requiring hospitalization.
  2. Patients with AKI stable enough to be managed as an outpatient with ongoing dialytic support.
    a. These patients cannot find placement in a chronic dialysis center because they have an "acute" process.
    b. These patients continue to require follow-up and intermittent hemodialysis and vascular access catheter care.

G. Patients needing TPE treatments.
  1. Inpatients requiring ongoing TPE treatments for an acute illness.
  2. Outpatients with recurring admissions to receive TPE treatments on a regularly scheduled basis.

V. Approach to program management. In the acute care setting, program management will vary significantly from one location to another depending on the size of the program, the services provided, and the employment relationship between nephrology and other care providers.

A. Contracts.
  1. Establish contracted rates for all nephrology nursing care services and required participation in hospital specific orientation, including that deemed necessary for credentialing contracted staff. For example:
     a. 1:1, 1:2, or 2:1 nursing-staff-to-patient ratio.
     b. Hemodialysis; slow, low-efficiency daily dialysis (SLEDD); or continuous renal replacement therapy (CRRT) treatments in the ICU.
     c. CRRT treatment initiation, daily maintenance, and discontinuation of therapy.
     d. Restarting a treatment after a clotted system.
     e. On-call treatments.
     f. Delayed and canceled treatments.
     g. Hourly rates for treatments over 5 hours.
     h. Nephrology nursing consultation.
     i. Peritoneal dialysis treatment initiation and daily maintenance.
     j. Education classes provided for the hospital personnel.
     k. Rates for storage space if not provided under the contract.
  2. Delineate responsibilities of nephrology and hospital personnel. For example:
     a. Transportation of dialysis patients.
     b. Administration of medications.
     c. Transporting blood specimens to the lab.
     d. Picking up blood products from the blood bank that are to be administered during the treatment.
     e. Submitting charge forms or entering charges in a computer for nephrology services provided.
     f. Housekeeping duties.
     g. Plant operations and maintenance of water and electrical services.
  3. Specify communication channels between the hospital and nephrology staff, including the management level with an assigned liaison.
  4. Define expectation for reporting of quality monitoring, water system records, etc., including when reports are due and the person(s) to whom reports are submitted.
  5. Provide a safe and secure working environment for contracted employees.

B. Staffing.
  1. Staffing patterns.
     a. A ratio of at least one RN to one patient (1:1) is typical for acute hemodialysis for the critically ill patient in the intensive care unit, emergency department, all bedside treatments, and for pediatric patients.
     b. Apheresis treatments are also usually performed with a 1:1 RN-to-patient staff ratio.
     c. Additionally, continuous renal replacement therapy (CRRT) is normally a ratio of one RN to one patient (1:1) and frequently requires two RNs to one patient (2:1) depending on the patient's condition.
     d. Depending on the severity of the patient's condition (not necessitating admission to a critical care unit), a higher level of care may be required for certain patients who are dialyzed in the dialysis treatment room or unit.
     e. An RN to patient ratio of 1:2 or 2:4 when performing hemodialysis in the dialysis treatment room or unit is typical in consideration of patient acuity.
  2. Hemodialysis nurses and dialysis technicians or patient care technicians.
     a. They are assigned based on total workload factors and according to their state's scope of practice laws and the acute facility's policies.
     b. If technicians perform dialysis at the bedside in a patient's room on a hospital unit, a competent hemodialysis trained nurse must also be on the unit and available to assist with any complications.
     c. Some facilities require that a minimum of two dialysis staff personnel are present in the dialysis treatment room or unit at all times while dialysis is being conducted. One of the staff must be a dialysis-trained professional nephrology nurse.
  3. Some facilities require that a physician be physically present in the hospital when dialysis is being conducted.
  4. The patient care staff must meet the credentialing requirements of the hospital or agency contracting the acute dialysis service, which may include a payment of required fees for processing the application for Allied Health Privileges.
  5. The agency providing the contracted service must provide the level of professional personnel required by each contract.
  6. The agency providing the contracted service must notify the hospital of changes in personnel.
  7. The contracting agency or hospital must provide the nephrology personnel with the necessary identification (ID) badge, parking permit, keys, and computer access as appropriate for each facility contracted.
  8. The agency providing the contracted service must provide education for nephrology personnel to ensure quality patient care.
     a. Complete orientation at hire.

(1) Plan for a minimum of 6 to 8 weeks of orientation for nurses hired from an ICU or chronic dialysis unit.

(2) Longer orientation may be needed for those with a general nursing background.

(3) Appropriate orientation time varies with the individual and the hospital's policies.

(4) Regular review and documentation of the orientee's progress, including regular meetings with the nurse manager and preceptor, with documentation of the education plan to move forward.

(5) Provide the same orientation process for traveling RNs who come in on a temporary contract to ensure consistent quality of care is being provided.

b. Provide and document training for any new procedure, new equipment, or upgrades prior to implementation.

c. Provide learning opportunities to enhance professional development.

d. Use annual performance reviews to determine individual educational needs and to develop a plan for obtaining or providing the appropriate training.

e. Establish annual competency testing and a written plan to address any deficiencies discovered to ensure competent, safe, quality patient care.
(1) Written exams.
(2) Clinical simulations.
(3) Case studies.
(4) Observation of procedure performance.

9. Hospital policies and procedures for epidemiology should be followed in the acute dialysis treatment room or unit.

a. Specific dialysis policy and procedures (P&P) should be included and be part of the ongoing education of the staff.
(1) Machine cleaning and maintenance schedule.
(2) Water quality.
(3) Hepatitis screening and prevention.

b. Environmental.
(1) Dedicate supplies for single patient use.
(2) Safe handling of dialyzers and blood tubing.
(3) Separate clean areas from contaminated areas.
(4) Clean and disinfect the dialysis station and patient treatment area between patients.

c. Standard precautions.
(1) Hand hygiene.
(2) Personal protective equipment: gown, gloves, mask.
(3) Safe injection practices.

d. Patient practices.

(1) New patients should be screened for HBsAg and HBsAb.

(2) Patients who are seronegative for surface antigen and antibody must be tested once a month for HBsAg, either SGOT or SGPT, and once every 3 months for HBsAb.

(3) Patients admitted to the dialysis treatment room or unit with a communicable infection should be placed on precautions according to isolation guidelines outlined by the hospital policies and procedures.

(4) CHG/alcohol or CHG/iodine solutions (Chloraprep or Chlorasept) should be used for prepping venipuncture sites, injection sites, etc., and according to infection control Intravenous Site Care Guidelines (CDC, 2002).

(5) Patients should be taught hand washing practices.

e. In-service.
(1) All new personnel will be instructed in infection control policies, including, but not limited to, aseptic technique and sterile technique.

(2) Continuing education and review of the above will be scheduled on an annual basis.

(3) All personnel will receive annual training in accordance with OSHA's Bloodborne Pathogens Standard and CDC guideline. (CDC, 2011a; 2011b).

f. Staff competencies should be assessed upon hire and at least yearly in the following categories. *Note*: not all categories will be applicable to all staff.
(1) Gloving and hand hygiene (all staff) – includes recognition of appropriate situations for glove use, proper hand hygiene technique, proper use and removal of gloves, and the appropriate PPE for each patient condition and/or disease process.

(2) Catheter dressing change technique – includes correct performance of hand hygiene, use of gloves, and correct use of antiseptics (proper application, allow drying).

(3) Vascular access technique – includes correct performance of hand hygiene and use of gloves; catheter site and port/vascular access antisepsis, and aseptic technique.

(4) Safe injection and safe medication practices, including proper technique for parenteral medication preparation, handling, administration, and storage (e.g., not in patient station, etc.), use of aseptic technique, proper hand hygiene before preparing or administering medications or

infusions, and proper cleansing of medication injection ports and medication vial diaphragms. This should also include proper use and handling of single-use vials, bags, or bottles.

C. Recordkeeping.
1. Employee files.
   a. Application with education and job history.
   b. Random drug screen.
   c. References.
   d. Background check.
   e. Orientation completed.
      (1) Orientation checklist.
      (2) Skills checklist.
   f. Continuing education records.
      (1) Required continuing education.
      (2) Policy and procedure changes.
      (3) New equipment training.
   g. Verification of license records and history.
   h. BCLS/ACLS/PALS (Basic Cardiac, Advanced Cardiac Life Support, and Pediatric Advanced Life Support) training records.
   i. Records regarding certification and maintenance of certification.
   j Performance appraisal and annual competency completed.
   k. Annual blood work and testing.
      (1) Hepatitis screening.
      (2) Rubella and rubeola immunity testing.
      (3) Tuberculin (TB) skin testing.
2. The agency contracted to provide dialysis services will provide:
   a. Policy and procedure (P&P) manuals with copies available on site at each contracted facility or available electronically.
   b. Evidence of ongoing annual reviews and staff education regarding changes in the P&Ps.
   c. Education regarding access to applicable hospital's P&Ps, either paper or electronic, will be provided by the contracting agency to the staff providing the dialysis service.
3. Equipment and supply documentation.
   a. Hemodialysis, water treatment, and pheresis equipment use, repair, and preventive maintenance logbooks.
   b. Reports of equipment failure that result in patient injury or death and its subsequent investigation.
   c. Equipment recall notices.
   d. Electrical safety inspection reports of new equipment or equipment moved from one facility to another.
   e. Annual electrical safety inspection reports.
   f. Conductivity and pH meter calibration log.
   g. Refrigerator temperature record log.
   h. Inventory audit and supply ordering records.

4. Treatment records.
   a. Treatment log.
   b. Patient treatment flowsheets.
   c. Results of documentation audits.
   d. Billing records.
5. QAPI and research records.
   a. Primary purpose is to monitor, evaluate, or improve the quality and safety of healthcare delivery.
   b. The following entities have been involved and may contribute to development of QAPI hemodialysis assessement tools.
      (1) Association for Professionals in Infection Control.
      (2) Association for the Advancement of Medical Instrumentation.
      (3) Centers for Medicare and Medicaid Services.
      (4) Centers for Disease Control.
      (5) End Stage Renal Disease Networks.
      (6) Contracting agency's facility specific data collection plans.
      (7) Food and Drug Administration.
      (8) International Standardization Organizations.
      (9) Specific requirements for safe use of a manufacturer's piece of equipment.
      (10) Occupational Safety and Health Administration.
      (11) Organizations such as NKF, ANNA, KDOQI, etc.
      (12) The Joint Commission.
      (13) Health Care Financing Administration.
      (14) In the acute settings, the goals of the hospital quality improvement initiatives from the Hospital Consumer Assessment of Healthcare Providers and Systems (HCAHP) scores are followed within the dialysis treatment room or unit (see HCAHPS section).
   c. Dialysis-specific quality assurance (QA) is performed and may include but not be limited to a review of:
      (1) Monthly patient volume, including number/ratio of 1:1 treatments.
      (2) Number of times when the on-call dialysis staff are called in to do a procedure.
      (3) The amount of time it took from the call-in to when the RN arrived at the hospital.
      (4) Average length of stay (LOS), especially for the patients newly diagnosed with CKD stage 5.
      (5) The number of treatments provided in each of the modalities offered by that agency or hospital, such as IHD vs. CRRT vs. PD vs. apheresis.

(6) The number of patients with AKI vs. CKD that were treated.

(7) The number and percentage of patients with AKI who regained their kidney function vs. those that progressed to CKD.

(8) Access management.
   (a) Number of new patients with CKD stage 5 who underwent vein mapping prior to discharge.
   (b) Arteriovenous fistula (AVF), arteriovenous graft (AVG), or catheter placement.
   (c) Access issues such as catheter line reversal.

(9) Infections, especially related to vascular access, such as central-line-associated bloodstream infection (CLABSI), catheter-related bloodstream infection (CRBSI), and/or catheter-associated urinary tract infection (CAUTI).

(10) Water quality, including chemical and microbiologic testing.
   (a) Monthly water and dialysate cultures.
   (b) Monthly water LALs (limulus amebocyte lysate).
   (c) Water analysis, annually or semiannually, depending on regional water quality.

(11) Manage and track adequacy of dialysis.
   (a) Kt/V.
   (b) URR.
   (c) CRRT ordered dose vs. delivered dose.
   (d) Intermittent hemodialysis (IHD) treatment time ordered vs. time delivered.

(12) Fluid management.
   (a) Using Crit-Line®.
   (b) Fluid goal compliance.
   (c) Accurate scales, weighing the patient before and after on the same scale.

(13) Hypotensive episodes.
(14) Hand hygiene.
(15) Falls.
(16) Pressure ulcers.
(17) Restraint usage.
(18) Equipment failure/out of service.
(19) Rapid responses/codes.
(20) Adverse events and sentinel event reports.
(21) Compliance with policies and procedures.
(22) Research projects requiring data collection, including the Institutional Review Board (IRB) applications and data collection materials.
(23) Safety alerts and recalls.

6. Inspection by any credentialing or accrediting body, i.e., State Department of Health (DOH), Centers for Medicare and Medicaid Services (CMS), Occupational Safety and Health Administration (OSHA), The Joint Commission (TJC), and Magnet Recognition Program.
   a. Inspection report.
   b. Facility response.
   c. Plan of action.
   d. Progress reports toward correction of any deficiencies.

7. The QAPI team.
   a. May include the patient and/or patient family/caregiver(s), nurse manager, bedside nurse, clinical nurse specialist, nurse practitioner, social worker, medical director, nephrologist, and case manager, if applicable. Special guests could include epidemiology, vascular interventional radiology, or other physician specialties.
   b. Addresses any issues and decides on follow-up needed using the Plan, Do Check, Act (PDCA) cycle as part of the quality improvement process.
   c. Documents monitoring of problems and trends with corresponding corrective action plans.

D. Communication.
   1. Hospital or departmental liaison.
      a. Establish rapport.
      b. Anticipate and discuss issues.
      c. Plan for solutions when things are not at crisis level.
      d. Coordinate scheduling of educational offerings for hospital personnel regarding nephrology nursing and care of patients with kidney disease.
      e. Discuss budgetary planning for new equipment or upgrading current equipment.
   2. Hospital unit managers and charge nurses.
      a. Establish rapport.
      b. Use communication tools to ensure continuity of care.
   3. Direct care providers and/or primary nurses.
      a. Discuss the schedule for dialysis treatment and any other procedures the patient may have planned for the same day.
      b. Receive SBAR (situation, background, assessment, recommendation) report pretreatment.
      c. Ensure the patient's medical record is with the patient so medical information and records are available for the nephrology team during treatment.
      d. Complete accurate and timely medication and treatment charting in the medical record appropriate for each contracted facility.
      e. Inform primary nurse of significant changes in the patient's condition during dialysis treatment.
      f. Provide SBAR report to primary nurse after the

dialysis treatment, prior to the patient transport to patient's nursing unit.

4. Discharge planners, case managers, and social workers.
   a. Establish rapport.
   b. Identify ongoing patient needs for treatment as an outpatient.
      (1) Dialysis with specialty dialyzer.
      (2) Transportation to and from treatment.
      (3) Vascular access follow-up.
      (4) Patient's mobility and ability to self-transfer.
      (5) Need for special dialysis chair or scale.
      (6) Need for specialty dialysate bath.
   c. Communicate changes in patient status to facilitate transfer or discharge of patient.

5. Dietitians and dietary department.
   a. Establish rapport.
   b. Diet review.
   c. Establish kidney diet based on patient's current nutritional needs.
   d. Coordinate for patient education regarding diet as kidney function changes.
   e. Request that meal trays be delivered to the dialysis treatment room/unit or kept for the patient until after treatment.
   f. Record accurate intake and output (I & O) on the patient's record for his/her time in the dialysis unit.

6. Radiology and interventional radiology departments.
   a. Schedule procedures.
   b. Coordinate and prioritize procedures based on patient needs.

7. Surgery department. Schedule and coordinate procedures preoperatively or postoperatively.

8. Cardiac catheterization lab to coordinate dialysis treatments after a procedure.
   a. Need for treatment based on amount of dye used in the procedure.
   b. Monitor the groin or radial line site.
   c. Monitor changes in peripheral pulses.
   d. Maintain bed rest and flat position as prescribed.

9. Hospital laboratory, blood gas laboratory, and blood bank.
   a. Ensure correct collection and handling of samples.
   b. Receive accurate results in a timely manner to allow changes to treatment plan.

10. Pharmacy.
    a. Coordinate obtaining medications needed during the dialysis treatment.
    b. Some dialysis units have automated medication dispensing systems on-site.
    c. Some dialysis units keep narcotics on stock requiring counts and recordkeeping per pharmacy policy.
    d. Maintain a current supply of emergency drugs in the dialysis unit and replace when used or prior to their expiration dates.
    e. Coordinate maintaining a current stock of CRRT and peritoneal dialysis solutions in the pharmacy to ensure availability at all times, thereby avoiding treatment delays.
    f. Facilitate updating the hospital formulary with new medications related to nephrology as they are introduced on the market.

11. Housekeeping department.
    a. Communicate special cleaning needs and protection of housekeeping personnel due to potential contamination with blood or body fluids.
    b. Train personnel on safely moving dialysis equipment to facilitate adequate cleaning.

12. Central supply, materials management, supply distribution.
    a. Work with each facility's procedures to record and monitor par level inventory, order stock (routine or special order), and rotate stock on shelves and in distribution.
    b. Negotiate lowest prices for dialysis-related supplies in conjunction with dialysis vendors. Include contracted facilities in those rates if possible.

13. Architectural services or space planners.
    a. Consult for new space or remodeling of existing hospitals to incorporate adequate space for nephrology services.
    b. Plan for suitable square footage per station to accommodate the dialysis equipment in addition to the patient's bed and equipment (approximately 100 to 120 square feet per station).
       (1) While the CMS Conditions of Participation do not stipulate a minimum square footage requirement for each dialysis treatment station, surveyors would expect sufficient space be provided to:
          (a) Allow access of emergency equipment when needed.
          (b) Separate patient from another patient's splash zone.
          (c) Provide privacy for the patient's personal needs (Payne, 2014).
       (2) Recognize that state licensing rules for hospitals may address space requirements. Examples include:
          (a) California requires 110 square feet be allotted per each acute HD station (http://www.documents.dgs.ca.gov/bsc /prpsd_chngs/oshpd-02-07-et-rev.pdf).
          (b) Massachusetts, in Article 145.210, states there shall be space between beds, in addition to that necessary for

associated equipment, sufficient to allow access to the patient by at least two persons. In any unit constructed or undergoing major renovations after May 1, 1975, there shall be a minimum of 110 square feet of floor space per dialysis station (http://www.mass.gov/eohhs/gov/laws-regs/masshealth/provider-library/provider-manual/renal-dialysis-center-manual.html).

(c) Michigan requires a minimum of 100 square feet per bed/stretcher treatment station, a minimum head wall width of 8 feet per treatment station, and a minimum of 4 feet clearance around the treatment station (http://michigan.gov/documents/mdch/bhs_2007_Minimum_Design_Standards_Final_PDF_Doc._198958_7.pdf).

c. Water requirements.
(1) Selection of appropriate water treatment system based on water quality testing and use of a central or portable system.
(a) Reverse osmosis (RO).
(b) Deionization (DI) as backup or polisher.
(c) Carbon filtration.
(d) Softener.
(2) Adequate water pressure in pounds per square inch (PSI) to meet equipment requirements.
(3) Thermostatic mixing/blending valves.
(4) Back-flow preventer.
(5) Drains at correct height with capacity for adequate volume.
(6) Dedicated water hook-up in ICUs, other designated units, and patient rooms.
d. Electrical requirements.
(1) Dedicated 20-amp circuit for each dialysis machine station or the amperage required by the brand of equipment being used.
(2) Adequate number of regular outlets at each station to accommodate the patient's bed, several IV pumps, and other equipment.
e. Adequate and secure square footage for storage of equipment when not in use, as well as the large volume of supplies required.
f. Location in the facility with preference to proximity to the ICU, telemetry floor, kidney floor, or the cardiac floor to enhance support for an emergency in the dialysis unit.
g. Request a dedicated dialysis treatment room, as opposed to performing treatments at bedside, to increase efficiency of staffing in the dialysis unit.
14. Plant operations, facility management, and maintenance.

a. Maintain water resources and quality for central or portable reverse osmosis (RO) water treatment system.
b. Maintain electrical resources for equipment needs.
15. Information technology and telecommunication departments.
a. Develop electronic medical record templates for dialysis procedures.
b. Maintain access to electronic records while preserving patient privacy with user access codes and passwords.
c. Maintain electronic backup of all electronic records.
d. Provide and maintain adequate equipment for communication (faxes, copiers, computers, phones, pagers, Vocera).
e. Supply and maintain current electronic entry access cards.
f. Communicate nephrology personnel's on-call schedule to the telecommunications center or answering service.

VI. Challenging issues facing practitioners in the acute care setting.

A. Communication with chronic outpatient dialysis clinics.
1. Share information regarding patient's hospitalization including any surgical procedures, changes in vascular access, and/or adjustment of dry weight to enhance continuity of care.
2. Inform outpatient dialysis unit of doses of antibiotics and/or iron therapy given, the number of doses needed, and the schedule for continuing administration.
3. Notify outpatient dialysis units when a patient presents to the hospital with a vascular access infection or sepsis related to the access.
4. Ensure the patient has a functional vascular access prior to discharge to prevent frequent readmissions.
5. Share information to facilitate completion of the CMS 2728 form by the chronic dialysis unit and coordinate placement of a new chronic dialysis patient in the outpatient setting.
a. Date of first dialysis.
b. Electrocardiogram.
c. Chest x-ray.
d. Blood chemistry prior to first dialysis treatment.
e. Complete blood count prior to first dialysis treatment.
f. Lipid panel (within last year of ESRD episode).
g. TB skin test if done.
h. Hepatitis panel.
i. Hemoglobin A1C.

6. Provide predialysis modality training to a hospitalized patient.
7. Communicate the next scheduled outpatient treatment day and time to the patient in cooperation with the outpatient unit to avoid missed treatments immediately after discharge.
8. Ideally, the patient should be discharged in a timely manner so the patient can keep a regularly scheduled chronic dialysis unit appointment. When that cannot be achieved, dialyze the patient on the day of discharge when needed to get the patient back on or keep on the regular outpatient schedule.
9. Collaborate with agencies preparing for and particiating in community disaster planning.
   a. Participate in the hospital warning system and plan for moving and/or relocating of patients.
   b. Develop telephone calling tree for alerting dialysis staff when assistance is needed and at what location.
   c. Conduct an annual review of disaster polices and procedures including terminating treatment
   d. Participate in drills to practice evacuation of patients.
   e. Coordinate backup facility plans in local area for sending and/or receiving additional patients, including medical records and treatment histories.

B. Staffing challenges.
   1. Orienting to multiple therapies with different machines.
   2. Maintaining competency in low-volume, high-complexity treatments.
   3. Variability of caseloads and work hours.
   4. RN supervision of unlicensed personnel.
   5. Distance between facilities when contracting with multiple hospitals.
   6. Orientation to multiple facilities with varying expectations and different standard procedures.
   7. Limited recruitment options due to high skill level required.
   8. Financial issues.
      a. Pay per hour or per case.
      b. Overtime pay.
      c. Bonus payment systems.
         (1) Shift and weekend differential.
         (2) On-call treatments.
         (3) On-call time availability.
         (4) Charge/coordinator nurse.
         (5) Preceptor.
      d. Working the day after being on-call and working through the night.
      e. Benefits.

9. Safety in the workplace.
   a. Working conditions.
   b. Violent and/or hostile patients.
   c. Arriving and leaving from facilities unescorted after dark.

C. Equipment.
   1. Completing machine repairs in a timely manner.
   2. Transporting machines between facilities and units.
   3. Performing routine disinfection and preventive maintenance on equipment in remote or low use locations.
   4. Not enough machines or support equipment at every facility.
   5. Multiple machines out of service at one time for cultures and *Limulus* amebocyte lysate (LAL) and preventive maintenance (PM), and/or machines sequestered for radioactive or infectious (Hepatitis B, Ebola, etc.) patient treatments, causing a longer workday for staff.

D. Contracted employees.
   1. Credentialing process.
      a. Length of time to complete process.
      b. Amount of documentation required.
   2. Relationships with facility personnel.
      a. Communication.
      b. Coordination of care.
      c. Support services.
      d. Different practice methodologies in multiple facilities.
      e. Education regarding the special needs of the dialysis team to foster safe, quality patient care.
      f. Involvement in patient care decisions.
      g. Nursing care challenges.

E. Relationships with healthcare providers.
   1. Conflicts with scheduling treatments for multiple physician groups.
      a. Establishing policy regarding prioritization.
      b. Avoiding late day add-ons for nonemergent care.
      c. Negotiating scheduling of nonemergent treatments on major holidays.
   2. Negotiating physician cooperation to establish consistent policies and procedures in all facilities.
   3. Interactions showing aggressive and/or disrespectful behaviors.
   4. Disagreement among physician specialists regarding patient plan of care.
   5. Participation in coordination of care with hospital units or outpatient clinics and acute nephrology staff.
   6. Nonemergent treatments performed by on-call personnel for physician convenience.

F. Information on impact of affordable care organizations (ACO).
    1. ACOs are provider organizations formed to assume responsibility for the overall total cost and quality of an assigned patient population. Primary care physicians are always included and may or may not include specialists and hospitals. ACOs can pursue contracts with public or private payers, who will reward them for controlling the cost of care, provided that quality metrics are met.
        a. Hospitals preparing to join both federal and private-sector ACO programs may need to assess and potentially revise their existing contracts with other providers that are also taking part in the ACO.
        b. Implementing the ACO concept may require hospitals, physicians, and other providers to accept one payment for all services and share financial incentives.
        c. Nonprofit hospitals would need to determine whether their involvement with participating, for-profit physician practices as part of an ACO complies with Internal Revenue Service (IRS) guidelines for nonprofit institutions.
        d. Hospital and health systems considering ACO participation should assess their capabilities in several key core competencies that will likely be necessary for successful ACO implementation, including:
            (1) Information technology (IT) infrastructure.
            (2) Resources for patient education.
            (3) Team-building capabilities.
            (4) Strong relationships with physicians and other providers.
            (5) The ability to monitor and report quality data.
        e. Study the formation of organizations that may become ACO partnerships or joint venture arrangements between hospitals and physicians and professionals.
        f. Consider the implications of the hospital employing physicians and professionals and the associated responsibilities.
    2. Challenges related to ACOs.
        a. Governance of establishing an entity that can manage risk and balance and that interests various organizations and individuals involved to create a shared vision for the best care.
        b. Physician participation is important, including recruitment and retention for both primary and specialty physicians.
        c. Ensuring all the data is fulfilling ACO objectives: adopt technology to incorporate health information, enabling ACO participants leverage to existing information systems to exchange data, facilitate care coordination, and

perform quality reporting.
        d. Educating patients for consumer acceptance to show the benefit of coordinated care and reassuring them that the ACO will provide the best care.
    3. Benefits to hospitals participating in ACO.
        a. Better and demonstrated clinical outcomes.
        b. Enhanced reputation for quality.
        c. Physician loyalty.
        d. Decreased costs of doing business.
        e. Increased efficiency.
        f. Improved affinity with the healthcare community.
        g. Patient satisfaction/engagement.
    4. Benefits to patients participating in ACO.
        a. Increased access to care.
        b. Improved communication and coordination, especially chronic care management.
        c. Unnecessary care eliminated: the possibility of fewer medical tests, since ACOs are based on pay-for-quality or fee-for-service models, and provider is less likely to order unnecessary or duplicative tests.
        d. Reduction in administrative processes: less paperwork; electronic health record allows access to all providers.
        e. Single point of contact: you will have one member of the care team to contact.
    5. Benefits to physician participating in ACO.
        a. Ease of entry to value-based payments. Medicare has roadmaps for ACOs.
        b. Patient retention and loyalty due to well-managed care and experiencing better outcomes.
        c. Physician-determined risk. Ability to earn Medicare incentives: fee-for-service; eligible for bonuses; no financial risk of cost of care increase in 3-year contract period.
    6. Impact to nephrologists participating in ACO.
        a. Patient Protection and Affordable Care Act and Center for Medicare and Medicaid regulations preclude renal-specific ACOs.
        b. Nonphysician, nonhospital providers (e.g., dialysis providers) are not eligible to form an ACO.
        c. The pathway for the CMS Innovation is a viable mechanism by which renal-specific ACOs may be created and tested under support of the broad renal community.
        d. In a renal-specific ACO, nephrologists would have responsibility for coordinating their patients' care and would be able to share the savings generated for caring for a group of high-cost Medicare patients. By contrast, in a primary-care-led ACO, patients with kidney disease may be seen as costly problems when compared with the majority of other patients.

G. Interactions with patients.
   1. Angry, hostile, violent patients.
      a. Psychiatric diagnoses vs. recreational drug abuse vs. response to life's issues.
      b. Establish parameters for acceptable behavior and when treatment will be discontinued due to violation of those parameters.
      c. Hospital or family to provide a "sitter" at the bedside during treatment.
      d. Healthcare provider to manage chemical or physical restraint choices, including documentation of patient responses.
      e. Security officer available or onsite when needed.
   2. Cultural and religious diversity.
      a. Staff education about respecting diversity.
      b. Language barriers.
         (1) Hospital-based translator.
         (2) Computer or telephone translator availability.
         (3) http://www.Babelfish.com
         (4) Provide written educational materials in patient's language.
         (5) Provide consent for treatment(s) in patient's language.
         (6) Blood or blood products – acceptable or not?
         (7) Native healers and traditional ceremonies.
         (8) Evaluating quality of life in consideration of end-of-life care, including the influence of cultural and religious leaders.
         (9) Complementary or alternative therapies.
   3. Nonadherence to schedule and fluid management in chronic treatment setting, leading to frequent emergent treatments in the acute setting.
   4. Financial issues.
      a. Underinsured.
      b. Uninsured.
      c. Disposition during the 90-day waiting period for Medicare coverage at outpatient dialysis clinic.
   5. Legal complexities.
      a. Undocumented residents.
      b. No durable power of attorney for health care (DPAHC) or conservator.

H. Interactions with patient's family.
   1. Family willingness to adhere to patient's decision.
   2. Overwhelming family involvement at the bedside.
      a. Boisterous or argumentative.
      b. Disruptive to patient or roommate.
      c. Attention seeking for their own issues over the patient's needs.
   3. No family available to make decisions.
   4. Family members contesting plan of care.
   5. Who makes decisions in the absence of a DPAHC?
   6. Evaluation of patient's quality of life.
   7. Participation in planning end-of-life care.

I. Hospital Consumer Assessment of Healthcare Providers and Systems (HCAHPS).
   1. Beginning in 2002, CMS partnered with the Agency for Healthcare Research and Quality (AHRQ), another agency in the federal Department of Health and Human Services, to develop and test the HCAHPS survey.
   2. The HCAHPS is the first national, standardized, publicly reported survey of patients' perspectives of hospital care. This 27-item instrument and data collection methodology measures patients' perceptions of their hospital experience.
   3. In May 2005, the HCAHPS survey was endorsed by the National Quality Forum (NQF), a national organization that represents the consensus of many healthcare providers, consumer groups, professional associations, purchasers, federal agencies, and research and quality organizations.
   4. In December 2005, the federal Office of Management and Budget (OMB) gave its final approval for the national implementation of HCAHPS for public reporting purposes.
   5. CMS implemented the HCAHPS Survey in October 2006, and the first public reporting of HCAHPS results occurred in March 2008. The survey, its methodology, and the results it produces are in the public domain.
   6. Enactment of the Deficit Reduction Act of 2005 created an additional incentive for acute care hospitals to participate in HCAHPS.
   7. Since July 2007, hospitals subject to the Inpatient Prospective Payment System (IPPS) annual payment update provisions (subsection [d]) must collect and submit HCAHPS data in order to receive their full annual payment update.
   8. IPPS hospitals that fail to publicly report the required quality measures, which include the HCAHPS Survey, may receive an annual payment update that is reduced by 2.0 percentage points.
   9. Non-IPPS hospitals, such as Critical Access Hospitals, may voluntarily participate in HCAHPS.
   10. Since 2008, HCAHPS has allowed valid comparisons to be made across hospitals locally, regionally, and nationally.
   11. Publicly reported HCAHPS results are based on four consecutive quarters of patient surveys.
   12. CMS publishes HCAHPS results on the Hospital Compare website (http://www.medicare.gov/hospitalcompare/search.html) four times a year, rolling the oldest quarter of patient surveys off and the newest quarter on each time.
   13. Eight HCAHPS measures are employed in hospital value-based purchasing within which system these are termed "dimensions" (http://www.hcahpsonline.org/home.aspx).

Patient Self–Determination Act (PSDA)

On November 5, 1990, Congress passed this measure as an amendment to the Omnibus Budget Reconciliation Act of 1990. It became effective on December 1, 1991. The Patient Self-Determination Act (PSDA) requires many Medicare and Medicaid providers (hospitals, nursing homes, hospice programs, home health agencies, and HMOs) to give adult individuals, at the time of inpatient admission or enrollment, certain information about their rights under laws governing advance directives, including: (1) the right to participate in and direct their own healthcare decisions; (2) the right to accept or refuse medical or surgical treatment; (3) the right to prepare an advance directive; (4) information on the provider's policies that govern the utilization of these rights. The act also prohibits institutions from discriminating against a patient who does not have an advance directive. The PSDA further requires institutions to document patient information and provide ongoing community education on advance directives.

Source: Ascension Health. (2005). Retrieved from www.ascension health.org/ethics/public/issues/patient_self.asp. Used with permission.

a. The six HCAHPS composites.
   (1) Communication with nurses.
   (2) Communication with doctors.
   (3) Staff responsiveness.
   (4) Pain management.
   (5) Communication about medicines.
   (6) Discharge information (http://www.hcahpsonline.org/Facts.aspx).
b. One new composite that combines the hospital cleanliness and quietness survey items.
c. One global item (Overall Rating of Hospital).
14. Used to calculate the Patient Experience of Care Domain score is the percentage of a hospital's patients who chose the most positive, or "top box," survey response to these HCAHPS surveys in these HCAHPS dimensions.
15. The incentive for IPPS hospitals to improve patient experience of care was further strengthened by the Patient Protection and Affordable Care Act of 2010 (P.L. 111-148), which specifically included HCAHPS performance in the calculation of the value-based incentive payment in the Hospital Value-Based Purchasing program, beginning with discharges in October 2012.

J. Ethical dilemmas.
  1. Definitions to consider.
     a. Respect for autonomy: the right of people to make choices.
     b. Beneficence: the obligation to help people in need.
     c. Nonmalificence: the duty to do no harm.
     d. Justice: treating everyone fairly.
     e. Distributive justice: all must receive a reasonable level of medical care.
  2. Examples of patient and staff concerns and issues.
     a. Initiating kidney replacement therapy on a patient with a Do Not Resuscitate (DNR) plan in place.
     b. Treatment of undocumented residents knowing they will be unable to receive adequate follow-up care in this country.
     c. Patients who have been discharged from the outpatient dialysis clinic due to violent and aggressive behavior now come to the acute care setting regularly. What do the acute care providers do to address continued behavior issues when there is no alternative for the patient to receive treatment?
     d. Patients who have verbalized clearly their end-of-life care to the acute care staff. Family arrive and demand the staff "do everything to save" their loved one.
  3. Factors to consider.
     a. Patient Self Determination Act (PSDA)(see Table 1.1).
        (1) Shared decision making includes physician, nurses, patient, and family in healthcare decisions.
        (2) Informed consent or refusal of treatment based on understanding of the personal decision.
     b. Emergency Medical Treatment & Labor Act (EMTALA) (see Table 1.2).
        (1) Obligation to treat everyone.
        (2) Staff must take precautions to minimize their personal risk.
  4. Resources available in the acute care setting.
     a. Ethics committee.
     b. Palliative care team.
     c. Pastoral care.
     d. Patient representative.
     e. Patient care team.
     f. Nephrologist.
     g. End-Stage Renal Disease (ESRD) Networks.
     h. Kidney End-of-Life Coalition at http://www.kidneysupportivecare.org/Home.aspx
     i. ANNA's Ethics Committee.
     j. Hospital liaison.
     k. Case managers and/or social workers.
     l. Dialysis unit leadership.
     m. Mental Health Advanced Practitioner.
     n. Complementary or alternative therapist.
     o. Hospice.

Table 1.2

Emergency Medical Treatment and Labor Act

In 1986, Section 1867 of the Social Security Act imposed specific obligations on Medicare participating hospitals that offered emergency services to provide a medical screening examination (MSE) when a request is made for examination or treatment for an emergency medical condition (EMC), including active labor, regardless of an individual's ability to pay. Hospitals were then required to provide stabilizing treatment for patients with EMCs. If a hospital is unable to stabilize a patient within its capability, or if the patient requests, an appropriate transfer should be implemented (Center for Medicare & Medicaid Services, 2006).

Source: Centers for Medicare and Medicaid Services. (2006). *Medicare coverage for ESRD patients, section 1881* (42 U.S.C. 1395rr). Retrieved from http://www.ssa.gov/OP_Home/ssact/title18/1881.htm. Used with permission.

References

Centers for Disease Control (CDC). (2002). *Guidelines for the prevention of intravascular catheter-related infections.* Retrieved from http://www.cdc.gov/mmwr/preview/mmwrhtml/rr5110al.htm

Centers for Disease Control (CDC). (2011a). *Bloodborne infectious diseases: HIV/AIDS, hepatitis B, hepatitis.* Retrieved from http://www.cdc.gov/niosh/topics/bbp

Centers for Disease Control (CDC). 2011b). *State by state provisions of state needle safety regulations.* Retrieved from http://www.cdc.gov/niosh/topics/bbp/ndl-law-1.html

Payne, G. (2014). Personal communication.

Appendix 1.1. Sample Patient Education Brochure (page 1 of 2)

Source: Creighton Nephrology, Creighton University, Omaha, Nebraska.

DIALYSIS CLINIC, INCORPORATED

OMAHA, NEBRASKA

ACUTE RENAL FAILURE

Acute Hemodialysis Service

1995 Margaret Nusser-Gerlach, BSN, RN, CNN

1998 Jina Bogle, RN

Transfusions

If the kidneys stop secreting erythropoietin, the patient will become anemic and may need blood transfusions.

Skin Care / Infection

It will be important to prevent pressure sores and infections. Nonfunctioning kidneys make patients prone to infection and prolong healing time.

Please minimize contact if you have been exposed to a contagious disease or have a cold or flu.

Appendix 1.1. Sample Patient Education Brochure (page 2 of 2)

NORMAL KIDNEY FUNCTION
Healthy kidneys have many important functions:
- Filter waste products from metabolism (creatinine) and protein foods *blood urea nitrogen (BUN)
- Removal of excess fluids
- Regulate chemicals and minerals
- Regulate bone metabolism
- Regulate balance of acid/base in blood and lungs
- Regulate blood pressure and sodium
- Secrete erythropoietin, a hormone that tells the bone marrow to make new red blood cells

KIDNEY INJURY AND DAMAGE
Many situations can injure or damage kidneys:
- Trauma/crushing injury to organs and muscles
- Large blood loss
- Prolonged low blood pressure
- Burns
- Infections in the blood stream (sepsis)
- Heart or blood vessel operation
- Liver failure
- Diabetes
- Too much or any drug – prescription or street drugs
- Dyes or toxic chemicals

Acute Renal Failure
The kidneys have millions of microscopic blood vessels that need a large blood supply. Any problem that interferes with the blood supply may injure or damage the filtering part of the kidneys.

A sudden injury causing loss of kidney function is called **acute renal failure**. Acute renal failure can be temporary, and may be reversible if the kidneys are able to heal. During this time, waste products and extra fluid will build up in the blood stream. They are toxic and cause death unless filtered out another way. Special treatments called **Hemodialysis** or **Continuous Renal Replacement Therapy (CRRT)** can be done.

Vascular Access
Neither hemodialysis nor CRRT can be performed without a way to obtain a blood flow of 200–400 mL (about 6–13 ounces) a minute through a dialyzer. A vein cannot supply that much blood in one minute for three to four hours. There are several ways to obtain this blood supply. They are called vascular accesses.

A large intravenous catheter with a wall down the middle and holes on the end is called a **dual lumen hemodialysis catheter**. A physician inserts the catheter into the subclavian (under the collarbone), jugular (in the neck), or femoral (in the groin) vein. The physician decides the best place to insert the catheter. Local anesthetic is used, and the catheter is stitched into place. A chest x-ray makes sure the catheter is in the right place.

Special dressings will cover the insertion site and should not get wet. The lumens will be clamped while not being used for dialysis. The catheter may be used to infuse medications between dialysis treatments. The catheter is removed when dialysis is no longer needed.

Hemodialysis
A dialysis machine uses an artificial kidney called a dialyzer to filter the waste products and extra fluid from the blood. Tubing is attached to the vascular access for three to five hours. The patient cannot feel the actual dialysis treatment.

The treatment is monitored continuously by a specially trained RN who brings the machine and supplies to the ICU/CCU. The Dialysis RN may transfuse blood, proteins, or medications during the treatment, and works with ICU/CCU RN to manage patient care.

Patients who are not in ICU/CCU and are medically stable can be transported to the Inpatient Hemodialysis Unit 5316 on the 5th floor at Creighton University Medical Center. There, dialysis nurses work together to dialyze one to four patients at a time. Patients are dialyzed in their rooms in all other CDI contracted hospitals.

Continuous Renal Replacement Therapy
The Nephrologist may order a slower continuous waste and fluid removal system, using an automated pump-assisted machine and artificial kidney. This therapy requires a dual lumen catheter to be placed in a large vein to provide vascular access for blood purification. The dialysis RN will initiate the therapy and work with the Critical Care RN to manage the patient's care while receiving CRRT. After the CRRT machine is functioning and the system is working the Critical Care RN takes over monitoring the machine, system, and patient care. The Dialysis RN is available 24 hours a day for support and problem solving. The Dialysis RN checks the machine system twice daily and periodically changes the artificial kidney. Every 24 hours, the Nephrologist will instruct the Dialysis RN to make changes in the therapy, continue or end the therapy.

Treatment Schedule
There is no way to predict how long a patient will need hemodialysis. The Nephrologist will check lab value daily to determine how often dialysis is needed. The patient is monitored closely for signs of returning kidney function.

Nutrition
While the kidneys are functioning, dietary protein, potassium, sodium, and fluids will be restricted to decrease the kidneys' workload and to keep toxic levels as low as possible. A special IV mixture called hyperalimentation may be infused for food/calories. Tube feedings or supplements may be ordered. A special renal dietitian will work with the Nephrologist.

If you have any questions or concerns, please ask to talk to the Nephrologist or Dialysis Nurse. We want to help you understand Acute Renal Failure and the hemodialysis process.

CHAPTER **2**
Acute Kidney Injury

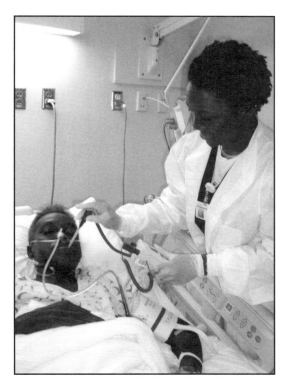

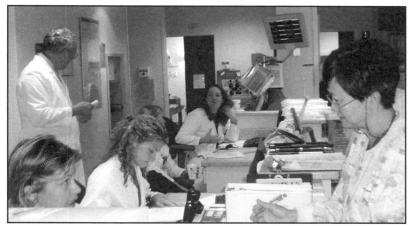

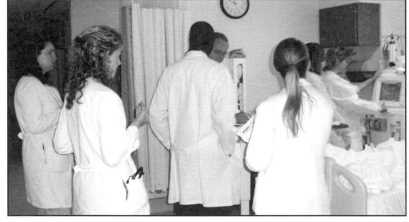

Chapter Editor
Helen F. Williams, MSN, BSN, RN, CNN

Authors
Susan Fallone, MS, RN, CNN
Ann Beemer Cotton, MS, RDN, CNSC

CHAPTER **2**

Acute Kidney Injury

This offering for **1.7 contact hours** is provided by the American Nephrology Nurses' Association (ANNA).

American Nephrology Nurses' Association is accredited as a provider of continuing nursing education by the American Nurses Credentialing Center Commission on Accreditation.

ANNA is a provider approved by the California Board of Registered Nursing, provider number CEP 00910.

This CNE offering meets the continuing nursing education requirements for certification and recertification by the Nephrology Nursing Certification Commission (NNCC).

To be awarded contact hours for this activity, read this chapter in its entirety. Then complete the CNE evaluation found at **www.annanurse.org/corecne** and submit it; or print it, complete it, and mail it in. Contact hours are not awarded until the evaluation for the activity is complete.

Example of reference for Chapter 2 in APA format.

Fallone, S., & Cotton, A.B. (2015). Acute kidney injury. In C.S. Counts (Ed.), *Core curriculum for nephrology nursing: Module 4. Acute kidney injury* (6th ed., pp. 19-54). Pitman, NJ: American Nephrology Nurses' Association.

Interpreted: Chapter authors. (Date). Title of chapter. In …

Cover photos by Sandra Cook.

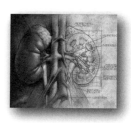

CHAPTER 2

Acute Kidney Injury

Purpose

The purpose of this chapter is to describe acute kidney injury and the etiology, pathology, assessment, and nursing care specific to this group of patients.

Objectives

Upon completion of this chapter, the learner will be able to:
1. Describe the debate surrounding the definition of acute kidney injury.
2. Describe the at-risk and special populations and their nursing care needs.
3. Describe the etiology, pathophysiology, assessment findings, presentation, and care management of patients with prerenal, intrarenal, and postrenal acute kidney injury.

I. **Definitions and descriptions of acute kidney injury and acute kidney failure.**

A. Traditional definitions.
   1. Sudden, rapid deterioration of kidney function.
   2. Potentially reversible.
   3. Associated with:
      a. Oliguria: < 500 mL/day (International System [SI] = 0.5 L/day).
      b. Nonoliguria: > 800 mL/day (SI = 0.8 L/day).
      c. Oliguria indicates a more severe insult to the kidney compared to nonoliguria. Usually associated with azotemia (retention of nitrogenous substances in the blood), although the actual levels of accumulation, as indicated by serum creatinine levels, that are necessary to be considered acute kidney injury are still under extensive debate.
   4. AKI may be defined as any of the following:
      a. An increase in serum creatinine (Cr) by 0.3 mg/dL within 48 hours, *or*
      b. An increase in serum Cr to 1.5 times baseline, which is known or presumed to have occurred within the prior 7 days, *or*
      c. Urine volume of 0.5 mL/kg/hr for 6 hours.
      d. These criteria have been incorporated into a three-tier staging of AKI presented in the KDIGO Guidelines of 2012 (see Table 2.1 KDIGO AKI Guidelines).
   5. The concern and attempt to define staging is directly related to the reality that AKI is common, is increasing in incidence, and is associated with considerable morbidity and mortality.

6. Mild alteration in kidney function to overt organ damage injury may exist without kidney impairment.
7. Some patients experience similar problems with fluid and electrolyte imbalances as those patients with chronic kidney disease, but not usually the profound neurologic and musculoskeletal disorders that develop over time.

Table 2.1

Staging of AKI

STAGE	SERUM CREATININE	URINE OUTPUT
1	1.5–1.9 baseline OR ≥ 0.3 mg/dL (≥ 26.5 µmol/L increase)	< 0.5 mL/kg/h for 6–12 hours
2	2.0–2.9 times baseline	< 0.5 mL/kg/h for ≥ 12 hours
3	3.0 baseline OR Increase in creatinine to ≥ 4.0 mg/dL (≥ 353.6 µmol/L) OR Initiation of renal replacement therapy OR In patients < 18 years, decrease in eGFR to < 135 mL/min per 1.73 m²	< 0.3 mL/kg/h for ≥ 24 hours OR Anuria for ≥ 12 hours

Used with permission from KDIGO (2012). Clinical practice guideline for acute kidney injury. Retrieved from http://kdigo.org/home/guidelines/acute-kidney-injury

B. Patients at risk for acute kidney injury.
1. The elderly.
2. Postsurgical patients, especially cardiovascular.
3. Patients who develop sepsis.
4. Patients who experience major trauma that results in significant blood loss and muscle damage.
5. Patients with multiple organ dysfunction syndrome (MODS), also called multisystem organ failure (MSOF).
6. Patients with hepatorenal syndrome.
7. Patients with complications from medications.
8. Patients with obstructive uropathy.
9. People with compromised underlying kidney disease that acquire a serious illness or suffer an exposure to a nephrotoxic agent.
   a. Develop what is known as "acute on chronic" kidney failure.
   b. It is important to preserve blood vessels for future vascular access placement.
   c. Avoid placement of PICC (peripherally inserted central catheter) lines if possible to preserve vessels.
   d. Exercise extra vigilance in monitoring to prevent and/or intervene quickly at first sign of AKI.

C. Incidence data.
1. The development of AKI increases the mortality associated with any primary disease.
2. AKI develops in 13% to 18% of all hospitalized patients.
3. One in 5 adults and 1 in 3 children experience AKI during a hospitalization (Susantitaphong et al., 2013).
4. 58% of these patients will require another hospitalization within a year (USRDS, 2013).
5. Approximately 20% to 60% of hospitalized patients who develop AKI require dialysis treatment.
6. Older age, male sex, and black race are associated with higher incidence of dialysis-requiring AKI (USRDS, 2013).
7. Of patients developing AKI, 50% to 60% will regain most, if not all, of their kidney function.
8. Depending on the severity of the kidney injury, mortality averages 50% to 80%.
9. Infection accounts for 75% of deaths in patients with AKI and is the primary cause of AKI.
10. Cardiorespiratory complications are the second most common cause of death.
11. Incidence and prevalence of AKI are significantly increased in the elderly.
12. AKI occurs in 1 of every 2000 to 5000 pregnancies.
13. Probably most transplant recipients have some degree of AKI.
    a. A conservative estimate of the incidence of AKI following nonrenal organ transplantation is 50%.
    b. Following cardiac transplant, early AKI (in the immediate postoperative period of 0 to 30 days) incidence is approximately 50%; late AKI (occurring after 30 days) has an incidence of 1% to 2%.

D. Search for consensus in AKI research.
1. Numerous studies have looked at treatment modalities, outcomes, prevention, and management of ARF/AKI over the past 5 decades.
2. Since the studies have used different criteria for defining what acute renal failure/acute kidney injury is, the results have limited generalizability to other locations and patient populations.
3. The PICARD (Program to Improve Care in Acute Renal Disease) experience, a large multicenter international study, confirmed the wide variation in definition of ARF/AKI and the practice patterns for management of care and choice of kidney replacement therapy.
4. Scoring systems available in the acute setting to predict patient outcomes.
   a. APACHE II.
      (1) Acute Physiology and Chronic Health Evaluation II score.
      (2) Designed to measure the severity of disease for patients (age 16 or more) admitted to intensive care units (ICUs).
      (3) A point score is calculated during the first 24 hours from 12 routine physiologic measurements, information about previous health status, and information obtained at admission.
      (4) The calculated score is used to establish a predicted death rate.
      (5) There are differing opinions about whether this tool is effective in patients with acute renal failure/acute kidney injury.
   b. SOFA score.
      (1) Sequential Organ Failure Assessment score.
      (2) A score is assigned to each of six organ systems (respiratory, cardiovascular, hepatic, coagulation, renal, and neurologic) with a grade range from 0 to 4.
      (3) Calculated on admission and then daily or every 48 hours to evaluate changes.
      (4) The initial, highest, and mean SOFA scores are evaluated to predict mortality rate.
      (5) Has been used successfully to evaluate and predict mortality in acute renal failure/acute kidney injury patients in the ICU.
   c. ATN-ISS.
      (1) Acute Tubular Necrosis Individual Severity score.
      (2) Produces a percent likelihood of mortality on the basis of several physiologic and

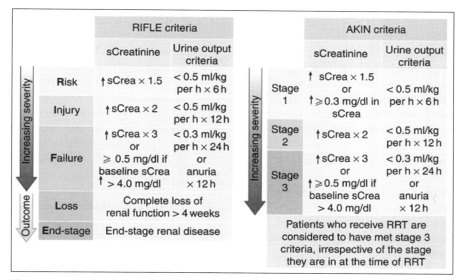

Figure 2.1. Comparison of RIFLE (risk, injury, failure, loss, and end-stage) and Acute Kidney Injury Network (AKIN) Criteria for the diagnosis of AKI.

Open source paper. Used with permission from Seller-Pérez, G., Herrera-Gutiérrez, M.E., Maynar-Moliner, J., Sánchez-Izquierdo-Riera, J.A., Marinho, A., & Luis do Pico, J. (2013). Estimating kidney function in the critically ill patients. *Critical Care Research and Practice.* doi:10.1155/2013/721810

laboratory parameters.
(3) Limited to patients with acute tubular necrosis (ATN); does not address other forms of ARF/AKI.
d. SHARF scores.
(1) Stuivenberg Hospital Acute Renal Failure scores.
(2) Factors included in the formula: age, serum albumin, and partial thromboplastin time (PTT) lab values. Respiratory support (vent) and heart failure are given a numeric value as absent (0) or present (1).
(3) Measurements calculated at both Time 0 (T0) and Time 48 hours (T48) were found to improve the predictive value of the model.
e. RIFLE (see Figure 2.1).
(1) Risk, Injury, Failure, Loss, and End-stage kidney failure.
(2) Product of the Acute Dialysis Quality Initiative group (ADQI).
(3) Patients classified based on estimated glomerular filtration rate (GFR) ranges and/or urine output in mL/kg/hr.
(4) May prove helpful in deciding timing of initiation of KRT as well as offering a prediction of prognosis for consideration in allocation of financial and personnel resources.
(5) A limitation of this method is that a baseline serum creatinine (SCr) is necessary but frequently unknown, resulting in use of an estimation using the

Modification of Diet in Renal Disease (MDRD), which is validated in CKD patients but not AKI patients.
f. AKIN staging system for AKI.
(1) Acute Kidney Injury Network, an international interdisciplinary group.
(2) Modification to RIFLE criteria.
(3) A highly sensitive staging system based on data indicating a small change in serum creatinine influences outcome and early detection of mild AKI.
(4) May identify patients with underlying CKD that may be missed by the RIFLE criteria (Murugan & Kellum, 2011).
(5) A limitation of this method is that it requires at least two SCr within 48 hours; it does not allow the identification of AKI when the SCr occurs greater than 48 hours.
g. KDIGO.
(1) Kidney Disease Improving Global Outcomes.
(2) Combined RIFLE and AKIN in order to establish one classification of AKI for practice (refer to Figure 2.1).

II. Prevention of further acute kidney injury/acute kidney failure.

A. Maintaining hydration.
1. May require placement of pulmonary artery catheter to measure filling pressures, cardiac output, and systemic vascular resistance to determine patient volume.

2. Preoperatively.
   a. Prevent kidney hypoperfusion and ischemia.
   b. Prophylactic dopamine should not be used specifically for prevention of AKI/ARF since studies have not supported any protective effect on kidney outcome or mortality.
3. In patients receiving nephrotoxic drugs.
   a. Adjust the initial drug dose based on the patient's GFR.
   b. Monitor serum levels and adjust doses accordingly.
   c. Avoid daily dosing in the presence of elevated creatinine level.
4. Prior to radiographic studies being conducted.
   a. The potential associated pathology may involve kidney vasoconstriction.
   b. Hydration with saline has shown improved kidney outcomes.
   c. Mannitol and furosemide infusions increase urinary output, but do not reduce the risk of worsening kidney function.
   d. Acetylcysteine (Mucomyst®) administration orally the day before and the day of administration of contrast.
      (1) Is an inexpensive alternative treatment.
      (2) May have some benefit in protecting kidney function.
      (3) Has antioxidant and vasodilatory properties.
      (4) May minimize vasoconstriction and oxygen-free radical generation from radiocontrast materials.
      (5) Use of low-osmolar or iso-osmolar contrast media.
5. Normal saline administration.
   a. Aggressive in patients with rhabdomyolysis to maintain urine output of 200 to 300 mL/hr.
   b. For patients with other risk factors, administration of saline to achieve a rate of urine output of 150 to 200 mL/hr is adequate.
6. Furosemide (Lasix®) use should be limited to times when diuresis is needed. Using as a prophylactic approach to prevent AKI/ARF may actually worsen kidney outcomes.

B. Maintaining kidney perfusion.
   1. Vasoactive agents.
      a. Low-dose dopamine is no longer shown to improve, and may actually decrease, return of kidney function. It can also contribute to adverse complications, such as cardiac arrhythmias, myocardial infarction (MI), and gastrointestinal (GI) ischemia.
      b. Calcium channel blockers may be effective in reducing the incidence and severity of AKI/ARF following cadaveric kidney transplantation.

   c. Atrial natriuretic peptide (ANP) has been shown to increase (GFR), reverse kidney vasoconstriction, and block sodium reabsorption in animal studies. At this point in the studies, it is not recommended to prevent or treat AKI (KDIGO, 2012).
   2. Volume expanders. The comparable effectiveness of crystalloids vs. colloids continues to be debated.
      a. Crystalloids: 0.9% saline (normal), 0.45% saline (half normal), dextrose 5% in water (D5W), and lactated Ringer's solution (LR), isotonic sodium bicarbonate solution (KDIGO, 2012).
      b. Colloids: albumin, dextran, and hetastarch.

C. Minimizing exposure to nephrotoxins.
   1. Antibiotics.
      a. Aminoglycosides are well-recognized nephrotoxins.
      b. Kidney hypoperfusion or kidney ischemia predisposes this nephrotoxicity.
   2. Radiocontrast materials.
   3. Nonsteroidal antiinflammatory drugs (NSAIDs).

D. Infection control.
   1. Skin care.
   2. Respiratory care.
   3. Management of indwelling lines and exit-site care.
   4. Removal of indwelling urinary catheters as soon as possible.

E. Nutritional support to maintain the building blocks for cellular reproduction and to mitigate the response to the stress and insult of acute illness.

F. Continual assessment and monitoring of kidney function to facilitate early interventions.

G. When to initiate dialysis in patients with AKI.
   1. Ideally, to minimize morbidity, treatment should be initiated prior to the onset of complications due to kidney failure.
   2. Indications include one or more of the following.
      a. Refractory fluid overload.
      b. Hyperkalemia (serum potassium concentration > 6.5 mEq/L) or rapidly rising potassium levels.
      c. Metabolic acidosis (pH < 7.1).
      d. Azotemia with BUN > 80 to 100 mg/dL (29 to 30 mmol/L).
      e. Signs of uremia.
         (1) Pericarditis.
         (2) Bleeding disorders from uremia platelet dysfunction.
         (3) Neuropathy or an otherwise unexplainable decline in mental status.
            (a) Asterixis.
            (b) Tremor.
            (c) Seizures.

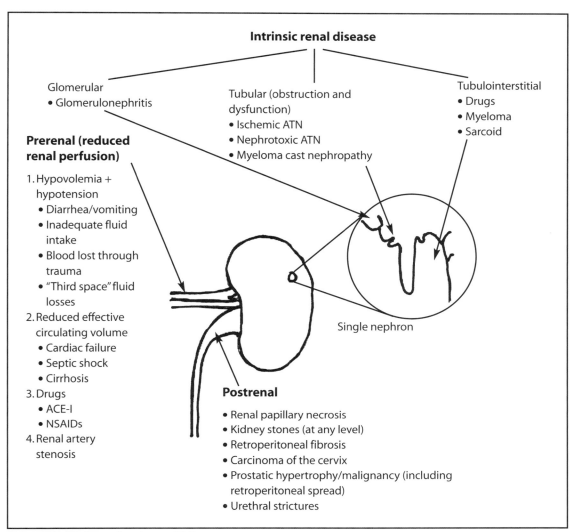

Intrinsic renal disease

Glomerular
• Glomerulonephritis

Tubular (obstruction and dysfunction)
• Ischemic ATN
• Nephrotoxic ATN
• Myeloma cast nephropathy

Tubulointerstitial
• Drugs
• Myeloma
• Sarcoid

Prerenal (reduced renal perfusion)

1. Hypovolemia + hypotension
    • Diarrhea/vomiting
    • Inadequate fluid intake
    • Blood lost through trauma
    • "Third space" fluid losses
2. Reduced effective circulating volume
    • Cardiac failure
    • Septic shock
    • Cirrhosis
3. Drugs
    • ACE-I
    • NSAIDs
4. Renal artery stenosis

Single nephron

Postrenal

• Renal papillary necrosis
• Kidney stones (at any level)
• Retroperitoneal fibrosis
• Carcinoma of the cervix
• Prostatic hypertrophy/malignancy (including retroperitoneal spread)
• Urethral strictures

Figure 2.2. Etiology of acute renal failure.

Source: Fry, A.C., & Farrington, K. (2006). Management of acute renal failure. *Postgraduate Medicine Journal, 82*, 106-116. Used with permission.

f. Severe dysnatremias with serum sodium levels < 120 mEq/L or > 155 mEq/L.
g. Hyperthermia.
h. Overdose with a dialyzable drug or toxin.
3. Less common indications.
    a. Drug intoxication requiring hemoperfusion.
    b. Hypothermia.
    c. Hyperurcemia.
    d. Hypercalcemia.
    e. Metabolic alkalosis requiring a special dialysis solution.

III. Causes, pathology, and management of acute kidney injury and acute kidney failure.

A. Prerenal acute renal failure.
    1. Incidence: approximately 35% of cases of ARF

depending on the definition of ARF used (see Figure 2.2).
2. Etiology.
    a. Decreased blood flow to the kidneys.
        (1) Intraoperative.
        (2) Blood vessel obstruction.
    b. Decreased intravascular volume (hypovolemia).
        (1) Sepsis and systemic inflammatory response syndrome (SIRS).
        (2) Hemorrhage.
        (3) Dehydration.
        (4) Over-diuresis.
        (5) Vomiting.
        (6) Diarrhea.
        (7) Peritonitis.
        (8) Integumentary loss from burns.
    c. Decreased effective circulating volume to the

kidneys related to decreased cardiac output or altered peripheral vascular resistance.
   (1) Congestive heart failure.
   (2) Myocardial infarction.
   (3) Cardiac tamponade.
   (4) Cardiac dysrhythmias.
   (5) Cirrhosis or hepatorenal syndrome.
   (6) Nephrotic syndrome.
   (7) Cardiogenic shock.
   (8) Vasodilatation.
   (9) Anaphylactic reactions.
   (10) Neurogenic shock.
   (11) Systemic septic shock.
   (12) Drug overdose.
 d. Impaired kidney blood flow because of exogenous agents.
   (1) Angiotensin-converting enzyme inhibitors (ACE).
   (2) NSAIDs.
 e. Impaired kidney blood flow because of kidney artery disorders.
   (1) Emboli.
   (2) Thrombi.
   (3) Stenosis.
   (4) Aneurysm.
   (5) Occlusion.
   (6) Trauma.
3. Pathophysiology.
 a. The parenchyma is initially undamaged.
 b. Kidneys respond as if volume depletion has occurred, using adaptive mechanisms of autoregulation and release of renin.
   (1) Autoregulation: afferent arteriole dilation and efferent arteriole constriction in an attempt to increase kidney blood flow and maintain normal GFR.
   (2) Release of renin.
     (a) Renin activates the angiotensin-aldosterone system, which results in peripheral vasoconstriction and increased sodium reabsorption, decreasing urinary sodium.
     (b) Increased plasma sodium causes the release of antidiuretic hormone (ADH) that enhances vasoconstriction and increases water reabsorption, thus decreasing urinary output and increasing circulating blood volume.
     (c) With increased sodium and water reabsorption, urea reabsorption increases. Therefore, blood urea nitrogen (BUN) increases.
     (d) These mechanisms attempt to maintain systemic and kidney perfusion to protect kidney function.
 c. If kidney hypoperfusion persists and exceeds

the capabilities of the kidney's adaptive mechanisms, AKI/ARF develops from ischemia.
 d. In congestive heart failure (CHF), decreased kidney blood flow can be caused by over diuresis or by hypervolemia that causes elevated filling pressures in the left ventricle and leads to decreased cardiac output.
 e. ACE inhibitors and angiotensin receptor blocking (ARB) agents reduce angiotensin II production or block its action on kidney tissue.
   (1) Angiotensin II constricts the efferent arteriole. Blocking the effect of angiotensin II on kidney tissue reduces the pressure on the glomerulus by allowing the efferent arteriole to dilate.
   (2) This effect is desired in many patients and reduces proteinuria.
   (3) However, patients with kidney artery stenosis should avoid ACE I's and ARB agents, as kidney failure can result when the efferent arteriole dilation drops the pressure in the glomerulus and decreases the GFR.
 f. NSAIDs block prostaglandin production, allowing constriction of the afferent arteriole, decreasing kidney perfusion, and potentially lowering GFR.
4. Assessment.
 a. History: collect data that could indicate poor kidney perfusion and/or poor systemic perfusion.
   (1) Surgery.
   (2) Fever.
   (3) Multiple tests that require no oral intake (NPO) and/or bowel preparation.
   (4) Acute myocardial infarction.
   (5) Anaphylactic drug or transfusion reaction.
   (6) Cardiac arrest with successful resuscitation.
   (7) Low sodium diets with fluid restriction, diuretics, and antihypertensives.
   (8) Exposure to consecutive days of hot, humid weather, with or without exercise.
   (9) Penetrating or nonpenetrating abdominal trauma.
 b. Physical assessment: findings related to fluid volume depletion vary depending on the etiology and need to be correlated with laboratory and history findings.
   (1) Dry mucous membranes.
   (2) Poor skin turgor.
   (3) Reduced jugular venous pressure.
   (4) Hypotension.
   (5) Weight loss.
 c. Laboratory findings.

(1) Decreased urine output (oliguria).
(2) Increased urine osmolality and specific gravity
   (a) Prerenal acute renal failure > 500 mOsm.
   (b) Intrinsic acute renal failure 250–300 mOsm.
(3) Decreased urine sodium and urea due to decreased capacity to reabsorb sodium.
(4) Increased blood urea nitrogen (BUN).
(5) Plasma creatinine usually normal
(6) The ratio of BUN to plasma creatinine increases to > 20:1 for prerenal acute renal failure and < 20:1 for intrinsic acute renal failure.
(7) Urinary sediment usually normal
(8) Fractional excretion of sodium
   (a) Is less than 1% in most prerenal acute renal failure patients.
   (b) Is > 3% in most patients with intrinsic acute renal failure.
(9) Calculation: 100 x (urine sodium/serum sodium)/(urine creatinine/serum creatinine) (Agrawal & Swartz, 2000).

5. Use of biomarkers to predict AKI.
  a. The role of biomarkers is to assess overall disease risk, early noninvasive screening, detection, and response to treatment.
  b. The loss of kidney function is most easily detected by measuring serum creatinine which is used to measure GFR. It is a suboptimal biomarker for diagnosing AKI. It is a late finding and is not used in early detection of AKI (Bonventre, 2007; KDIGO, 2012).
  c. Different urinary and serum proteins have been intensely studied to detect early diagnosis of AKI.
  d. Examples of diagnostic biomarkers.
    (1) Urinary tubular enzymes consist of proximal renal tubular epithelial antigens released from the proximal tubule epithelial cells 12 hours to 4 days earlier than a rise in serum creatinine. However, it cannot distinguish between prerenal and ATN.
    (2) Urinary low molecular weight proteins are produced at different sites in the kidney, filtered at the glomerulus, and reabsorbed by the proximal tubule with no secretion. They may distinguish prerenal from ATN disease but may not indicate persistent or irreversible damage.
    (3) Neutrophil gelatinase-associated lipocalin (NGAL) shows promise as an early detector to diagnose ATN. It also can differentiate between prerenal disease and ATN after renal ischemia (Haase et al., 2011).

  e. For biomarkers to be used clinically, they need to be validated in different settings of AKI, such as cardiac surgery, sepsis, contrast induced nephropathy, pediatric population, and at different medical centers.
  f. There also needs to be the development of testing of rapid assays, and further development of several biomarkers.
  g. Investigational biomarkers have not been approved for clinical use in the United States (Bonventre, 2007).
  h. Promising biomarkers for AKI include:
    (1) Neutrophil gelatinase-associated lipocalin (NGAL).
    (2) Kidney injury molecule-1 (KIM-1).
    (3) Urinary Interleukin-18 (IL-18).
    (4) Urinary angiotensinogen may be useful as a prognostic marker for severe AKI (Bonventre, 2009; KDIGO, 2012).

6. Goal of treatment: early restoration of kidney perfusion to shorten the ischemic time and prevent parenchymal injury.
  a. Treat the underlying disorder.
  b. Administer fluids to increase circulatory blood volume: 500 mL (SI = 0.5 L) over 30 minutes and repeat if no increase in urine volume.
  c. Achieve and maintain euvolemia.
  d. Eliminate causative agents.

7. Nursing care interventions by hospital staff.
  a. When administering fluid bolus/es, monitor for cardiovascular response to the increased intravascular volume, expecting an increase in blood pressure (BP) and central venous pressure (CVP).
  b. Measure and document accurate intake and output (I & O).
  c. Exercise infection control measures.
  d. Review medications for nephrotoxins.
  e. Monitor volume status, including I & O, body weight, BP, heart rate, jugular venous distention (JVD), and edema (periorbital, sacral, pretibial, and peripheral).

8. Nursing care interventions by dialysis staff.
  a. In most cases, the acute dialysis staff will not be involved with this patient's care because early intervention on the part of nephrology staff will resolve the problems before kidney replacement therapy (KRT) is needed.
  b. If the conditions are not resolved in a timely manner, the patient will progress to intrarenal kidney damage, for which nursing care will be addressed in that section.

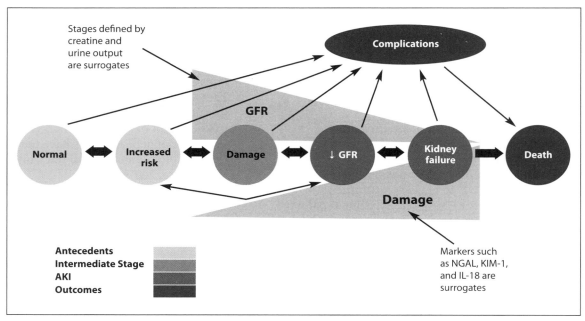

Figure 2.3. Conceptual model of acute kidney injury (AKI).

Source: Murray et al. (2008). A framework and key research questions in AKI diagnosis and staging in different environments. *Clinical Journal of the American Society of Nephrology, 3*(3), 864-868. Used with permission.

B. Intrarenal acute renal failure.
1. Incidence.
   a. Approximately 50% of cases of AKI/ARF.
   b. Patients at risk include the elderly and those with diabetes, congestive heart failure (CHF), or chronic kidney disease (CKD).
2. Etiology: usually caused by intrarenal ischemia or toxins or both.
   a. Tubular disease: acute tubular necrosis (ATN) (refer to Figure 2.2).
      (1) Ischemia.
         (a) Failure to reverse hypovolemia due to prolonged prerenal azotemia.
         (b) Perfusion injury and/or prolonged ischemia in transplanted kidney.
      (2) Nephrotoxic agents.
         (a) Drugs: antineoplastics, anesthetics, antimicrobials, anti-inflammatory agents, and immunosuppressants.
         (b) Radiocontrast agents.
         (c) Poisons.
            i. Environmental agents: pesticides and organic solvents.
            ii. Heavy metals: lead, mercury, and gold.
            iii. Plant and animal substances: mushrooms and snake venom.
            iv. Some herbal agents.
         (d) Blockage of tubules.
            i. Pigments: myoglobin in

rhabdomyolysis, hemoglobin with hemolysis.
            ii. Tumor products in myeloma.
   b. Interstitial disease: acute interstitial nephritis (AIN).
      (1) Patients frequently present with fever, rash, and eosinophilia.
      (2) Allergic reaction to drugs.
         (a) Antibiotics: cephalosporins, penicillins, sulfonamides.
         (b) NSAIDs.
         (c) Diuretics.
         (d) Allopurinol (Zyloprim).
      (3) Some herbal agents: mutong and fang chi contain aristolochic acid, which causes focal interstitial nephritis.
      (4) Autoimmune disease.
         (a) Systemic lupus erythematosus (SLE).
         (b) Mixed connective tissue disease.
      (5) Pyelonephritis.
      (6) Infiltrative disease.
         (a) Lymphoma.
         (b) Leukemia.
   c. Glomerular disease.
      (1) Characterized by hypertension, proteinuria, and hematuria.
      (2) Rapidly progressive glomerulonephritis.
         (a) Systemic lupus erythematosus.
         (b) Small vessel vasculitis.
            i. Wegener's granulomatosis.

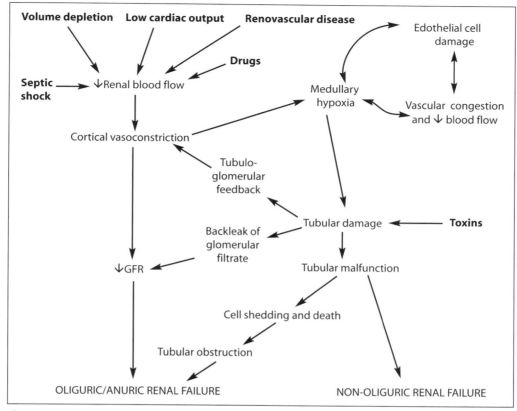

Figure 2.4. Mechanisms of acute tubular necrosis.

Source: Fry, A.C., & Farrington, K. (2006). Management of acute renal failure. *Postgraduate Medicine Journal, 82,* 106-116. Used with permission.

ii. Polyarteritis nodosa.
(c) Henoch-Schonlein purpura (immunoglobulin A nephropathy).
(d) Goodpasture syndrome.
(3) Acute proliferative glomerulonephritis.
(a) Endocarditis.
(b) Poststreptococcal infection.
(c) Postpneumococcal infection.
d. Vascular disease.
(1) Present with microangiopathic hemolysis and acute renal failure.
(2) Microvascular disease.
(a) Thrombotic thrombocytopenia purpura (TTP).
(b) Hemolytic uremic syndrome (HUS).
(c) HELLP syndrome (hemolysis, elevated liver enzymes, and low platelets).
(d) Atheroembolic disease (cholesterol-plaque microembolism).
(3) Macrovascular disease.
(a) Renal artery occlusion.
(b) Severe abdominal aortic disease (aneurysm).
(c) Renal vein thrombosis.

e. Systemic and vascular disorders.
(1) Wilson disease.
(2) Malaria.
(3) Multiple myeloma.
(4) Sickle cell disease.
(5) Malignant hypertension.
(6) Diabetes mellitus.
(7) Systemic lupus erythematosus.
(8) Pregnancy related disorders.
(a) Septic abortion.
(b) Preeclampsia.
(c) Abruptio placenta.
(d) Intrauterine fetal death.
(e) Idiopathic postpartum kidney failure.
3. Pathophysiology.
a. Ischemic intrarenal acute kidney failure (ischemic ATN).
(1) The ischemic event refers to prolonged hypoperfusion and ischemia of the kidneys with a sustained mean arterial pressure (MAP) of less than 75 mmHg.
(2) Kidney autoregulation fails and the sympathetic nervous system (SNS) response, renin-angiotensin system (RAS),

and possibly endothelin cause severe afferent arteriole constriction.

(3) These mechanisms cause decreased glomerular blood flow, glomerular hydrostatic pressure, and GFR.

(4) The amount and degree of renal cellular damage depends on the length of the ischemic episode.

   (a) Ischemia of 25 minutes or less causes reversible mild injury.

   (b) Ischemia of 40 to 60 minutes causes more severe damage that may recover to some extent in 2 to 3 weeks.

   (c) Ischemia lasting 60 to 90 minutes usually causes irreversible damage.

   (d) Cellular damage often continues after MAP and kidney perfusion are restored.

   (e) Renal blood flow can be reduced by 50% after an episode of ischemia; this is termed no reflow phenomenon.

   (f) The kidneys are unable to synthesize vasodilating prostaglandins without which the ischemic injury may be exacerbated.

(5) Sympathetic nervous system (SNS) stimulation and angiotensin II redistribute blood flow from the cortex to the medulla. This further decreases glomerular capillary flow and worsens tubular ischemia because these structures are located primarily in the cortex.

(6) With kidney ischemia, the nutrients and oxygen for basic cellular metabolism and tubular transport systems within the kidney are diminished.

   (a) Production of adenosine triphosphate (ATP) by kidney cell mitochondria decreases significantly.

   (b) Without adequate oxygen and ATP, kidney cell metabolism shifts from aerobic to anaerobic. There is a corresponding kidney tissue extracellular and intracellular acidosis that alters kidney function.

(7) Ischemia causes a decrease in kidney cellular potassium, magnesium, and inorganic phosphates, and an increase in intracellular sodium, chloride, and calcium.

   (a) Sodium (Na)/calcium (Ca) exchange is abnormal owing to low ATP, altered Ca-ATPase, and increased cellular sodium. As a result, there is an increase in cellular calcium, which increases cell injury.

   (b) During reperfusion after a prolonged kidney ischemic event, the formation of oxygen-free radicals further exacerbates cellular damage.

(8) As the final outcome of prolonged tubular ischemia, tubular cells swell and become necrotic, altering the function of the basement membrane.

   (a) Tubular obstruction occurs from sloughed necrotic cells and cast formation.

   (b) The tubular obstruction increases tubular hydrostatic pressure and Bowman's capsule hydrostatic pressure, which opposes the glomerular hydro-static pressure and decreases GFR.

   (c) Injury to the basement membrane increases tubular permeability and allows tubular filtrate to leak back into the interstitium and peritubular capillaries, further decreasing tubular filtrate.

(9) Ischemic ATN is usually associated with oliguria because of extensive nephron injury (see Table 2.2). Other clinical indications include:

   (a) Decreased urea excretion and elevated BUN.

   (b) Decreased creatinine clearance and elevated plasma creatinine (Cr).

   (c) Abnormal kidney handling of sodium. Usually there is sodium loss with urinary sodium equal to sodium filtered into the tubule from the glomerulus.

   (d) Inability to concentrate urine. Urinary osmolality approximates plasma osmolality or 300 to 320 mOsm/L (SI = 300 to 320 mOsm/L), a condition called isosthenuria.

b. Toxic intrarenal acute kidney failure (toxic ATN).

(1) The toxic event refers to toxic products of organisms and/or nephrotoxic agents, which begin by causing injury to the tubular cells.

(2) There is tubular cell necrosis, cast formation, tubular obstruction, and altered GFR.

   (a) The basement membrane is usually intact, and the injured necrotic areas are more localized than with ischemic ATN.

   (b) Nonoliguria occurs more often with toxic ATN than with ischemic ATN.

(3) The injury with toxic ATN can be less than with ischemic ATN. Therefore, the healing

Table 2.2

Typical Findings in Prerenal and Intrarenal Acute Renal Failure

	Prerenal	Intrarenal Renal
Volume	Oliguria	Oliguria or nonoliguria
Urinary sediment	Normal (hyaline and granular casts)	RBC casts Cellular debris
Specific gravity	High	Low
Osmolality (mOsm/Kg H_2O)	High	Low (Isosthenuria)
Ratio Osm Urine to Osm Plasma	> 1.5	< 1.2
Urine Na (mEq/L)	Low (< 20)	Increased over prerenal (> 20)
Urine urea (g/24 hrs)	Low (15)	Low (5)
Urine creatinine (g/24 hrs)	Normal (> 1.0)	Low (< 1.0)
Ratio urine creatinine to plasma creatinine	> 15:1	< 10:1

Source: Lancaster, L.E. (1990). Renal response to shock. *Critical Care Nursing Clinics of North America, 2*(2), 221-223. Used with permission.

process can be more rapid with toxic ATN.

(4) Reasons the kidney is so susceptible to toxic damage.

(a) Blood circulates through the kidney approximately 14 times a minute. Therefore, the kidney is repeatedly exposed to all components in the blood.

(b) The kidney is the major excretory organ for toxic substances, and as these substances await transport, they are held within kidney cells where they can disrupt cellular function.

(c) The liver usually detoxifies substances, and with liver disease, the kidney can be overloaded with under detoxified substances.

(d) The kidney transforms many substances. Some of these new metabolites can be toxic to the kidney.

(e) The countercurrent mechanism (the method in which the sodium pump concentrates urine as it travels through the hairpin turns made by the loop of Henle, folding back on itself, creating a higher osmotic gradient between the descending and ascending flows) concentrates bodily substances as well as other substances. This increased concentration can result in toxicity to the kidney.

4. Assessment.

a. History. Collect data that identify an event, series of events, agent, or agents that have caused kidney injury, especially those related to ischemia or toxins.

(1) Exposure to nephrotoxins.

(2) Radiologic tests that require administration of a dye.

(3) Hypersensitivity reaction to a drug or dye.

(4) Recent infections.

(5) Sepsis.

(6) Recent trauma.

(7) Antineoplastics with or without irradiation.

(8) Multiple myeloma.

(9) Pregnancy.

(10) History of cardiac, kidney, or liver disease.

b. Physical assessment. No one specific finding pinpoints intrarenal azotemia. Correlate all findings with history and laboratory findings.

c. Laboratory findings and other considerations

for differentiating prerenal azotemia from ATN.

(1) Because prerenal problems often correspond with the onset phase of ATN, and because prerenal is a reversible phase, it is essential for diagnosis and aggressive management to begin early in the course of prerenal problems.

(2) Urinalysis, microscopic examination of the urine, and laboratory plasma values provide important data for differentiating prerenal azotemia from intrinsic.

(3) In prerenal problems, the urinary specific gravity and osmolality are high and the urinary sodium is low because of decreased kidney blood flow and decreased GFR, which the kidneys interpret as a state of dehydration. As a response, under the influence of aldosterone and ADH, maximal sodium and water are reabsorbed from the distal tubule and collecting duct into the peritubular capillary plasma. Thus, a small amount (oliguria) of very concentrated urine with high specific gravity and high osmolality is excreted.

(a) Although maximal sodium is reabsorbed, the urine is concentrated due to urea or other solutes.

(b) Urinary and plasma creatinine levels often show wide variation in the prerenal period.

(4) In contrast to prerenal problems, ATN is characterized by parenchymal damage that causes impaired sodium reabsorption.

(a) This results in an increase in urinary sodium, greater than 20 mEq/L (SI = 20 mmol/L). The serum sodium varies, depending on the state of hydration.

(b) The fractional excretion of sodium is > 3% and urine osmolality between 250 and 300 mOsm.

(c) Oliguria is usually associated with post ischemic ATN, whereas nephrotoxic ATN can be associated with either oliguria or nonoliguria, as explained above.

(d) The creatinine clearance is severely decreased and the plasma creatinine rises at a rate of about 1 to 3 mg/dL/day (SI = 88 to 264 mmol/L/day) in ATN.

(e) The urine to plasma creatinine ratio is less than 10 to 1 in ATN compared to more than 15 to 1 in prerenal.

(5) Another distinguishing factor between prerenal and ATN is the response to therapy.

(a) In prerenal illness in which no actual nephron damage has occurred, the kidney's response to therapy aimed at correcting the underlying problem is often rapid with return to normal urine output and normal blood chemistries.

(b) In ATN, which indicates nephron damage, response to therapy aimed at the underlying cause of the damage is minimal. ATN requires additional interventions aimed at correcting the abnormalities resulting from the inability of the kidneys to maintain their functions.

5. Goals of treatment.
   a. Correct the primary disorder.
   b. Correct fluid and electrolyte disorders.
   c. Prevent infection.
   d. Maintain optimal nutrition.
   e. Treat systemic effects of uremia.
   f. Provide education and support to patient and family.

6. Treatment.
   a. Must be tailored to address the specific presentation of the AKI/ARF.
   b. Pharmacologic interventions, clinical interventions, medical and nursing treatments, and laboratory monitoring all play a role in sustaining the patient through this acute illness.

7. Nursing care interventions by hospital staff.
   a. Monitor closely volume status including I & O, body weight, BP, heart rate, jugular venous distention (JVD), and edema (periorbital, sacral, pretibial, or peripheral).
   b. Concentrate IV infusions.
   c. Use medication protocols, such as Lasix®.
   d. Monitor changes in mental status that can indicate an electrolyte imbalance or hypoxemia.
   e. Monitor lab values for electrolyte imbalances.
   f. Increase awareness of nephrotoxic agents, such as contrast media and antibiotics.
   g. Provide skin care for rash, ischemia ("purple toes"), and tissue integrity.
   h. Monitor dialysis access site for infection.

8. Nursing care interventions by dialysis staff.
   a. Educate patient and family.
   b. Educate hospital staff.
   c. Comprehensive nursing assessment, including lab values, changes in weight and fluid status, mental status changes, cardiac and respiratory condition, prior to initiating kidney replacement therapy.
   d. Report assessment findings and collaborate with nephrologist/APRN/PA to tailor the treatment plan for optimal patient treatment outcomes.

e. Collaborate with hospital staff caring for patient.
  (1) Receive report prior to initiating KRT and incorporate information into assessment and treatment plan.
  (2) Review medications for nephrotoxins, dialyzability, and impact on hemodynamics.
  (3) During treatment, advise hospital staff of changes in condition and interventions used to respond to changes.
  (4) Participate in infection control procedures.
  (5) Perform dialysis access catheter care, inform hospital staff of assessment, and document condition of site.
  (6) Assist with skin care and turning when appropriate.
  (7) Following treatment, report to hospital staff regarding patient's response to treatment, amount of fluid removed, posttreatment vital signs, medications given, blood products administered, access status, and plan for next treatment if known.
f. Avoid hypotension during dialysis treatments.
g. Document patient education provided.
h. Evaluate dialysis treatment outcome and communicate need to modify next treatment to supervisor and/or provider as appropriate.

C. Postrenal acute renal failure.
  1. Incidence: 5% to 10% of cases of AKI/ARF.
  2. Etiology.
    a. Interference with flow of urine from the kidneys to the exterior of the body.
    b. Most often due to obstruction of the lower urinary tract.
    c. Obstruction.
      (1) Ureteral, bladder neck, or urethral obstruction.
        (a) Calculi, neoplasms, or sloughed papillary tissue.
        (b) Strictures, trauma, or blood clots.
        (c) Congenital or developmental abnormalities.
        (d) Foreign objects or inadvertent surgical ligation.
      (2) Benign prostatic hypertrophy or prostatic cancer.
      (3) Cervical cancer.
      (4) Retroperitoneal fibrosis.
      (5) Intratubular obstruction (crystals or myeloma light chains).
      (6) Pelvic mass or invasive pelvic malignancy.
      (7) Intraluminal bladder mass.
      (8) Neurogenic bladder.
      (9) Pregnancy.
      (10) Drugs, such as antihistamines and ganglionic blocking agents.
  3. Pathophysiology.
    a. Obstruction of urine outflow may lead to a sudden decrease in urine output.
    b. Obstruction in the urinary tract causes an increase in pressure near the obstruction due to the continued production of urine by glomerular filtration.
    c. The increased pressure from the obstruction is transmitted retrograde through the collecting system to the nephron.
    d. When the pressure in the tubule exceeds the pressure in the glomerulus, glomerular filtration is stopped.
      (1) Increased reabsorption of sodium, water, and urea results in decreased urinary sodium, increased urine osmolality, and increased BUN.
      (2) Decreased GFR results in a decreased creatinine clearance and increased plasma creatinine.
    e. Prolonged obstruction can result in:
      (1) Dilation of the collecting system and compression of parenchymal tissue.
      (2) Increased tubular hydrostatic pressure.
      (3) Kidney interstitial edema.
      (4) Reduced kidney blood flow.
      (5) Secondary tubular damage.
    f. Temporary obstruction results in little dilation of the collecting system and little or no loss of kidney tissue.
    g. The obstruction can be total or partial with resulting symptoms depending on the amount of change in GFR.
  4. Assessment.
    a. History. Collect data that indicate obstruction or disruption of the urinary tract.
      (1) History of change in urine volume and/or urinating pattern.
      (2) History of prostatic disease or abdominal neoplasms.
      (3) History of urinary tract stones or nephralgia.
      (4) Pregnancy.
      (5) Recent abdominal surgery.
      (6) Paralysis (quadriplegia).
    b. Physical assessment. Findings vary with etiology and need to be correlated with laboratory and history findings.
    c. Laboratory findings.
      (1) Urine volume variable: may be oliguria or polyuria, or abrupt anuria.
      (2) Urine osmolality variable: increases or may be similar to plasma osmolality.
      (3) Urine specific gravity: variable.
      (4) Urine sodium variable: decreases (often similar to plasma sodium).

(5) Urine urea decreases.

(6) BUN and plasma creatinine increase: ratio normal to slightly increased.

(7) Urinary sediment usually normal, unless urinary tract infection is present.

d. Diagnostic studies that may be used.

(1) X-ray of kidneys, ureters, and bladder (KUB) to determine size, shape, and placement of kidneys.

(2) Intravenous pyelogram (IVP) to detect location and/or type of obstruction.

(3) Radionuclide studies to screen for tumors, cysts, and blood flow.

(4) Ultrasound, computed tomography (CT), or magnetic resonance imaging (MRI) to screen for hydronephrosis and location of obstruction.

5. Goals of treatment.

a. Relieve the obstruction as soon as possible. The potential for recovery of kidney function is often inversely related to the duration of the obstruction.

b. Ongoing prevention and detection of urosepsis.

6. Treatment.

a. Bladder catheterization can be both diagnostic and therapeutic in bladder or urethral obstruction.

b. Other treatments may include percutaneous nephrostomy, lithotripsy, ureteral stenting, and urethral stenting.

7. Nursing care interventions by hospital staff.

a. Stoma and skin care.

b. Nephrostomy and urostomy care and dressing changes.

c. Appliances.

d. Identify early stent tissue overgrowth.

8. Nursing care interventions by dialysis staff.

a. Resource and support for hospital staff.

b. Provide KRT options for potential acute complications.

IV. Complications of acute kidney injury/acute renal failure. Not all patients with AKI experience all of these complications, but they can occur in some natural sequence.

A. The diagnosis of AKI/ARF.

1. Signs and symptoms of kidney impairment are present, such as decreased urine volume.

2. Treatment goals are to determine the cause of the AKI/ARF and establish a treatment plan based on the etiology.

3. Nursing care interventions are supportive and responsive to signs and symptoms.

B. Oliguria or nonoliguria.

1. If it occurs, it usually lasts from 5 to 15 days, but it can persist for weeks.

2. Approximately 50% of AKI/ARF patients are nonoliguric, which may indicate a less severe insult to the kidney than patients who are oliguric.

3. Kidney pathology.

a. Kidney healing occurs.

(1) Tubular cells regenerate.

(2) Destroyed basement membrane is replaced with fibrous scar tissue.

(3) Tubules are clogged with inflammatory products.

b. Functional changes.

(1) Decreased glomerular filtration.

(2) Decreased tubular transport of substances.

(3) Decreased urine formation.

(4) Decreased kidney clearance.

c. When ARF persists for weeks or longer, kidney endocrine functions are altered, including decreased secretion of erythropoietin.

4. Frequent causes of death are cardiac arrest due to hyperkalemia, gastrointestinal bleeding, and infection.

5. Treatment goals are to keep the patient alive until the kidney damage heals.

6. Signs, symptoms, and related nursing (hospital and nephrology) care interventions.

a. Increased susceptibility to infection (especially urinary and respiratory) related to altered immune, nutritional, biochemical status, as well as hospitalization.

(1) Implement infection preventive measures.

(a) Avoid invasive procedures, especially urinary bladder catheters.

(b) Use aseptic technique for all invasive procedures and dressing changes.

(c) Wash hands before and after contact with patient.

(d) Turn, cough, and deep breathe; provide incentive spirometry equipment for regular use.

(e) Frequent position changes and skin care to prevent skin breakdown.

(f) Remove catheters, tubings, and lines as soon as possible. Hospitals may choose to perform daily assessment of catheters, tubings, and lines, including dialysis accesses, to evaluate the necessity for change or removal as soon as possible.

(2) Instruct patient on increased susceptibility to infection.

(a) Signs and symptoms to report.

(b) Avoid contact with people who have infections.

(c) Importance of hand washing.

(d) Encourage level of activity tolerated to facilitate deep respirations.

(3) Assess for changes in infection status.

   (a) Assess vital signs for elevated temperature, increased respiratory rate, increased heart rate, and/or decreased BP.

   (b) Monitor lung sounds and productivity of cough.

   (c) Monitor lab values: white blood cell count (WBCs), blood culture results.

   (d) Review reports of chest x-rays.

   (e) Observe dialysis access catheter exit sites for infection, and remove sutures from new tunneled catheter exit sites two weeks after placement.

   (f) Perform dressing changes per protocol using aseptic technique.

b. Fluid volume excess related to decreased kidney excretion of water, inappropriate fluid intake, and/or sodium retention.

(1) Instruct patient and family on appropriate fluid intake and dietary restrictions.

(2) Monitor intake and output (I & O) accurately.

(3) Weigh patient daily using correctly calibrated scale.

(4) Observe for BP changes, orthostatic hypotension, and increased heart rate.

(5) Observe for JVD or, when available, elevated CVP.

(6) Observe for edema (periorbital, sacral, pretibial, or peripheral).

(7) Observe skin turgor.

(8) Check lab values of brain natriuretic peptide (BNP) and for hyponatremia.

c. Hyperkalemia related to decreased kidney regulation and excretion of potassium, increased endogenous production of potassium, increased potassium intake, tissue breakdown, and/or metabolic acidosis (see Figure 2.5).

(1) Instruct patient and family on dietary potassium and its effect on the heart.

(2) Monitor electrocardiogram (EKG) for signs of hyperkalemia.

   (a) Tall, peaked T waves.

   (b) Prolonged PR interval.

   (c) ST depression.

   (d) Widened QRS.

   (e) Loss of P wave.

(3) Monitor for signs and symptoms of hyperkalemia.

   (a) Irritability.

   (b) Anxiety.

   (c) Abdominal cramping.

   (d) Diarrhea.

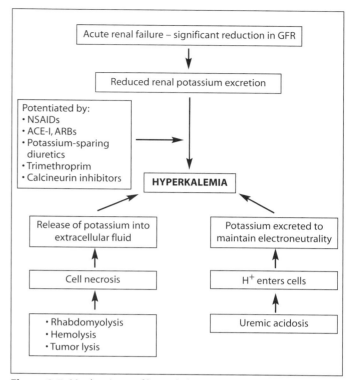

Figure 2.5. Mechanisms of hyperkalemia in acute renal failure.

Source: Fry, A.C., & Farrington, K. (2006). Management of acute renal failure. *Postgraduate Medicine Journal, 82*, 106-116. Used with permission.

   (e) Weakness, especially of lower extremities.

   (f) Paresthesias.

(4) Administer blood products during hemodialysis treatments if possible to remove extra potassium resulting from cell breakdown in handling and administration.

(5) Monitor signs of tissue breakdown and/or GI bleeding and report to nephrologist or appropriate medical doctor (MD).

(6) Administer emergency medications as needed while waiting for initiation of hemodialysis: insulin and glucose, calcium, and/or resin exchange products (Kayexalate®).

(7) Use apple or cranberry juice to treat hypoglycemia instead of the traditional orange juice to prevent hyperkalemia. For more rapid response, dextrose 50% can be given IV.

d. Hyperphosphatemia related to decreased kidney excretion and regulation of phosphate, increased or continued intake of phosphate, and tissue breakdown, especially muscle tissue.

(1) Monitor for signs and symptoms of hyperphosphatemia. Most of the symptoms are related to the development of hypocalcemia.

(a) Anorexia.
(b) Nausea.
(c) Vomiting.
(d) Muscle weakness.
(e) Hyperreflexia.
(f) Tetany.
(g) Tachycardia.
(2) Instruct patient and family on dietary phosphorus and its relationship to calcium in maintaining good balance.
(3) Administer phosphate binders with meals to increase effectiveness.
e. Metabolic acidosis related to decreased kidney excretion of acid load, decreased regeneration of bicarbonate, increased tissue catabolism, and endogenous production of acids.
(1) Administer sodium bicarbonate and/or other medications for electrolyte repletion as needed.
(2) Coordinate schedule of KRT to correct electrolyte imbalances.
f. Potential for GI bleeding related to stress, uremia resulting in retention of metabolic wastes and end products, altered capillary permeability, and platelet dysfunction.
(1) Instruct patient and family to report any signs of GI bleeding.
(2) Monitor lab values for changes in hematocrit (Hct) and hemoglobin (Hgb).
(3) Monitor vital signs to detect volume loss.
(4) Guaiac test nasogastric (NG) drainage, emesis, and stool for occult blood.
(5) Administer erythropoiesis-stimulating agents (ESAs) during hemodialysis treatments and/or as ordered, subcutaneously (SC) or intravenously (IV).
g. Alteration in nutrition.
(1) Review diet prescription for appropriateness.
(2) Address uremia-caused anorexia, nausea, and vomiting.
(3) Provide antiemetic medications prior to mealtime as needed.
(4) Encourage dietary selection of foods that are appealing to patient.
(5) If meals are missed due to tests or treatments, arrange for snacks between meals.
(6) Avoid scheduling other activities (exercise, dressing changes, etc.) at mealtimes.
(7) Dietary supplements, tube feedings, and/or total parenteral nutrition (TPN) may be necessary to meet caloric and protein needs while this catabolic state persists.
(a) Mild degree of catabolism.
    i. Urea nitrogen appearance (UNA) level < 5 g/24 hours. UNA is measured as the amount of urea excreted in urine plus the net amount accumulated in body water (Maroni formula).
    ii. Adequate nutritional support can usually be achieved with oral intake alone.
    iii. Caloric needs: 30 to 35 cal/kg edema free body weight.
    iv. Protein needs: 0.6 to 0.8 mg/kg provided as both essential and nonessential amino acids.
    v. Fluid and electrolyte restrictions usually not indicated.
(b) Moderate degree of catabolism.
    i. Urea nitrogen appearance level 5 to 10 mg/24 hours.
    ii. Nutritional support is by tube feeding or TPN.
    iii. Caloric needs: 30 to 35 cal/kg edema free body weight.
    iv. Protein needs: 1.0 to 1.2 g/kg provided as both essential and nonessential amino acids.
    v. Fluid requirements adjusted for intake and output and dialysis losses.
    vi. Electrolytes usually limited unless lab results indicate otherwise.
(c) Severe degree of catabolism.
    i. Urea nitrogen appearance level greater than 10 g/24 hours.
    ii. Nutritional support most often TPN as GI dysfunction occurs frequently in this setting.
    iii. During the first 24 to 48 hours after injury, nutrition support should be withheld. Infusion of large quantities of amino acids or glucose during this time can increase oxygen demand and further aggravate tubular damage.
    iv. Caloric needs: 35 to 45 cal/kg edema free body weight.
    v. Protein needs: 1.5 to 2.0 g/kg provided as essential and nonessential amino acids.
    vi. Fluid requirements adjusted for intake and output and dialysis losses.
    vii. Electrolytes are usually limited unless laboratory results indicate otherwise.
    viii. Hyperkalemia and hyperphosphatemia can be

significant secondary to catabolism of lean body mass as well as secondary to impaired excretion and should be monitored closely.

    ix. Maintain normoglycemic state using frequent bedside glucose monitoring and insulin IV drip or sliding scale injections.

h. Medical nutrition therapy (MNT) by AKI stage (Gervasio & Cotton, 2009).

(1) Stage 1 – Etiologies commonly only prerenal or postrenal.

  (a) Postrenal usually requires only correction of obstruction with little or no MNT, provide adequate energy and protein, no electrolyte restrictions.

  (b) Prerenal – assess volume status.

    i. Inadequate hydration/dehydration – provide resuscitation and an adequate intake of energy and protein.

    ii. Volume overload – monitor response to diuretic therapy, Na, and fluid restriction may be necessary.

(2) Stage 2 – Etiologies include postrenal, prerenal, and tubulointerstitial.

  (a) Multiple etiologies may be involved.

  (b) Correct obstruction if postrenal and provide adequate energy and protein.

  (c) Correct volume status if prerenal, adding sodium and fluid restriction if indicated with volume excess.

  (d) Investigate the use of high-dose ascorbic acid or other alternative therapies related to nephrotoxicity.

  (e) Provide oral diet adequate in energy and protein.

    i. Energy: 30 to 35 kcal/kg.

    ii. Protein: 1.0 to 1.2 g/kg.

  (f) Oral supplements if oral intake < 75% or estimated needs.

  (g) Oral diet restrictions per labs and/or urine output. If UOP < 1L, potassium restriction may be necessary.

  (h) Kidney replacement therapy (KRT) not needed.

(3) Stage 3 – Etiologies include postrenal, prerenal, and tubulointerstitial.

  (a) Multiple etiologies may be involved.

  (b) Often AKI on chronic kidney disease.

  (c) KRT required when:

    i. Hypervolemia with oliguria or anuria.

    ii. Hyperkalemia.

    iii. Metabolic acidosis.

  (d) If stable nonventilated, provide oral diet.

    i. Energy: 30 to 35 kcal/kg.

    ii. Hemodialysis: 1.2 to 1.3 g/kg protein.

    iii. Potassium, phosphorus, and fluid restrictions as indicated.

  (e) If critically ill/ventilated, 25 to 30 kcal/kg.

    i. Hemodialysis 1.2 to 1.3 g/kg protein.

    ii. Continuous renal replacement therapy (CRRT) 2.0 to 2.2 g/kg protein. A higher level of protein is needed to correct for protein and amino acid losses over CRRT filter.

    iii. Enteral nutrition when oral diet not possible.

      [a] Renal formula if hyperkalemia present.

      [b] High protein, lower volume formula with CRRT.

    iv. Prescribe renal-specific vitamin to replace water-soluble vitamin losses related to KRT/CRRT. Vitamin C intake should not exceed 200 mg to avoid oxalate accumulation and irreversible AKI.

i. Potential for drug toxicity and nephrotoxicity related to inability of kidney to excrete all drugs, continued administration of drugs excreted by the kidney, and nephrotoxic drugs.

(1) Adjust doses of medications by clinical pharmacist based on patient's residual kidney function as well as the type of dialytic therapy and the membrane characteristics being used.

(2) Review medications for kidney toxicity prior to administration.

(3) Review serum drug levels (digoxin, antibiotics) prior to administering the next dose to be sure they are not in a toxic range.

(4) Monitor pain medications to avoid oversedation due to decreased metabolism and/or excretion.

(5) Do not administer medications prior to the hemodialysis treatment that will be removed by the dialytic process.

(6) Hold medications that will lower the patient's blood pressure prior to his/her scheduled hemodialysis treatment.

(7) Do not withhold pain medications from patients on dialysis because they may be partially removed by the treatment. Arrange for an extra dose if necessary to respond effectively to the patient's pain level.

(8) Hospital staff and nephrology nurses will collaborate to provide appropriate

medication administration during the dialysis treatment.

j. Potential for skin breakdown related to bed rest, fluid/electrolyte imbalances, metabolic products and toxin accumulation, edema, disrupted hemostasis and increased capillary fragility, repeated venipunctures, and other invasive procedures.

   (1) Maintain skin cleanliness and dry bedding at all times.

   (2) Treat skin breakdown with appropriate protective agents; consult wound care nurse if needed.

   (3) Turn patient and provide skin care regularly.

   (4) Position patient off bony prominences.

   (5) Consider the possibility of allergy to soaps, and request extra-rinse, nonallergenic linens if needed.

   (6) Use linen and pads appropriate for the specific therapeutic bed, when one is in use.

   (7) Consider the fragility of the patient's skin when selecting the kind of tape to use on a wound or exit-site dressing.

k. Disturbances in self-concept related to loss of bodily function, dependency, separation from family and friends, fatigue, inability to meet personal and professional responsibilities, confusion, lack of knowledge, hopelessness, and loss of control.

   (1) Provide support to patient and family as they transition through the various stages of their acute illness experience.

   (2) Provide education at the bedside and use printed materials to increase level of understanding and to provide an element of hope.

   (3) Use the expertise of the nephrology nurse at the bedside to educate hospital staff, patients, and family members about the AKI/ARF process.

   (4) Allow patients to make as many decisions about their care as possible to return some element of control to them while they are in a world where many things are beyond their control.

   (5) Allow frequent rest periods with opportunities for naps.

   (6) Encourage family involvement in care and decision making when possible.

   (7) Provide regular reorientation to place and time.

l. Disturbances in sleep pattern related to biochemical disruption, anxiety, hospitalization, isolation from family and friends, fear regarding lack of recovery of kidney function, multiple tests, and/or dietary and fluid restrictions.

   (1) Encourage a realization of time of day by using "dark hours" for sleep during the night shift.

   (2) Administer sleeping medications when needed to facilitate a good night's sleep.

   (3) Minimize interruptions of patient's sleep when only related to staff convenience for performing procedures.

   (4) Encourage family and friends presence at the bedside within the hospital's visitation policies.

   (5) Develop a professional relationship of listening and supporting to help alleviate the patient's anxiety, fear, and uncertainty.

m. Lack of knowledge related to kidney function, diagnostic tests, pathogenesis of AKI/ARF, effects of AKI/ARF on all body systems; course, management, prognosis, complications, and prevention of AKI/ARF.

   (1) Explain all tests, procedures, and interventions prior to performing them.

   (2) Consult nephrologist and nephrology nurses for intervention and education related to return of kidney function.

   (3) Review lab tests and other measures of potential return of function with the patient and family so they know what to be aware of and to know the level of progress.

C. Diuresis.

1. If it occurs, it usually lasts from 1 to 2 weeks, but can persist for many weeks.

2. Oliguric patients have a greater diuresis than nonoliguric patients.

3. Self-limiting diuresis occurs because:

   a. Kidney tubular patency is restored.

   b. Retained substances (e.g., urea and sodium) act as osmotic agents.

   c. Nephron's ability to concentrate urine is not recovered.

4. With continued kidney healing, the kidney regains most of its lost function except its concentrating ability. The amount regained is dependent on the degree of initial injury and of permanent basement membrane loss.

5. Frequent causes of death are infection and gastrointestinal bleeding.

6. Treatment goals are to keep the patient alive until the kidney lesion heals.

7. Signs, symptoms, and related nursing (hospital and nephrology) care interventions.

   a. Signs and symptoms of azotemia gradually diminish.

   b. Fluid volume deficit related to increased kidney excretion of water, inadequate fluid intake, sodium loss, continued use of diuretics/dialysis, and fluid loss through nonrenal sources.

(1) Perform fluid status assessment: edema, JVD, hypotension (including orthostatic), heart rate, lung sounds, skin turgor, mucous membranes, constipation and/or hard stool, and weight changes.

(2) Weigh patient daily on a correctly calibrated scale.

(3) Record accurate I & O.

(4) Correlate the physical assessment with the weight and I & O to determine fluid status: balanced, deficit, or overload.

(5) Educate the patient and family about the kidney's response to the diuresis, including the need for increased fluid intake.

(6) Develop fluid plan for the day with the patient and coordinate with dietitian.

(7) Adjust fluid intake to approximate fluid losses to protect the returning kidney function, increasing or decreasing as the kidney responds.

(8) Provide for excretory needs, keeping commode, urinal, or bedpan within easy access of the patient.

(9) Avoid procedures that require the patient to have nothing by mouth (NPO) or to have a bowel preparation until diuresis subsides. Or initiate intravenous therapy to maintain fluid balance.

c. Hypokalemia related to increased excretion of potassium, decreased potassium intake, metabolic alkalosis, continued administration of diuretics or resin exchangers, intravenous fluid without potassium, and GI fluid losses.

(1) Educate the patient and family regarding the risk of hypokalemia, as well as the signs and symptoms they should report.

(2) Review lab values for serum potassium levels.

(3) Assess for decreased neuromuscular irritability, constipation, weakness, and/or diminished reflexes; severe hypokalemia can lead to ineffective breathing due to weakness or paralysis of respiratory muscles.

(4) Monitor EKG for signs of hypokalemia.
   (a) ST segment depression.
   (b) Flattened T wave.
   (c) Presence of U wave.
   (d) Ventricular arrhythmias.

(5) Consult dietitian for adequate dietary intake of potassium.

(6) Administer potassium parenterally if unable to ingest adequate dietary potassium.

(7) Prevent metabolic alkalosis because of hydrogen-potassium cellular exchange; discontinue bicarbonate infusions.

(8) Control GI losses.

(9) Avoid medications that cause potassium loss (e.g., diuretics).

8. The following problems, described in the oliguria/nonoliguria section, persist and require continued nursing monitoring and interventions.
   a. Increased susceptibility to infection.
   b. Gastrointestinal bleeding.
   c. Alteration in nutrition.
   d. Skin breakdown.
   e. Drug toxicity and nephrotoxicity.
   f. Disturbances in sleep patterns.

9. The problems of hyperphosphatemia and metabolic acidosis gradually resolve during diuresis as kidney function improves; the kidneys are once more able to regulate and excrete hydrogen and phosphate and to reabsorb bicarbonate ions.

D. Recovery of kidney function.
   1. If it occurs, the process usually lasts several months to 1 year.
   2. Healing process completed.
      a. Contractile scar tissue replaces damaged basement membrane.
      b. Nephrons are maximally patent and tubular cells regenerated.
      c. Probably some scar tissue remains in all AKI/ARF kidneys, but the functional loss is not always clinically significant.
      d. Maximal kidney functions return (e.g., concentrating ability) and kidneys respond to body's needs through regulatory and excretory mechanisms.
      e. Urine osmolality increases, urine volume stabilizes, plasma substances normalize, body fluids balance, and uremia resolves.
   3. No special form of treatment is required other than general healthy living.
   4. Major patient issues requiring nursing (hospital and nephrology) care and intervention.
      a. Lack of knowledge regarding the AKI/ARF episode, including follow-up care and prevention of another episode.
      b. Educate the patient and family about the ARF episode and interventions to prevent another episode.
         (1) Avoid nephrotoxins.
         (2) Drink plenty of water.

V. Manifestations of frequently occurring acute kidney injury processes.

A. Acute tubular necrosis (ATN).
  1. The most common cause of intrinsic AKI/ARF, responsible for 38% to 76% of cases.
  2. Can be the result of septic, toxic, or ischemic insults.
  3. Mortality rate in patients requiring dialysis is between 50% and 80%.
  4. Presentation and assessment.
     a. Lab values show increased urine sodium concentration and fractional excretion of sodium.
     b. ATN is a part of a catabolic illness, making nutritional support critical, including administration of essential amino acids.
     c. Use of enteral feeds rather than parenteral is recommended when possible.
  5. Nursing interventions and collaborative treatments.
     a. Continuous or intermittent forms of KRT may be used.
     b. The avoidance of hypotension is the key with either modality.

B. Rhabdomyolysis is necrosis of skeletal muscle.
  1. Clinical presentation.
     a. Local features.
        (1) Muscle pain.
        (2) Tenderness.
        (3) Swelling.
        (4) Bruising.
        (5) Weakness.
     b. Systemic features.
        (1) Tea-colored urine.
        (2) Fever.
        (3) Malaise.
        (4) Nausea.
        (5) Emesis.
        (6) Confusion.
        (7) Agitation.
        (8) Delirium.
        (9) Anuria.
  2. It is the cause of 7% to 10% of AKI/ARF.
  3. It can occur from direct traumatic injury or nontraumatic (compression or exertional) injury.
  4. The most common causes are alcohol abuse, muscle overexertion, muscle compression, and the use of certain medications or illicit drugs.
     a. When injured, muscle cells release myoglobin,

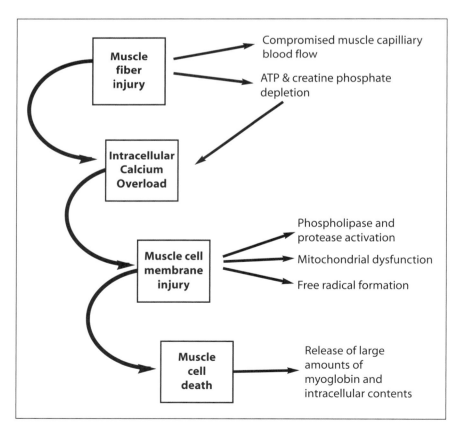

Figure 2.6. Pathogenesis of exertional rhabdomyolysis.

Source: Russell, T.A. (2005). Acute renal failure related to rhabdomyolysis: Pathophysiology, diagnosis, and collaborative management. *Nephrology Nursing Journal, 32*, 409-417. Used with permission.

which enters the circulation (see Figure 2.6).
- (1) Myoglobin is normally filtered by the glomerulus, but when excessive amounts damage the kidney tubule cells, glomerular filtration is overwhelmed.
- (2) The myoglobin also precipitates and forms casts, which can obstruct flow through the tubules. AKI/ARF can occur.
  - b. CPK (creatine phosphokinase) is also released from damaged muscle.
    - (1) The level of CPK can indicate the likelihood of complications.
    - (2) AKI/ARF usually occurs with creatine kinase "MM" isoenzyme (CK-MM) levels of more than 15,000, but treatment may be initiated at a lower level.
  - c. Large amounts of fluid can accumulate in the necrotic muscle tissues, leading to hypovolemia, which is one of the causes of AKI/ARF in these patients.
  - d. Compartment syndrome can occur, requiring fasciotomy to prevent secondary tissue necrosis.
  - e. Disseminated intravascular coagulation (DIC) and multiorgan dysfunction syndrome (MODS) can also occur.
  - f. Hyperkalemia, hyperphosphatemia, and lactic acidosis are other electrolyte disturbances likely to occur.
  - g. Changes in the urine are also evident (see Table 2.3).
- 5. Nursing interventions and collaborative treatments.
  - a. Treatment includes aggressive attempts to maintain high urine volume with IV infusions at 200 to 300 mL/hr.
  - b. Continuous or intermittent forms of KRT may be used depending on the severity of the necrosis and catabolism, electrolyte imbalances, and hemodynamics.

C. Acute interstitial nephritis (AIN).
1. Causes approximately 10% to 15% of ARF.
2. For many years, AIN was known as the complication of streptococcal infections.
3. With increased development and use of antibiotics, AIN became the complication of antibiotics and other drugs.
4. It is an immune-mediated cause of AKI/ARF that is identified on kidney biopsy as inflammatory cell infiltrates in the interstitium of the kidney.
5. Most frequently caused by drug hypersensitivity reactions that create an allergic reaction within the interstitium, but the tubules can also be involved.
6. NSAIDs and antibiotics are the most frequent

Table 2.3

Urinalysis Findings in Rhabdomyolysis

Color	Dark (cola-colored)
pH	Acidic

Blood
  Benzidine reagent
  Microscopy
	3+ to 4+
	Less than 5 RBCs per high power field

Sediment	Pigmented brown granular casts Renal tubular epithelial cell
Urinary sodium concentration	> 20 mEq/L
FE_{NA}	> 1%

FE_{NA} = fractional excretion of sodium

Source: Russell, T.A. (2005). Acute renal failure related to rhabdomyolysis: pathophysiology, diagnosis, and collaborative management. *Nephrology Nursing Journal, 32*, 409-417. Used with permission.

source of the reaction. Other medications that have been found to induce AIN include analgesics and diuretics.
7. The elderly are the age group most at risk of experiencing this complication due to their increased use of prescription drugs and the reduced ability of their kidneys to clear drugs.
8. Presentation and assessment.
  a. Classic symptoms on presentation are fever, rash, and eosinophilia.
  b. Other symptoms can include oliguria, arthalgia, and loin pain.
9. Nursing interventions and collaborative treatments.
  a. The treatment of choice is removal of the causative agent.
  b. KRT support is frequently needed.
  c. Corticosteroids are often used in treatment based on the assumption of an immune system response in this disease process.
  d. Current studies are bringing the effectiveness of this use of steroids under scrutiny.

D. Goodpasture syndrome.
1. It is characterized by pulmonary hemorrhage and crescentic glomerulonephritis.
2. It is a disease of serum antibodies attacking the

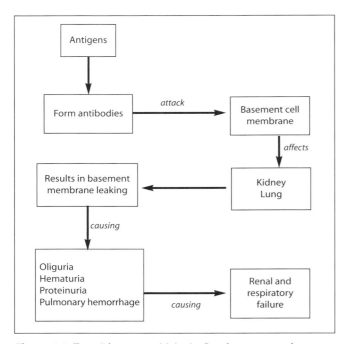

Figure 2.7. Type II hypersensitivity in Goodpasture syndrome.

Source: Bergs, L. (2005). Goodpasture syndrome. *Critical Care Nurse, 25,* 50-58. Used with permission.

glomerular and alveolar basement membranes (see Figure 2.7).
3. Presentation and assessment.
   a. Initially the patient may exhibit flu-like symptoms with malaise and a rapid onset of microscopic hematuria and proteinuria.
   b. 50% to 75% of patients exhibit pulmonary symptoms, such as cough, mild shortness of breath, and hemoptysis.
   c. The pulmonary symptoms may occur days, weeks, or months before the kidney symptoms present.
4. Nursing interventions and collaborative treatments.
   a. Pulmonary hemorrhage can be severe and lead to iron deficiency anemia and a significant increase in mortality.
   b. Airway management and pulmonary failure with increasing oxygen needs must be closely monitored.
   c. Therapeutic plasma exchange (TPE) is performed to decrease the circulating antibodies.
   d. To prevent exacerbation of pulmonary hemorrhage, fresh frozen plasma is used as the replacement fluid for TPE to replace the clotting factors lost by the removal of the patient's plasma.

    e. Immunosuppression is used to prevent further antibody formation. Acute renal failure may develop, requiring KRT treatments.
    f. Heparin should be avoided during KRT.

E. Sepsis and SIRS (systemic inflammatory response syndrome).
   1. Definition of terms for the septic state.
      a. Bacteremia or fungemia – blood cultures positive for bacteria or fungi.
      b. SIRS – a syndrome characterized by at least two of the following:
         (1) Hyperthermia or hypothermia (oral temp > 38°C or < 36°C.
         (2) Hyperventilation (respiratory rate > 20 breaths/min.
         (3) Tachycardia (> 90 beats/min).
         (4) Leukocytosis (> 12,000 uL) or leukopenia (< 4,000 u/L).
      c. Sepsis – SIRS of suspected or proven microbial origin.
      d. Severe sepsis – sepsis with organ dysfunction or lactic acidosis.
      e. Septic shock – sepsis with systolic blood pressure < 90 mmHg or 40 mmHg below patient's baseline that is unresponsive to fluid resuscitation.
      f. MODS – dysfunction of more than one organ (e.g., lungs, kidney, heart, liver, CNS).

   2. Infectious causes are bacteria and fungi. Noninfectious causes include pancreatitis, burns, and trauma. SIRS is the term used to refer to noninfectious causes.
   3. Presentation and assessment.
      a. The pathophysiology of sepsis is, at least in part, an inappropriate and overwhelming inflammatory response: increased production of pro-inflammatory cytokines and decreased production of cytokines that normally inhibit inflammation.
      b. The clotting cascade is activated and fibrinolysis is inhibited, frequently leading to development of disseminated intravascular coagulation (DIC).
      c. Peripheral vasodilation occurs resulting in decreased systemic vascular resistance (SVR). At the same time, catecholamines and angiotensin II are elevated, as evidenced by resistance of the vascular smooth muscles to constrict, leading to poor response to vasopressors.
      d. Early in sepsis, cardiac output (CO) is increased and is able to maintain blood pressure in spite of the reduced afterload that results from the vasodilation.

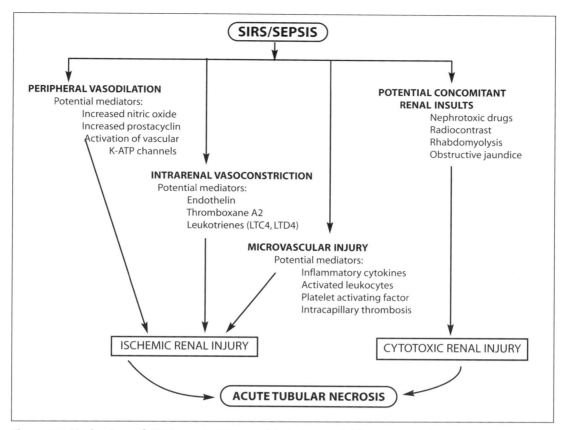

Figure 2.8. Mechanisms of ATN in sepsis. ATN associated with sepsis is largely caused by ischemic injury. Renal hypoperfusion is the combined result of peripheral vasodilation, intrarenal vasocontriction, and microvascular injury to the renal vasculature. These events commonly cause renal ischemia in sepsis even in the absence of hypotension. When septic shock develops, the incidence of ATN markedly increases. Because patients with sepsis often are subject to nephrotoxic events, cytotoxic injury to tubular cells often compounds the ischemic damage associated with sepis. LTC4 = leukotriene: C4: LTD4 = leukotriene: D4: K-ATP = ATP-sensitive potassium channels.

Source: Abernathy, V.E., & Lieberthal, W. (2002). Acute renal failure in the critically ill patient. *Critical Care Clinics, 18*, 203-222. Used with permission from Elsevier.

e. As sepsis progresses, myocardial function becomes impaired and cardiac output (CO) decreases.

f. Intravascular fluid loss occurs because of capillary leak syndrome and third spacing.

g. There is decreased preload due to vasodilation and loss of intravascular volume due to increased vascular permeability. The combination of all these factors leads to hypotension.

h. Sepsis and SIRS are often associated with MODS.

i. The cause of ATN in sepsis is renal hypoperfusion and ischemic injury to proximal tubule cells (see Figure 2.8).

4. Nursing interventions and collaborative treatments.

a. Intensive insulin therapy to keep blood glucose level between 140 and 180 has resulted in lower morbidity and mortality rates in critically ill patients with sepsis (Jacobi et al., 2012).

(1) The protective mechanism of insulin is unknown.

(2) Correcting hyperglycemia may improve the bacterial phagocytic action of neutrophils that is impaired in sepsis.

b. Volume resuscitation to optimize preload, afterload, and contractility of the heart in patients with severe sepsis has improved the likelihood of survival.

(1) Use of crystalloid, vasoactive agents, and transfusions of red blood cells to increase oxygen delivery have all been found to have positive influence.

(2) Monitors for adequacy of oxygen delivery include normalizing values of mixed venous oxygen saturation, lactate concentration, base deficit, and pH.

c. KRT support is provided as needed.

Table 2.4

Diagnostic Criteria for TTP–HUS to Initiate Therapeutic Plasmapheresis Exchange

Classic pentad of symptoms TTP-HUS	Current dyad of symptoms TTP-HUS (in the absence of another apparent cause)
Microangiopathic anemia (MAHA) Thrombocytopenia purpura Neurologic disease Renal disease Fever	Microangiopathic anemia (MAHA) Thrombocytopenia purpura

Adapted from George, J.N., Gilcher, R.O., Smith, J.W., Chandler, L., Duvall, D., & Ellis, C. (1998). Thrombotic thrombocytopenic purpura-hemolytic uremic syndrome: Diagnosis and management. *Journal of Clinical Apheresis, 13*, 120-125. Printed in Myers, L. (2002). Thrombotic thrombocytopenia purpura-hemolytic uremic syndrome: Pathophysiology and management. *Nephrology Nursing Journal, 29*, 171-182. Used with permission.

F. TTP (thrombotic thrombocytopenia purpura) and HUS (hemolytic uremic syndrome).
1. This is a disorder in which microthrombi occlude the terminal ends of arterioles and capillaries.
2. It leads to ischemia in various organs, including the kidneys.
3. Presentation and assessment.
   a. Classic symptoms of TTP and HUS include microangiopathic hemolytic anemia, thrombocytopenia, fever, neurologic changes, and kidney failure (see Table 2.4).
   b. The occluding lesions in the terminal arterioles and capillaries consist of platelet aggregation and von Willebrand Factor (vWF) of unusually large molecular weight.
   c. Metalloproteinase is an enzyme that normally breaks up large clumps of vWF but seems to be decreased or ineffective in patients with TTP-HUS.
   d. Thrombocytopenia with counts dropping below 10,000/mm^3 is classic.
   e. LDH (lactic dehydrogenase) is the primary indicator of intravascular red cell destruction (hemolysis).
   f. TTP and HUS are often difficult to differentiate.
      (1) In general, patients who develop kidney failure are described as having HUS. Compared to patients with TTP, they may have less severe thrombocytopenia, less elevation in LDH, and fewer schistocytes on smear. Kidney failure develops due to infarction and kidney cortical necrosis, leading to occlusion of tubular lumina with the debris of the necrosis, fibrin, and hemolyzed red blood cells (RBCs).
      (2) TTP patients may arrive more acutely ill than HUS patients, with signs of systemic platelet aggregation causing ischemia involving the central nervous system and/or the GI system. They will also have extreme thrombocytopenia, significantly elevated LDH, and more schistocytes on smear in comparison to HUS patients.
      (3) When the diagnosis of TTP or HUS is unclear, TPE may be used initially; AKI/ARF may also develop, requiring treatment with both TPE and hemodialysis to support full recovery.
   g. There are several variations of TTP and HUS.
      (1) Acute idiopathic TTP.
         (a) Single episode occurs without a known cause in late adolescence and middle life with no recurrence.
         (b) Reoccurs now and then up to 8 years after the initial illness.
      (2) Chronic relapsing TTP: rare, congenital condition of infancy or early childhood with frequent episodes of hemolysis that respond to infusions of fresh frozen plasma (FFP) to replace the metalloproteinase.
      (3) Chronic unremitting TTP: adult patients with persistent elevations of LDH, elevated reticulocytes, and thrombocytopenia despite treatment.
      (4) Acquired HUS: occurs after GI infection with *E. coli* or other gram-negative organisms.
      (5) Childhood HUS: most occur before age 6 months and present with bloody diarrhea; usually self-limiting with intravenous (IV) fluids and supportive care.
      (6) Atypical HUS (complement-mediated HUS): rare condition with defect in genes for the complement-proteins C3, factors H, B, I, and CD46, with a high mortality rate, recurrence rate, and the development of chronic kidney failure.

(7) Eculizumab (Soliris®) is the first treatment approved by the U.S. Food and Drug Administration (FDA) (September 2011) for adults and children with atypical hemolytic uremic syndrome (aHUS) (Soliris® packet insert).

4. Nursing interventions and collaborative treatments for TTP.
   a. Treatment of choice is therapeutic plasma exchange (TPE).
   b. Increasing platelet count and decreasing LDH are markers of successful treatment.

G. HELLP (Hemolysis, Elevated Liver enzymes, Low Platelets).
   1. A potentially fatal syndrome for the mother related to a progression of severe preeclampsia.
   2. The problems of vasospasm in preeclampsia (Pellitteri, 2002).
      a. Vascular effects.
         (1) Vasoconstriction.
         (2) Poor organ perfusion.
         (3) Increased blood pressure.
      b. Effects on kidney.
         (1) Decreased glomerular filtration rate.
         (2) Increased permeability of glomerular membranes.
         (3) Increased serum blood urea nitrogen, uric acid, and creatinine levels.
         (4) Decreased urine output.
         (5) Proteinuria.
      c. Interstitial effects.
         (1) Diffusion of fluid from bloodstream to interstitial tissue.
         (2) Edema.
   3. Can also decrease perfusion of the placenta and threaten the fetus with a potential for hypoxia, malnutrition, small size for gestational age, acidosis, mental disabilities, or death.
      a. Presentation and assessment.
         (1) Hemolysis is a microangiopathic hemolytic anemia.
         (2) Elevated liver enzymes are related to obstruction of hepatic blood flow by fibrin deposits.
         (3) Thrombocytopenia (low platelets) is a result of increased consumption and/or increased destruction of platelets.
      b. This syndrome can begin in the third trimester of pregnancy or as late as 7 days after delivery.
      c. HELLP can be ranked into three classes.
         (1) Class 1 = Platelet count < 50,000/mm³.
         (2) Class 2 = Platelet count 50,000 to < 100,000/mm³.
         (3) Class 3 = Platelet count 100,000 to 150,000/mm³.

   d. Lab values.
      (1) Tend to worsen following delivery and then start to normalize after 3 or 4 days.
      (2) Monitor LDH and platelet count to determine changes in disease process.
   4. Nursing interventions and collaborative treatments.
      a. In Class 1, expediting delivery of the fetus (within 48 hours) is the treatment of choice.
      b. In Class 2 and 3, more conservative management can be considered based on gestational age along with close monitoring of the condition of the mother and the fetus.
      c. TPE has been effective in treating HELLP patients with severe lab values, such as platelet count less than 30,000/mm³ and persistent elevation of LDH.
      d. TTP-HUS can occur in complicated pregnancies, causing AKI/ARF and requiring treatment with both TPE and hemodialysis to support full recovery.

H. Patients with drug intoxication.
   1. Aspirin (ASA) intoxications (Merck Manual, 2015).
      a. One of our oldest medications and is widely used.
      b. Rapidly metabolized when ingested into salicylic acid.
      c. Most common cause of death is acute noncardiogenic pulmonary edema.
      d. Other sources of salicylate products.
         (1) Wart remover compounds.
         (2) Oil of wintergreen (methyl salicylate) is the most concentrated and toxic form of salicylate, which is a component of some creams used for musculoskeletal pain and solutions used in hot vaporizers.
         (3) Some herbal remedies.
      e. Presentation and assessment.
         (1) Early symptoms.
            (a) Tinnitus and vertigo.
            (b) Nausea and vomiting.
            (c) Hyperventilation.
            (d) Alteration in mental status.
            (e) Noncardiogenic pulmonary edema.
            (f) Fever.
         (2) Later symptoms.
            (a) Hyperactivity.
            (b) Fever.
            (c) Confusion.
            (d) Seizures.
            (e) Rhabdomyolysis, acute kidney failure, and respiratory failure may eventually develop.
            (f) Hyperactivity can change to lethargy.

(g) Hyperventilation can progress to hypoventilation with mixed respiratory alkalosis-metabolic acidosis and respiratory failure.

f. Diagnostic evaluation.
  (1) Salicylate level, arterial blood gas, basic metabolic panel, chest x-ray.
  (2) Significant salicylate toxicity is suggested by serum levels much higher than therapeutic (10–20 mg/dL), particularly 6 hours after ingestion.
  (3) Repeat salicylate level every 2 hours until level declining.
  (4) Repeat blood gas every 2 hours until acid-base status stable or improving.

g. Treatment.
  (1) Activated charcoal as soon as possible and if bowel sounds are present.
  (2) Alkaline diuresis to a urine pH equal to or above 8.
      (a) IV solution of 1 L of D5W, three 50 mEq ampules of $NaHCO_3$, and 40 mEq of KCl at 1.5 to 2 times the maintenance IV fluid rate.
      (b) Hypokalemia may interfere with alkaline diuresis; potassium and glucose levels should be monitored closely.
      (c) Do not use acetazolamides to alkalinize the urine because they will worsen metabolic acidosis and decrease blood pH.
  (3) Hemodialysis is indicated for the patient with:
      (a) Acute pulmonary or cerebral edema even with an ASA level not at a toxic level.
      (b) Profoundly altered mental status.
      (c) Renal insufficiency that interferes with salicylate excretion.
      (d) Fluid overload that prevents the administration of sodium bicarbonate.
      (e) A plasma salicylate concentration > 100 mg/dL (7.2 mmol/L).
      (f) Clinical deterioration despite aggressive and appropriate supportive care.

h. Nursing interventions and collaborative treatment.
  (1) Monitor for bleeding and use no heparin during hemodialysis.
  (2) Draw serial serum salicylate levels peripherally rather than from a dialysis access catheter to avoid recirculation that could alter serum drug levels.
  (3) Consult with nephrologist to discontinue bicarbonate IV solution prior to initiating HD treatment to prevent overcompensating for metabolic acidosis.
  (4) Volume resuscitation and glucose supplementation may be needed in severe intoxication, which can impact the hemodialysis treatment.

2. Ethylene glycol.
  a. An ingredient of automotive antifreeze, windshield wiper fluid, and solvents, which may produce lethal serum levels with only a 100 mL ingestion.
  b. Toxicology and nephrology physicians collaborate to determine the most efficient course of treatment.
  c. Presentation and assessment.
    (1) Serum ethylene glycol level exceeding 50 mg/dL indicates toxicity.
    (2) Manifestations.
        (a) Confusion.
        (b) Drunkenness.
        (c) Convulsions.
        (d) Tachypnea.
        (e) Pulmonary edema.
        (f) Severe high anion gap with metabolic acidosis.
        (g) Coma.
        (h) Myocarditis.
        (i) Increased plasma osmolar gap.
    (3) AKI/ARF occurs due to urine oxalate precipitation that delays excretion of toxic metabolites.
  d. Nursing interventions and collaborative treatment.
    (1) Hemodialysis is required to remove the toxic metabolites using a large surface area dialyzer (> 1.5 m²), a blood flow rate of 300 mL/min or greater, and a bicarbonate dialysate bath.
    (2) Fomepizole IV rapidly and competitively inhibits alcohol dehydrogenase, more potently than alcohol. It is the antidote of choice for ethylene glycol and methanol intoxication (Keyes & Kagawalla, 2012).
        (a) To compensate for fomepizole elimination during dialysis, clarify fomepizole dosing with nephrologist.
        (b) The frequency of dosing should be increased to every 4 hours during HD.
        (c) Administer an additional dose at the beginning of dialysis if greater than 6 hours since the last dose.
        (d) During HD, administer fomepizole after blood pump in the infusion port of the venous chamber if no other central line or IV catheter is available.
    (3) Treat metabolic acidosis with sodium bicarbonate infusion. Clarify with

nephrologists if this infusion should be discontinued once HD is initiated.
- (4) If fomepizole is not available, ethanol should be used as an antidote to decrease the toxic effects of the poisoning. Once HD has been initiated, administer the ethanol infusion after blood pump in the infusion port of the venous chamber if no other central line or IV catheter is available.
- (5) Serial serum ethylene glycol levels should be monitored.
  - (a) HD should be continued until levels are less than 20 mg/dL.
  - (b) Rebound can be expected within 12 hours.
  - (c) Repeat HD treatment or initiate CRRT as needed to minimize rebound.
- (6) Monitor metabolic acidosis with arterial blood gases (ABGs). Continue HD until it is corrected.
- (7) If the lab is unable to perform timely ethylene glycol levels, HD treatment should continue for no less than 8 hours, depending on the serum level at initiation.
- (8) Systemic heparin anticoagulation during HD to prevent clotting the system is acceptable.
  - (a) These patients usually have normal hemoglobin and hematocrit levels.
  - (b) Reconsider if the patient has underlying chronic kidney injury or disease.
- (9) Forced diuresis with fluids and mannitol may preserve kidney function during ethylene glycol intoxication by preventing oxalate formation. However, if the patient develops pulmonary edema during HD:
  - (a) Mannitol may need to be discontinued due to its osmotic pull.
  - (b) Ultrafiltration rate should be clarified with the nephrologist.
- 3. Methanol.
  - a. A component of solvents, varnish, de-icing solutions, and other solutions containing wood alcohols to include "moonshine."
  - b. Mortality rate is 80% or greater in patients who present with seizures, coma, or pH < 7.0. Without these symptoms, the mortality rate is less than 6%.
  - c. Presentation and assessment.
    - (1) Serum methanol level greater than 50 mg/dL indicates toxicity.
    - (2) Methanol poisoning presents similarly to ethylene glycol poisoning.
      - (a) Early presentation is confusion.
      - (b) Metabolic acidosis begins 12 to 36 hours after ingestion.

- (c) Retinal involvement also occurs in 12 to 36 hours.
- (3) Manifestations include:
  - (a) Weakness.
  - (b) Nausea.
  - (c) Headache.
  - (d) Decreased vision.
  - (e) High risk of permanent blindness.
- (4) Nursing interventions and collaborative treatments are similar to ethylene glycol intoxication.
- 4. Lithium carbonate.
  - a. Mortality rate is approximately 25% with an acute overdose.
  - b. In patients intoxicated during maintenance therapy, 10% suffer permanent neurologic damage and the mortality rate is 9%.
  - c. Presentation and assessment.
    - (1) Serum lithium greater than 4.0 mEq/L indicates toxicity, regardless of the clinical status of the patient, and treatment with HD is indicated.
    - (2) Manifestations.
      - (a) Common characteristics.
        - i. Neuromuscular irritability.
        - ii. Nausea.
        - iii. Diarrhea.
      - (b) Other possible symptoms.
        - i. Muscle weakness.
        - ii. Increased deep tendon reflexes.
        - iii. Somnolence.
        - iv. T-wave flattening.
        - v. Coma eventually leading to death.
  - d. Nursing interventions and collaborative treatment.
    - (1) Primary medical management includes discontinuing diuretics and initiating 0.45% normal saline IV for rehydration.
    - (2) The initial HD treatment should last 6 to 8 hours, until the serum level is 0.6 mEq/L or lower.
    - (3) Hemodialysis is very effective at clearing lithium. However, levels may rebound within 12 hours of treatment.
    - (4) Consecutive HD should be performed until lithium levels stay at or below 1.0 mEq/L for 6 to 8 hours after treatment.
    - (5) CRRT may be an effective modality choice to minimize rebound.
- I. Hepatorenal syndrome/failure (HRS).
  - 1. Definition: a life-threatening medical condition that consists of rapid deterioration in kidney function in individuals with acute or chronic liver failure.
  - 2. Arterial vasodilation in the splanchnic circulation induced by portal hypertension plays a significant

role in changes in the hemodynamic status and decline in kidney function (Fisher & Brown, 2010).

3. Hepatorenal syndrome is characterized by type:
   a. Type 1: Most serious increase in serum creatinine, urine output less than 400 to 500 mL/day.
   b. Type 2: Kidney impairment less severe, ascites present due to resistance to diuretics (Ginès, 2009).

4. Causes.
   a. Acetaminophen toxicity.
   b. Ischemic hepatic injury.
   c. Hepatitis B.
   d. Wilson disease.
   e. Acute fatty liver of pregnancy/HELLP.
   f. Herpes simplex virus.
   g. Reye syndrome.
   h. Sepsis.
   i. Heat stroke.

5. Manifestations.
   a. Fatigue/malaise.
   b. Lethargy.
   c. Anorexia.
   d. Nausea and or vomiting.
   e. Pruritus.
   f. Jaundice.
   g. Abdominal distension from ascites.

6. Laboratory findings.
   a. Prolonged prothrombin time with INR > 1.5.
   b. Elevated aminotransferase levels.
   c. Elevated bilirubin level.
   d. Low Platelet count ($\leq$ 150,000/mm^3).
   e. Elevated BUN/creatinine.
   f. Elevated amylase and lipase.
   g. Hypoglycemia.
   h. Hypophosphatemia.
   i. Hypomagnesemia.
   j. Hypokalemia.
   k. Acidosis or alkalosis.
   l. Elevated ammonia level.
   m. Elevated LDH (actate dehydrogenase level).

7. Nursing interventions and collaborative treatment.
   a. Monitor and prevent complications of altered hemodynamic status.
   b. Monitor laboratory and diagnostic findings.

8. Therapy considerations.
   a. Fluid management goals are to achieve diuresis without further loss of sodium, and to maintain adequate circulatory volume and hemodynamic stability.
   b. The goal is to prevent over-constriction of the renal or systemic vasculature.
   c. IV fluid replacement may vary, based on patient's serum sodium level, to prevent additional sodium retention.
   d. Avoid hypertonic solutions to prevent rapid refilling from the interstitial fluid to the vascular space to prevent pulmonary edema.
   e. Albumin is recommended for low serum albumin levels for volume expansion not to exceed 100 grams.
   f. Paracentesis may be indicated in patients with impaired kidney function to reduce renal venous pressure for ascites.
   g. Kidney replacement therapy is indicated with CRRT preferred over hemodialysis because of reduced hemodynamic instability. Avoiding hypotension is important.
   h. Hemodialysis may be indicated for rapid correction of acidosis, hyperkalemia, uremic symptoms, or volume overload.

9. Pharmacologic management.
   a. The goal is to restore systemic and splanchnic vasoconstriction while promoting kidney dilatation, normal sodium levels, and normal fluid volume.
   b. The use of vasoconstrictive medications, such as norepinephrine or neosynephrine, along with albumin improved renal function.
   c. Midodrine and octreotide can also be used (Singh et al., 2012).
   d. Terlipressin therapy is used but not available in the United States (Velez & Nietert, 2011).
   e. Monitor toxicity and ensure medications are prescribed and adjusted to renal dose ranges.

10. Surgical management.
    a. TIPS Procedure: Transjugular intrahepatic portosystemic shunt is a procedure performed in which a shunt is placed between the portal and hepatic veins to manage refractory ascites.
    b. Liver/kidney transplant.

11. Prevention of infection.
    a. Standard precautions.
    b. Monitor for signs and symptoms of infection.

12. Nutrition.
    a. Maintain protein intake at normal levels unless severe malnutrition is present.
    b. Nutritional supplements include amino acids, low total fat, multivitamins, and minerals such as zinc.
    c. Monitor fluid restrictions.
    d. Monitor weight, intake and output, calorie intake.

J. Nephrogenic systemic fibrosis (NSF).
   1. NSF is a progressive and potentially fatal multiorgan system fibrosing disease only seen in patients with acute or chronic kidney failure. It has occurred in patients with ESRD primarily, but 20% of the cases reported occurred in patients with AKI or CKD stages 4 and 5 (Abu-Alfa, 2011).
   2. It is characterized by two primary features:
      a. Thickening and hardening of the skin overlying the extremities and trunk.

b. Fibrosis extending into other organ systems.

3. Most patients with this disorder are on hemodialysis but can also include patients on peritoneal dialysis, kidney transplant recipients with reduced allograft function, patients with advanced CKD, and patients with AKI not receiving dialysis.

4. As of January 2014, 400 cases of NSF have been reported to the International NSF registry at Yale University (Krefting, 2012).

5. Most cases are in adults, but children are affected, too.

6. NSF is caused by exposure of patients with advanced kidney failure to a new medication, infection, or exposure to contrast agents containing gadolinium.

 a. Gadolinium is a nonradioactive contrast agent primarily used for magnetic resonance imaging (MRI) or MR angiography studies.

 b. The FDA currently warns against the use of gadolinium-based contrast agents in patients with a GFR less than 30 mL/min per 1.73 m² (Schlaudecker & Bernheisel, 2009).

 c. Gadolinium is a heavy metal toxin that is chelated when administered. It is retained in the tissue.

 d. Kidney failure increases the duration of the gadolinium exposure through decreased clearance of free gadolinium. The deposits lead to fibrocytes, which along with the pro-inflammatory state it creates, causes tissue injury and further fibrocytes leading to NSF (Schlaudecker & Bernheisel, 2009).

7. Treatment.

 a. There is no proven treatment for NSF other than recovery of kidney function.

 b. Hemodialysis is effective at removing gadolinium from the body and should be done within 3 hours after exposure (Schalaudecker & Bernheisel, 2009).

 c. Physical therapy is recommended to prevent or reverse joint contractions.

VI. Special patient populations and AKI/ARF.

A. Pregnancy.

1. AKI/ARF occurs in 1 of every 2000 to 5000 pregnancies.

2. Presentation and assessment.

 a. Frequency distribution is bimodal.

 (1) First peak in early pregnancy: associated with septic abortion and shock or fluid and electrolyte imbalances from hyperemesis.

 (2) Second peak in final gestational month: associated with pre-eclampsia, hemorrhagic complications, and abruptio placentae.

 b. AKI/ARF also associated with prolonged intrauterine fetal death, disseminated intravascular coagulation (DIC), urinary tract obstruction from stones, and/or ureteral obstruction from size and position of the uterus.

3. Nursing interventions and collaborative treatment.

 a. Treatment similar to nongravidas with AKI/ARF.

 (1) Since urea, creatinine, and other substances cross the placenta, dialysis may need to be implemented early and performed more frequently to maintain a normal fetal environment.

 (2) Dialysate may need to be adjusted to lower levels of bicarbonate and higher levels of magnesium.

 b. Intradialytic monitoring to prevent hypotension and hypertension.

 c. Collaborate with obstetric (OB) nurses for fetal monitoring during hemodialysis treatments.

B. Gerontologic patients.

1. Changes in demographic characteristics due to increased life expectancy have brought increased occurrences of progressive renal failure in the aging population.

 a. Treatments, including noninvasive interventions, have improved expanding alternatives for the elderly patient while contributing to a reduction in morbidity and mortality.

 b. Decisions related to management of older adult care lead to additional moral and ethical considerations, including cost of dialysis therapy and scarcity of transplantable organs (Davison, 1998).

2. Older adults experience an increased incidence of AKI/ARF; prevalence is increased threefold.

3. Factors influencing the occurrence of AKI/ARF in the elderly.

 a. Increased systemic disease.

 b. Structural changes in the aging kidneys.

 c. Functional changes in the aging kidneys.

4. Anatomic and physiologic changes in the elderly kidney (Davison, 1998; Pascual et al., 1995).

 a. Reduction in renal mass up to 30% by the 8th decade.

 b. Development of focal sclerosis in a significant number of the remaining glomeruli.

 c. Reduction in the size and number of tubules.

 d. Significant deposition of connective tissue in the medulla.

 e. Thickening of the glomerular and tubular basement membrane.

f. Structural vascular changes leading to atrophy of the glomerulus.

g. Progressive decline in GFR at a decremental rate of 0.75 mL/min/year.

h. Development of diverticula of the distal nephrons.

i. Decreased ability to reabsorb sodium by the thickened ascending limb of the loop of Henle.

j. Impaired renal acid excretion with subsequent impaired buffering.

k. In spite of these changes, the aging kidney is capable of maintaining fluid and electrolyte balance under normal circumstances.

l. The aged kidney's adaptive capacity is impaired, so during episodes of systemic disease, hemodynamic or abrupt intravascular volume change, the administration of toxic drugs, or other insults, acute kidney failure may be a recurrent problem for the older adult.

5. Presentation and assessment.

a. Similar to younger patients, but more likely to be superimposed on underlying kidney insufficiency.

b. Presence of other comorbidities may interfere with expedient diagnosis in the elderly.

c. Interpretation of diagnostic data may vary in the elderly.

(1) Decreased ability to concentrate and dilute urine, resulting in impaired thirst mechanism, volume depletion, and hyponatremia.

(2) Serum creatinine can be maintained due to declining muscle mass and body weight.

(3) Tubular function decreases, causing less effective concentration and dilution of urine. An adult normal osmolality may be 1,109 mOsm/kg while the older adult may only be 882 mOsm/kg.

(4) Fractional Excretion of Sodium (FENa+) can be affected by the decreased ability to reabsorb sodium yielding unreliable values for discerning prerenal from intrinsic renal failure.

d. Up to 90% mortality in older adults in AKI/ARF occurring in an ICU and/or associated with sepsis.

e. Iatrogenic factors also put the older adult patient at risk for AKI/ARF.

(1) Aggressive treatment of congestive heart failure with diuretics, leading to volume contraction and decreased kidney perfusion.

(2) Salt restriction and diuretics for treatment of hypertension.

(3) Medication management.

(a) NSAIDs are frequently administered to treat rheumatic diseases, which are common in the elderly.

(b) ACE inhibitors.

(c) Combination of medications (e.g., NSAIDs, ACE inhibitors, diuretics).

6. Causes of acute prerenal failure in the elderly.

a. External losses of fluids with inadequate fluid replacement (dehydration).

(1) Decreased concentrating ability of the kidney.

(2) Inability of kidney to retain sodium.

(3) Impairment of thirst regulation.

b. Internal redistribution of volume from intravascular to interstitial space.

(1) Sepsis.

(a) Decreased urine output may precede temperature spike by hours.

(b) Absence of temperature spike is not unusual in the elderly.

(2) Hypoproteinemia.

(a) Nephrotic syndrome.

(b) Cirrhosis/hepatorenal failure.

(c) Malnutrition.

(d) Tissue injury (e.g., burns, pancreatitis).

(3) Decreased cardiac output.

(a) Myocardial dysfunction.

(b) Pericardial disease.

c. Drug-induced nephropathy, by altering intrarenal hemodynamics.

(1) ACE inhibitors.

(a) Mechanism: fall in blood pressure and efferent glomerular arteriolar tone that decreases transglomerular hydraulic pressure and thereby glomerular filtration rate (GFR).

(b) Used to treat hypertension, congestive heart failure, and secondary prevention of myocardial infarction.

(c) Risk factors.

i. The presence of bilateral renovascular disease.

ii. Arterial stenosis in a solitary kidney.

iii. Volume depletion.

iv. Concomitant treatment with diuretics.

v. Low salt diet.

vi. Cardiac failure.

vii. Combined treatment with NSAIDs.

viii. Presence of diabetes mellitus.

(d) Withdrawal of drug and volume repletion, if indicated, will result in kidney recovery.

(2) NSAIDs.

(a) Incidence of NSAID-induced uremia in patients with baseline kidney insufficiency may be as high as 30%.

(b) Mechanism A.
  i. NSAIDs inhibit cyclooxygenase-mediated arachidonic acid metabolites.
  ii. They, in turn, inhibit production of prostaglandins, leaving the vasoconstrictive hormones (norepinephrine and angiotensin II) unopposed.
  iii. Decrease in circulating volume may result in severe kidney vaso-constriction and a rapid decrease in renal blood flow and GFR.
(c) Mechanism B.
  i. Immunologically mediated nephrotic syndrome.
  ii. Release of lymphokines and eosinophil chemotactic factors cause a diffuse infiltration of the kidney interstitium by mononuclear inflammatory cells and eosinophils.
  iii. Leads to tubulitis.
(d) Risk factors.
  i. Heart failure.
  ii. Cirrhosis.
  iii. Nephrotic syndrome.
  iv. Volume depletion.
  v. Combined treatment with ACE inhibitors.
(e) Withdrawal of medication usually results in recovery of kidney function.
(3) Calcineurin inhibitors: cyclosporine and tacrolimas.
  (a) Mechanism: vasoconstriction of the afferent kidney arterioles caused by excessive endothelin-1 production.
  (b) Kidney function improves or recovers completely after reducing the dosage or discontinuing the drug.
7. Causes of acute renal parenchymal (intrarenal) failure in the elderly.
  a. Acute tubular necrosis (ATN).
    (1) Drug-induced nephrotoxicity occurrence is increased in the elderly.
    (2) Elderly patients have a longer recovery period.
    (3) Recovery may be compromised by the presence of comorbidities.
  b. Tubulointerstitial nephritis.
    (1) May be idiopathic or related to infection or a drug.
    (2) Increased incidence over age 60.
    (3) Discontinuation of medication will frequently result in return of kidney function.
  c. Acute glomerulonephritis (GN).

(1) Responsible for 19% of AKI/ARF in the elderly.
(2) Rapidly progressive glomerular nephritis (RPGN) is most common type in the elderly.
(3) Treatable glomerular and tubulointerstitial diseases are common in the elderly, underscoring the importance of early diagnosis.
(4) Kidney biopsy, the gold standard for establishing diagnosis of these diseases, is well tolerated by older adults.
  d. Atheroembolic kidney disease.
    (1) This age group makes up approximately 36% of reported cases.
    (2) Strong association between atrial fibrillation and atheroembolic kidney disease has been made.
  e. Cholesterol embolization.
    (1) The elderly make up 63% of the reported cases.
    (2) Prognosis is dependent on the extent of organ(s) involvement. Kidney function may recover even if a course of KRT is required during the acute stage.
8. Acute obstructive uropathy (postrenal acute kidney failure) in the elderly.
  a. Responsible for 10% to 15% of the cases of AKI/ARF in the elderly.
  b. Prostatic disease is the most common cause of obstructive uropathy in males.
  c. In females, bladder involvement and tumors of the pelvic organs are primarily responsible for obstruction.
  d. 4.5% of the elderly population with obstructive uropathy did not demonstrate upper tract dilation with ultrasound or CT scan.
    (1) This may be caused by a tumor encapsulating the kidneys and ureters.
    (2) Also may be present in patients with retroperitoneal fibrosa.
  e. Treatment will focus on relieving obstruction and providing supportive KRT until kidney function returns.
9. Nursing care and collaborative interventions.
  a. Older patients generally become symptomatic at lower levels of BUN and serum creatinine than younger patients.
  b. Symptoms the elderly patient may present.
    (1) Exacerbation of previously well-controlled heart failure.
    (2) Unexplained changes in mental status.
    (3) Changes in behavior.
    (4) Personality changes.
    (5) Change in sense of well-being.
  c. Indications for treatment.

(1) Pulmonary edema.

(2) Hyperkalemia.

(3) Severe acidemia.

(4) Catabolic state.

10. Modalities for treatment of elderly include intermittent hemodialysis, daily hemodialysis, peritoneal dialysis, transplantation, or withdrawal from treatment (Davison, 1998).

a. Hemodialysis.

(1) Some older adult patients have difficulty in establishing an adequate vascular access, requiring frequent procedures to address the complications.

(2) Fluid gains between treatment are frequently poorly tolerated.

(3) Vascular instability is common.

(4) Osmolality and fluid shifts associated with intermittent hemodialysis are not well tolerated by many older adult patients because of their altered compensatory mechanisms associated with the aging process.

(5) Many older adult patients are lonely, and going to the dialysis clinic three times a week can be good therapy.

(6) Evidence has shown that hemodialysis can be satisfactory for older adults, given that they have a good support system to help them maintain mobility, adequate nutrition, and mental functioning.

b. Peritoneal dialysis.

(1) CAPD can be demanding of time and energy, with several exchanges needing to be done every day.

(2) CCPD can be adjusted to fit the older adult's schedule.

(3) CCPD works well with older adult patients who cannot tolerate the rapid fluid removal of hemodialysis (e.g., heart failure).

(4) Nutritional status must be monitored closely due to loss of protein in the process of treatment.

c. Transplantation.

(1) Prior reluctance to transplant the elderly has become less of a barrier for this therapy.

(2) Patients may be transplanted into their 8th decade depending on their physical and mental likelihood of achieving benefit from the treatment.

(3) Scarcity of organs has raised ethical discussion of transplanting the elderly as opposed to transplanting a patient who would likely benefit from it for a longer period of time.

(4) Living related donor transplants might be confounded by the age of the potential donor who may also have significant comorbidities to consider for their own longevity.

d. Withdrawal from treatment.

(1) This is a process demanding careful and caring consideration.

(2) The desires of the patient who is of sound mind should be the basis of such a discussion with his or her medical and nursing care providers.

(3) An elder may decide that treatment is prolonging life but not supporting good living.

(4) Elders who are not of sound mind or who are psychiatrically unsound should be carefully evaluated with consideration of prior expressed desires, clinical deterioration, and communication with family and support systems for the decision.

e. Choice of treatment modality will depend on the clinical presentation of the patient as well as the patient's hemodynamic condition.

References

Abernathy, V.E., & Lieberthal, W. (2002). Acute renal failure in the critically ill patient. *Critical Care Clinics, 18*, 203-222.

Abu-Alfa A.K. (2011). Nephrogenic systemic fibrosis and gadolinium-based contrast agents. *Advances Chronic Kidney Disease, 18*(3) 188-198. doi:10.1053/j.ackd.2011.03.001

Agrawal, M., & Swartz, R. (2000). Acute renal failure. *American Family Physician, 61*, 2077-2088.

Bergs, L. (2005). Goodpasture syndrome. *Critical Care Nurse, 25*, 50-58.

Bonventre, J.V. (2007). Diagnosis of acute kidney injury: From classic parameters to new biomarkers. *Contributions in Nephrology, 156*, 213-219.

Bonventre, J.V. (2009). Kidney injury model (KIM-1): A urinary biomarker and much more. *Nephrology Dialysis and Transplant, 24*, 3265-3268.

Davison, A.M. (1998). Renal disease in the elderly. *Nephron, 80*, 6-16.

Fisher, E.M., & Brown, D.K. (2010). Hepatorenal syndrome. *AACN Advanced Critical Care, 21*(2), 165-186. doi:10.1097/NCI.0b013e3181d9261b

Fry, A.C., & Farrington, K. (2006). Management of acute renal failure. *Postgraduate Medicine Journal, 82*, 106-116.

George, J.N., Gilcher, R.O., Smith, J.W., Chandler, L., Duvall, D., & Ellis, C. (1998). Thrombotic thrombocytopenic purpura-hemolytic uremic syndrome: Diagnosis and management. *Journal of Clinical Apheresis, 13*, 120-125.

Gervasio, J.M. & Cotton, A.B. (2009). Nutrition support therapy in acute kidney injury: Distinguishing dogma from good practice. *Current Gastroenterologoy Reports, 11*(4), 325-331.

Haase, M., Haase-Fielitz, A., Belloma, R., & Mertens, P.R. (2011). Neutrophil gelatinase-associated lipocalin as a marker for acute reanal disease. *Current Opinion in Hematology, 18*(1) 11-18. doi:10.1097/MOH.0b013e3283411517

Jacobi, J., Bircher, N., Kinsley, J., Agus, M., Braithwaite, S.S., Deutschman, C., … Schunemann, H. (2012). Guidelines for use of an insulin infusion for the management of hyperglycemia in critically ill patients. *Critcal Care Medicine, 40,* 3251. doi:10.1097/CCM.0b013e3182653269

Kidney Disease: Improving Global Outcomes (KDIGO) Acute Kidney Injury Work Group. (2012). KDIGO clinical practice guideline for acute kidney injury. *Kidney International Supplement, 2,* 1-138. Retrieved from http://kdigo.org/home/guidelines/acute-kidney-injury/

Keyes, D.C., & Kagalwalla, A.A. (2012, August). *Ethylene glycol toxicity treatment and management.* Retrieved from http://emedicine.medscape.com/article/814701-treatment#a1126

Krefting, I. (2012). FDA. Personal communication. Presented at 5th Annual Scientific Symposium on NSF and Allied Fibrotic Disorders, May 20, 2011. Yale University School of Medicine, New Haven, CT.

Lancaster, L.E. (1990). Renal response to shock. *Critical Care Nursing Clinics of North America, 2*(2), 221-223.

Merck Manual, 2015. *Aspirin and other salicylate poisoning.* Retrieved from http://www.merckmanuals.com/professional/injuries _poisoning/poisoning/aspirin_and_other_salicylate_poisoning.html

Murray, P.T, Devarajan, P., Levey, A.S, Eckardt, K,U., Bonventre, J.V., Lombardi, R., Herget-Rosenthal, S., & Levin, A. (2008). A framework and key research questions in AKI diagnosis and staging in different environments. *Clinical Journal of the American Society of Nephrology, 3(3),* 864-868.

Murugan R., & Kellum, J.A. (2011). Acute kidney injury: What's the prognosis? *Nature Reviews Nephrology, 7*(4), 209-217.

Pascual, J., Liano, F., & Ortuno, J. (1995). The elderly patient with acute renal failure. *Journal of the American Society of Nephrology, 6*(2), 144-153.

Pillitteri, A. (Ed.) (2002). *Maternal & child health nursing* (4th ed.). Lippincott Williams & Wilkins.

Russell, T.A. (2005). Acute renal failure related to rhabdomyolysis: Pathophysiology, diagnosis, and collaborative management. *Nephrology Nursing Journal, 32,* 409-417.

Sauret, J.M., & Marinides, G. (2002). Rhabdomyolysis. *American Family Physician, 65,* 5, 907-912.

Schlaudecker, J.D., & Bernheisel, C.R. (2009) Gadolinium-associated nephrogenic systemic fibrosis. *American Family Physican, 80*(7), 711-714.

Singh, V., Dhungana, S.P., & Singh, B. (2012). Midodrine in patients with cirrhosis and refactory or recurrent ascities: A randomized pilot study. *Journal of Hepatology, 56*(2), 348-354.

Soliris (eculizumab) (2011). Package insert. Cheshire, CT: Alexion Pharmaceutical.[Full Text].

Susantitaphong, P., Cruz, D.N., Cerda, J., Abulfaraj, M., Algahtani, F., Koulouridis, I., … Acute Kidney Injury Advisory Group of the American Society of Nephrology. (2013). World incidence of AKI: A meta-analysis. *Clinical Journal of the American Society of Nephrology, 8*(9), 1482-1493. doi: 10.2215/CJN.00710113

Traub, S.J. (2007). ASA intoxication overview. In B.D. Rose (Ed.), *UpToDate.* Waltham, MA.

United States Renal Data System (USRDS). (2013). *2013 USRDS annual data report. Chapter 6: Acute kidney injury,* 95-106. Retrieved from http://www.usrds.org/2013/pdf/v1_ch6_13.pdf

Velez J.C., & Nietert, P.J. (2011). Therapeutic response to vasoconstrictors in hepatorenal syndrome parallels increase in mean arterial pressure: A pooled analysis of clinical trials. *American Journal of Kidney Diseases, 58*(6), 928-938. doi:10.1053/j.ajkd.2011.07.017

CHAPTER **3**

Hemodialysis in the Acute Care Setting

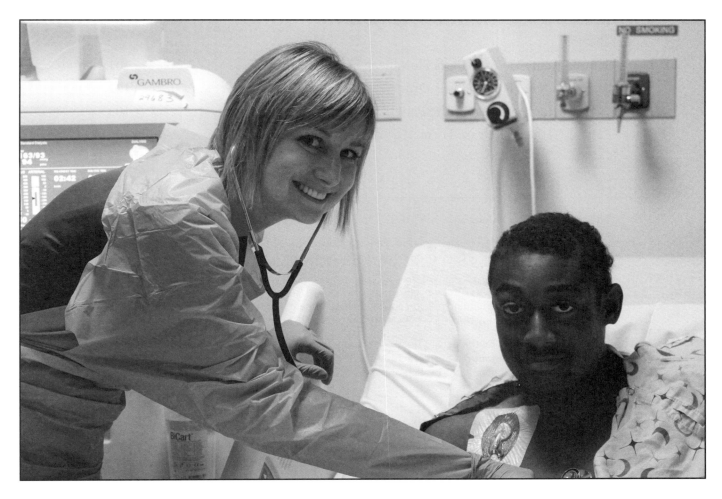

Chapter Editor
Helen F. Williams, MSN, BSN, RN, CNN

Author
Billie Axley, MSN, RN, CNN

CHAPTER **3**

Hemodialysis in the Acute Care Setting

This offering for **1.7 contact hours** is provided by the American Nephrology Nurses' Association (ANNA).

American Nephrology Nurses' Association is accredited as a provider of continuing nursing education by the American Nurses Credentialing Center Commission on Accreditation.

ANNA is a provider approved by the California Board of Registered Nursing, provider number CEP 00910.

This CNE offering meets the continuing nursing education requirements for certification and recertification by the Nephrology Nursing Certification Commission (NNCC).

To be awarded contact hours for this activity, read this chapter in its entirety. Then complete the CNE evaluation found at **www.annanurse.org/corecne** and submit it; or print it, complete it, and mail it in. Contact hours are not awarded until the evaluation for the activity is complete.

Example of reference for Chapter 3 in APA format. One author for entire chapter.

Axley, B. (2015). Hemodialysis in the acute setting. In C.S. Counts (Ed.), *Core curriculum for nephrology nursing: Module 4. Acute kidney injury* (6th ed., pp. 55-106). Pitman, NJ: American Nephrology Nurses' Association.

Interpreted: Chapter author. (Date). Title of chapter. In …

Cover photo by Counts/Morganello

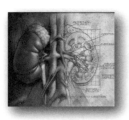

CHAPTER 3

Hemodialysis in the Acute Care Setting

Purpose

The purpose of this chapter is to describe the care of patients undergoing hemodialysis in the acute care setting.

Objectives

Upon completion of this chapter, the learner will be able to:
1. Develop a nephrology nursing care plan for hemodialysis patients in the acute care setting.
2. Discuss pharmaceutical and dialytic interventions for treatment of intradialytic hypotension and other complications experienced by patients in the acute care setting.
3. Describe tools available to the nephrology nurse in the acute setting to evaluate the care needs and patient responses to therapies.

I. Patients who need hemodialysis (HD) in the acute care setting.

A. Patients with acute kidney injury (AKI) with solute or fluid imbalance.

B. Patients with AKI superimposed on chronic kidney disease (CKD) ("acute on chronic") with solute or fluid imbalance.

C. Patients with CKD stage 5/end-stage renal disease (ESRD) in the acute care setting.
  1. Patients with a dialysis access-related event.
  2. Patients with a medical or surgical intervention or complication.
  3. Patients with comorbidity requiring hospital admission.
  4. Patients needing physical or mental rehabilitation.

II. Prehemodialysis patient assessment.

A. The purpose of an acute patient nephrology nursing assessment is to obtain baseline information relative to the patient's physical and/or mental status. This information provides a framework for the nephrology nurse to evaluate the patient for appropriate interventions to achieve an adequate and safe HD treatment.

B. An assessment of the patient must be done prior to initiation of every HD treatment and documented on the treatment record (see Appendix 3.1: Acute Hemodialysis Flowsheet).

C. Medicare guidelines and nursing scope of practice regulations designate a registered nurse as the appropriate professional to perform the following actions.
  1. Complete the prehemodialysis, intrahemodialysis, and posthemodialysis treatment assessment.
  2. Collaboratively formulate a treatment plan.
  3. Delegate care that does not require nursing judgment and ongoing nursing assessment to documented, trained, competent, and supervised unlicensed personnel when appropriate.
  4. Perform and oversee treatment interventions.
  5. Evaluate the patient's response to the HD treatment and interventions.

D. Patient history.
  1. Do not resuscitate (DNR) and advance directive status.
  2. Isolation precautions.
    a. Reason for isolation. Isolation precautions in the healthcare setting include patients with documented or suspected infection or colonization with transmissible, or

"epidemiologically-important organisms," which are defined as readily transmissible, difficult to treat, have a predisposition toward causing outbreaks, or may be associated with a severe outcome (Siegel et al., 2007).

b. Date and source of culture, the organisms cultured, and their sensitivity. Drug-resistant organisms (DROs) and multiple drug-resistant organisms (MDROs) such as methicillin-resistant *Staphylococcus aureus* (MRSA), vancomycin-resistant enterococcus (VRE), vancomycin-resistant *Staphylococcus aureus* (VRSA), extended-spectrum-beta-lactamase-producing gram-negative bacilli (ESBLs), and *Clostridium difficile* require additional precautions to prevent transmission (Siegel et al., 2007).

c. Type of isolation and necessary precautions.
   (1) Standard precautions apply to all patients.
      (a) Standard precautions are based upon the principle that all blood, body fluids, secretions (except sweat), nonintact skin, and mucous membranes may contain transmissible infectious agents (Siegel et al., 2007).
      (b) The Centers for Disease Control and Prevention (CDC) guidelines document for isolation precautions state, "Assume that every person is potentially infected or colonized with an organism that could be transmitted in the healthcare setting…" (Siegel et al., 2007).
   (2) Transmission-based precautions are used when route(s) of transmission are not completely interrupted by use of standard precautions (Siegel et al., 2007).
      (a) Contact precautions are used for patients with known or suspected infection or colonization with epidemiologically important microorganisms that can be spread by direct contact with the patient (direct transmission) and/or the patient's environment (indirect transmission). Resistant-organism precautions are implemented for infections/colonization caused by microorganisms resistant to several antimicrobial agents (MDROs) (Siegel et al., 2007).
      (b) Droplet precautions are intended to prevent transmission of pathogens spread through close respiratory or mucous membrane contact with respiratory secretions (Siegel et al., 2007).
         i. These airborne organisms generated during coughing, sneezing, singing, talking, suctioning, and bronchoscopy do not remain infectious over long distances.
         ii. Droplet precautions are used for droplets that are propelled a short distance (historically defined as 3 feet) in the air and are deposited on a host or in the environment (Park et al., 2004).
         iii. Investigations during the Global SARS outbreaks of 2003 suggest that droplets could reach 6 feet or more from their source.
         iv. The primary transmission method is respiratory droplet spread or by direct contact (e.g., influenza virus, rhinovirus, *N. meningitides*, group A *Streptococcus*) (CDC, 2012).
      (c) Airborne precautions are used to prevent transmission of infectious agents that remain infectious over long distances when suspended in the air (Siegel et al., 2007).
         i. The preferred placement for patients who require airborne precautions is in an airborne infection isolation room (AIIR) (e.g., *M. tuberculosis*, rubeola virus (measles), varicella virus (chickenpox) (Siegel et al., 2007).
         ii. Healthcare personnel caring for patients on airborne precautions wear a mask or respirator, depending upon the disease-specific recommendation that is applied prior to entering the patient's room (CDC, 2012).
         iii. Nonimmune healthcare workers (HCWs) should not care for patients with vaccine-preventable airborne diseases (e.g., measles, chickenpox, smallpox).
      (d) Empiric application of transmission-based precautions is a category of precautions that can be used in addition to standard precautions to call attention to an epidemiologically important organism (Siegel et al., 2007).
         i. Diagnosis of many infections requires laboratory confirmation that depends on culture techniques that often require 2 or more days for completion. Transmission-based precautions must be put into place while test results are pending based upon clinical presentation and likely pathogens.

ii. Isolation precautions implemented at the time a patient arrives at a healthcare facility with symptoms, or at the time a patient develops symptoms and/or signs of transmissible infection, reduces transmission opportunities.

iii. For diseases that have multiple routes of transmission, such as SARS and *Ebola* virus disease (EVD), more than one transmission-based precautions category may be used in combination.

[a] If patient has positive history of travel to an area with an ongoing outbreak of viral hemorrhagic fevers (VHF) (e.g., *Ebola, Lassa, Marburg* viruses), standard, contact, and droplet precautions are recommended (CDC, 2014).

[b] If the patient has other illnesses (e.g., tuberculosis, MDROs, etc.), additional infection control measures will be necessary (CDC, 2014).

(3) Protective environment neutropenic precautions are used when caring for patients with a compromised immune system (Siegel et al., 2007).

(a) Patients with a compromised immune system are at increased risk for numerous types of infections while in the healthcare environment.

(b) A protective environment is designed to protect a patient from infectious organisms that might be carried by people, on surfaces, and/or in the air.

(c) Patients at risk include both patients who have congenital primary immune deficiencies and patients with acquired disease (e.g., treatment-induced immune deficiencies).

3. Reason for admission.
   a. Identifies the specific event or events that brought the patient to the acute care setting.
   b. May be an exacerbation of a chronic condition or a new acute illness.

4. Current problem list.
   a. Current medical diagnosis. Examples of diagnosis of patients requiring renal replacement therapy may include the following.
      (1) CKD stages 1 to 5.
      (2) AKI.
      (3) Diabetes.
      (4) Hypertension.
      (5) Dyslipidemia.
      (6) Anemia.
      (7) Congestive heart failure.
      (8) Diastolic dysfunction.
      (9) Atrial fibrillation.
      (10) Atherosclerosis.
      (11) Systemic lupus erythematosis.
      (12) Cirrhosis.
      (13) Calcific uremic arteriolopathy, also known as calciphylaxsis (Santos et al., 2014).
      (14) Infection.
         (a) Dialysis access-related.
         (b) Diabetic wound/ulcer-related.
         (c) Pneumonia.
         (d) UTI.
         (e) Sepsis (Bagshaw & Bellomo, 2008).
      (15) Rhabdomyolysis (NIH, 2013).
      (16) Drug overdose.
         (a) Acetaminophen (Burns et al., 2014).
         (b) Heroin (Rice et al., 2000).
         (c) Bath salts/synthetic stimulants (McNeeley et al., 2012).
      (17) Trauma (deAbreu et al., 2010).
      (18) Hypovolemia (Himmelfarb et al., 2008).
   b. Recent surgical interventions.
      (1) Type and date of surgery. Examples of surgical procedures occurring for patients with concurrent renal replacement therapy needs would include the following.
         (a) Cardiac surgery-associated acute kidney injury (CSA-AKI) (Mao et al., 2013).
         (b) Coronary artery bypass graft (CABG).
         (c) Heart valve replacement.
         (d) Abdominal aortic aneurysm repair.
         (e) Left ventricular assist device (LVAD), right ventricular assist device (RVAD), or biventricular assist device (BiVAD) (Ochiai et al., 2002; Patel et al., 2012).
         (f) Kidney or other solid organ transplant.
         (g) Dialysis vascular access creation.
         (h) Ultrasound guided or open-kidney biopsy.
         (i) Amputation.
      (2) Intraoperative or postoperative events.
         (a) Length of surgery.
         (b) Hypotensive episode(s).
         (c) Blood loss.
         (d) Relative kidney hypoperfusion (e.g., cross-clamp time).
      (3) Wound healing considerations.
         (a) Minimize systemic anticoagulation.
         (b) Minimize edema.
         (c) Minimize uremic environment.
         (d) Optimize nitrogen balance with adequate nutrition and adequate dialysis.

(4) Ventilation.
    (a) Cough and deep breathe.
    (b) Mobilization at least every 2 hours, even while on renal replacement therapy.
    (c) Optimize fluid balance for good pulmonary function.
(5) Pain control.
c. Recent diagnostic procedures.
    (1) Chest x-ray.
        (a) Presence of pulmonary edema, effusion, and/or congestion.
        (b) Verify line placement.
    (2) Computed tomography (CT), interventional radiology (IR), or magnetic resonance imaging (MRI) scan.
        (a) Placement of tunneled dialysis catheter.
        (b) Dialysis vascular access study.
        (c) Coronary angiogram.
        (d) Other diagnostic studies.
            i. Rule out or define a tumor.
            ii. Define blood vessels anatomically or functionally.
            iii. Observe and define other systemic functions.
        (e) Exposure to contrast agents (see Chapter 2, Acute Kidney Injury).
        (f) FDA warns that gadolinium (MRI contrast agent) exposure is contraindicated in patients with reduced kidney function such as CKD stage 5/ESRD, due to risk of nephrogenic systemic fibrosis (NSF), also known as nephrogenic fibrosing dermopathy (NFD) (CDC, 2007).
    (3) Echocardiogram.
        (a) Heart size.
        (b) Ventricular function.
        (c) Vegetation on heart valves.
        (d) Pericardial effusion.
    (4) Ultrasound.
        (a) Rule out hydronephrosis.
        (b) Vein mapping in preparation for dialysis access placement.
        (c) Guidance for kidney biopsy.
    (5) Colonoscopy.
        (a) Evaluate patient for gastrointestinal bleeding.
        (b) Preventive health following recommended guidelines (CDC, 2013).
5. Medications.
  a. Review allergies with patient/family.
  b. Dose adjustment. Patients with compromised kidney clearance may need to have their medication doses adjusted (Cincotta & Schonder, 2008).

    (1) Medications that have a narrow therapeutic window and are subject to overdosing or underdosing.
    (2) Medications that rely on renal excretion.
  c. Medications that have significant clearance during HD may need administration after treatment or supplemental dosing to adjust for this clearance (Craig, 2008).
  d. Clearance of medications is affected by several factors (Cincotta & Schonder, 2008; Craig, 2008).
    (1) Molecular size.
    (2) Volume of distribution.
    (3) Water solubility.
    (4) Protein binding. If protein binding exceeds 90%, the medication will be minimally cleared with dialysis and does not need supplemental dosing.
  e. Examples.
    (1) Analgesics.
        (a) Narcotic analgesics produce sedation that may be more profound in patients with renal insufficiency.
        (b) The smallest effective dose should be used (Cincotta & Schonder, 2008).
        (c) Medications whose metabolites are normally excreted through the kidneys (e.g., meperidine) may accumulate and decrease the seizure threshold in patients with reduced kidney function. Morphine and codeine have an active metabolite that may accumulate (Cincotta & Schonder, 2008).
    (2) Anticoagulants.
        (a) Drugs used to reduce a patient's risk of clot formation or to prevent a clot that has formed from enlarging (Mayo Clinic, 2013a).
        (b) Anticoagulants inhibit clot formation by blocking the action of clotting factors at different points in the clotting cascade (Mayo Clinic, 2013a).
        (c) Heparin is the most common method of preventing clotting in the HD extracorporeal system (Amato et al., 2008). Heparin-induced thrombocytopenia (platelet count below 150,000) and heparin-dependent IgG antibodies are more commonly associated with the use of unfractionated heparin than with low-molecular–weight heparin (LMWH), such as dalteparin, enoxaprin, nadroparin, reviparin, and tinzaparin. LMWHs have varying pharmacokinetics that will affect their administration for

Table 3.1

Pressors and Their Actions

Pressors	Heart Rate (Chronotropic)	Contractility (Inotropic)	Vasoconstriction
Dopamine	+ +	+ +	+ +
Vasopressin	0	+/ -	+ + +
Neosynephrine	0	0	+ + +
Levophed (Norepi)	+ +	+ +	+ + +
Dobutamine	+	+ + +	- (Dilates)
Epinephrine	+ + +	+ + +	+ +

Source: Dr. Geraldine Corrigan, Western Nephrology Acute Dialysis Medical Director, Denver, Colorado (2005). Used with permission.

hemodialysis (Davenport, 2009; Shen & Winkelmayer, 2012; Warkentin et al., 1995).

(d) Anticoagulants such as warfarin (Coumadin®), dabigatran (Pradaxa®), and rivaroxaban (Xarelto®) are drugs used to prevent clots from forming in medical conditions such as atrial fibrillation, history of deep vein thrombosis (DVT), or pulmonary embolism (PE) (Bristol-Meyers Squibb, 2013; Mayo Clinic, 2013a).

   i. Warfarin requires lab (INR) monitoring, restriction in dietary intake of foods rich in vitamin K, and has potential for multiple medication interactions.

   ii. Patients with mechanical heart valves are generally placed on anticoagulant therapy to prevent valve thrombosis and thromboembolic events (Aurigemma et al., 2014).

(e) Patients may be on more than one form of anticoagulant, such as heparin and warfarin, affecting different points in the clotting cascade (Ogbru, 2014).

(f) Collaborate with nephrologist on anticoagulation for HD. Best practices continue to evolve as new information becomes available from data compiled after a drug gains FDA approval. For example, a study from the University of Pittsburgh in 2010–2011 showed that for those taking dabigatran (Pradaxa®), the risk of major bleeding was especially high among those with chronic kidney disease (Preidt, 2014).

A study by Chan et al. (2015) identified an increased risk of bleeding in patients on hemodialysis using dabigatran (Pradaxa®) and rivaroxaban (Xarelto®).

(3) Antiplatelet agents.

(a) Antiplatelet agents, including aspirin, clopidogrel, dipyramole, or ticlopidine work by inhibiting the production of thromboxane, a chemical that platelets release to signal other platelets to stick together and form a blood clot (Texas Heart Institute, 2013a).

(b) Administration of a combination of antiplatelet agents with different mechanisms of action may provide increased efficacy as compared to aspirin alone for prevention of vascular events (Albers & Amarenco, 2001; American Stroke Association, 2014).

(4) Antihypertensives. Administration of antihypertensive medications should be correlated to minimize hypotensive complications during hemodialysis (Cincotta & Schonder, 2008).

(5) Vasopressors (see Table 3.1).

(a) Type.

(b) Dose and recent titration.

(c) Patients with AKI require careful titration of fluids to maintain sufficient circulating intravascular volume for management of blood pressure and cardiac output; the use of vasoactive medications is done in conjunction with fluid management and hemodynamic monitoring (KDIGO, 2012).

(d) Binding of vasopressor agents to their receptors can be altered by hypoxia or acidosis, muting their clinical effect (Garg et al., 2012; Overgaard & Dzavik, 2008).

(6) Cardiovascular.
   (a) Digoxin (Lanoxin).
      i. Used to treat congestive heart failure (CHF) and atrial arrhythmias (Cincotta & Schonder, 2008; Texas Heart Institute, 2013b).
      ii. Cardiologic effects of digoxin include an increase in the force of myocardial systolic contraction (positive inotropic action) and slowing of the heart rate (negative chronotropic effect) (RxList, 2014).
      iii. In patients with kidney disease, digoxin is initiated at a reduced dose and maintained at a reduced dose (e.g., 0.125 mg every 2 to 3 days).
      iv. As clearance of digoxin correlates with creatinine clearance, patients with kidney impairment require careful titration of dosage based on clinical response and monitoring of serum digoxin concentrations (RxList, 2014).
      v. Digoxin has a narrow therapeutic/ toxic ratio whereby patient-level pharmacokinetics, metabolism, and clearance factors aggregate to introduce variability in the drug responsiveness (Chan et al., 2010).
      vi. Hypokalemia may enhance the toxicity of digoxin; low serum potassium predialysis and/or decline in serum potassium level during dialysis can potentiate digoxin toxicity (Chan et al., 2010).
   (b) Beta blockers.
      i. Used to treat hypertension, CHF, arrhythmias, and angina (Texas Heart Institute, 2012a).
      ii. Reduces the workload on the heart and relaxes blood vessels, resulting in the heart beating slower and with less force (Mayo Clinic, 2013b).
   (c) Calcium channel blockers.
      i. Used to control hypertension, angina, and arrhythmias (Texas Heart Institute, 2012b).
      ii. Relax the muscle of the blood vessels and may slow the heart rate (Mayo Clinic, 2013b).
   (d) Diuretics.
      i. The role of diuretics in optimal fluid management in AKI is complex (Grams et al., 2011).

      ii. Post-AKI diuretic therapy has been shown to have a favorable effect on mortality (Ejaz & Mohandas, 2014).
      iii. Larger doses are associated with more adverse events (e.g., ototoxicity) (NKF, 2002).
      iv. Potassium-sparing diuretics are not typically used in patients with a GFR < 30 mL/min because of the risk for hyperkalemia (Cincotta & Schonder, 2008).

(7) Antimicrobial agents.
   (a) This is a general term for drugs or chemicals that either kill or slow the growth of microbes (i.e., antibiotic agents/bacteria, antiviral agents/ viruses, antifungal agents/fungi, and parasite agents/parasites) (CDC, 2010).
   (b) Dose adjustments to antibiotics are common in patients who are dependent on kidney replacement therapy.
   (c) Therapeutic drug monitoring may be required to achieve a therapeutic drug level for the patient (e.g., vancomycin).
   (d) If significant clearance is expected with intermittent HD, the antimicrobial agent should be administered after dialysis, or a supplemental dose may be provided.

(8) Sedatives or hypnotics.
   (a) Patients with reduced kidney function taking a sedative or hypnotic experience excessive sedation as the most common adverse effect.
   (b) The etiology of somnolence or encephalopathy (e.g., uremic symptoms or oversedation) may be difficult to differentiate.

(9) Neuromuscular blocking agents (NMBA).
   (a) Group of drugs that prevent motor nerve endings from exciting skeletal muscle fibers such as D-tubocurarine and decamethonium (Drugs.com, 2014a).
   (b) Extreme caution should be taken in assessing mental status and respiratory effort on a patient dependent on kidney replacement therapy after NMBA administration due to prolonged half-life in the presence of CKD (Craig & Hunter, 2008).
   (c) Curarization is the induction of muscular relaxation or paralysis by administration of compounds that have the ability to block nerve impulse transmission at the myoneural

junction, the synaptic connection of motor nerve endings to skeletal muscle fiber (Drugs.com, 2014a, 2014c).

    (d) Curarization (usually with tubocurarine) is used to induce muscular relaxation by blocking activity at the myoneural junction.

    (e) Pancuronium should be avoided in patients dependent on kidney replacement therapy because of the potential for a prolonged recurarization effect.

(10) Antihyperglycemic agents.

    (a) Renal metabolism of insulin decreases with declining GFR (NKF, 2012).

    (b) Some oral agents used for the management of blood glucose in diabetes may result in hypoglycemia in patients with reduced kidney function.

    (c) Insulin infusion for blood glucose control in the ICU, ketoacidosis (ADA, 2004).

(11) Antidepressants or selective serotonin-reuptake inhibitors (SSRIs). Side effects may include tremors and changes to gastrointestinal motility, sleep patterns, appetite, and sexual response.

(12) Erythropoiesis stimulating agents (ESA) and iron.

    (a) Maintain outpatient dosing to avoid decrease in Hgb during hospitalzation.

    (b) Dose adjustment may be indicated for inflammatory block related to acute illness (Kalantar-Zadeh et al., 2004).

    (c) Iron repletion is ordered based upon iron, ferritin, and TSAT lab results.

(13) Immunosuppressants.

    (a) Maintain transplanted organ.

    (b) Suppress autoimmune disease activity.

E. Physical assessment.

  1. General assessment.

    a. Perform the physical assessment, documenting findings on the treatment record, and compare them to previous treatment records to determine any changes in patient's clinical status that may require further evaluation and reporting.

    b. Assess patient for changes in energy and overall well-being.

  2. Vital signs.

    a. Blood pressure (BP).

     (1) Noninvasive blood pressure (NIBP).

      (a) The middle of the blood pressure cuff should be level with the patient's right atrium, at the midpoint of the atrium; if the upper arm is below the level of the right atrium, readings will be too high; if the upper arm is above the right atrium, the readings will be too low (AHA, 2005).

      (b) To avoid inaccurate readings taken from an arterial pulsation site other than the brachial artery in the antecubital fossa, ensure the site is supported at the heart level; for example, for patients with arm circumference greater than 50 cm, the cuff is wrapped around the forearm, supported at the heart level, and the radial pulse felt at the wrist (AHA, 2005).

      (c) To measure blood pressure for children, there are various positions of cuff placement and auscultation areas. For example, placing the limb at the level of the heart, place cuff around the upper arm and auscultate at the brachial artery.

       i. If using the lower arm, position the limb at the level of the heart, place the cuff above the wrist, and auscultate the radial artery.

       ii. For measurement using the thigh, place the cuff above the knee and auscultate the popliteal artery.

       iii. To obtain blood pressure on the calf or ankle, place the cuff above the malleoli or at midcalf and auscultate the posterior tibia or dorsal pedal artery (Kyle, 2008).

       iv. For children with elevated measurements, leg blood pressure may be measured by auscultation over the popliteal fossa with the use of a thigh cuff or oversized arm cuff (AHA, 2005).

     (2) Arterial BP (ABP).

      (a) The arterial catheter is inserted into the radial, brachial, or femoral artery and connected to a continuous flush transducer system leveled to heart level (technically the level of the left atrium) and zeroed to atmosphere (McGhee & Bridges, 2002). The transducer is connected via pressure tubing to a pressurized flush system.

      (b) Provides continuous blood pressure monitoring and calculated mean arterial pressure (MAP) reading: MAP = [(2 x diastolic BP) + systolic BP]/3 (GlobalRPh, 2012).

      (c) An arterial line can be used for blood gas analysis or other laboratory test blood specimen sampling. Verify that the pressure line is anticoagulant-free if

test results will be impacted by the presence of an anticoagulant.
- (d) Obtain NIBP readings for comparison to the ABP for accuracy at least once per shift.
- (e) Flush and observe the arterial line waveform to evaluate accuracy of reading.
- (f) Components of normal ABP waveforms and waveform morphology can be found at http://ccn.aacnjournals.org/content/22/2/60.full.pdf+html (McGhee & Brides, 2002).

(3) Obtain both sitting and standing BPs as patient condition permits to observe for orthostatic changes.
- (a) For the immobile patient, prior to any repositioning, ensure repositioning will not compromise the patient's condition.
- (b) If not contraindicated, sitting and standing can be simulated by taking the BP with the head of the bed (HOB) down and then with the HOB elevated at an 80–90-degree angle.
  - i. Keep the patient's head of bed at ≥ 30 degrees for patients with elevated intracranial pressure (ICP) to minimize intracranial pressure.
  - ii. Patients who are ventilator dependent or receiving a tube feeding are at risk for aspiration of secretions or feeding and should not be left in an HOB down position.
- (c) Orthostatic changes are defined as a systolic BP decrease > 20 mmHg, a diastolic decrease > 10 mmHg, or a pulse increase > 20 beats per minute between position changes.
- (d) Orthostatic changes in BP and/or pulse readings taken within 2 minutes of the position change may reflect hypotension and/or vascular disease, which could be volume and/or medication related including beta-blockers, calcium channel blockers, ACE inhibitors, nitrates, and angiotensin II blockers (Cleveland Clinic, 2013).

(4) Elevated diastolic pressures along with other clinical manifestations may indicate right heart failure.

(5) Auscultating the patient's blood pressure may be difficult when a patient is hypotensive, experiencing atrial fibrillation, or has vascular anomalies such

as multiple vascular surgeries. Palpable BPs may be necessary with those patients to estimate systolic pressure.
- (a) To palpate the blood pressure, place a cuff on the upper arm.
- (b) Palpate the brachial pulse or the radial pulse.
- (c) Inflate the cuff until the pulse is no longer felt.
- (d) Slowly deflate the cuff, noting the point at which the pulse is felt again; this is the systolic pressure.
- (e) *Example*: If patient's blood pressure was palpated at 90 mmHg, document "90/P."
- (f) If the patient's arm is too swollen or BP is so low that a pulse cannot be palpated, a Doppler may be used to obtain systolic BP readings and documented as "90/P obtained from Doppler."

b. Temperature.
- (1) Uremic patients often manifest a body temperature < 37°C. Setting the dialysis solution temperature higher than the patient's temperature can cause vasodilation and increase potential for the incidence of hypotension (Pergola et al., 2004).
- (2) Elevated temperature may indicate infection, malignancies, or other illness. Alterations of the febrile response of patients with kidney failure can occur; therefore, fever cannot be relied on for diagnosis of infection in some dialysis patients (Lentino & Leehey, 1994; Lewis, 1992). A rise in temperature above the patient's baseline and according to specific unit guidelines can direct additional assessment.
- (3) Elevated temperature will cause an increase in insensible fluid loss.

3. Fluid balance.
a. Intake and output (I/O).
- (1) Intake.
  - (a) IV infusions.
  - (b) Oral (PO) intake.
  - (c) Gastric tube feeds.
- (2) Output.
  - (a) Urine.
  - (b) Ultrafiltrate removed.
  - (c) Stool.
  - (d) Drains (e.g., chest tube, nasogastric suction, and wounds).
  - (e) Insensible losses related to burns, wounds, ventilation, or temperature elevation.

b. Weight.
  (1) Patients on kidney replacement therapy should be weighed at the same time daily to increase the likelihood of meaningful data.
  (2) Weights performed using a bed scale must be done using standardized linen on the bed at the time of weighting and the bed position.
  (3) Compare daily weight to the prescribed estimated "dry" weight obtained from the outpatient setting records if available, or to the hospital admission weight, for an additional assessment of volume status.

c. Edema.
  (1) May be classified by grading 1 to 4, based on amount of edema (Merck Sharp & Dohme Corporation, 2014). Also see http://wps .prenhall.com/wps/media/objects/2791/28 58109/toolbox/Figure18_24.pdf (Pearson Education, 2007).
    (a) 0 = No pitting.
    (b) 1+ = Trace.
    (c) 2+ = Mild.
    (d) 3+ = Moderate.
    (e) 4+ = Severe
  (2) Assess dependent areas for edema as fluid may shift to this position.
    (a) Sacral for supine patients.
    (b) Legs, feet, and scrotum for sitting or ambulatory patients.
    (c) Facial or periorbital in the prone or reclined patient.
    (d) Facial and upper extremity edema may indicate blockage of venous return from occluded subclavian and jugular veins (Baskin et al., 2009).
  (3) "Pitting" edema is the presence of fluid in tissue that mobilizes with pressure and does not rapidly refill after applied pressure is released.
  (4) "Brawny" (nonpitting) edema presents with dark-colored skin (percutaneous hyperpig-mentation) that appears distended but is resistant to pressure. The skin is so tight due to the excess fluid that the fluid cannot be displaced (Merck Sharp & Dohme Corporation, 2014; Phelps, 1990).
  (5) Anasarca is generalized edema.
  (6) Severe edema with venous stasis may result in skin ulceration and can develop into "eczematous dermatitis" (Phelps, 1990).

d. Ascites.
  (1) Fluid third-spaced in the peritoneal cavity.
  (2) Related to increased portal vein pressure, inflammation, and/or malignancy.
  (3) Ascitic fluid has relatively high protein content, resulting in high oncotic pressure, making it difficult to mobilize fluid into the vasculature for removal with ultrafiltration during HD.

e. Neck vein distention.
  (1) If not contraindicated, have patient sit up to a 45-degree angle.
  (2) Have patient turn head to one side.
  (3) Locate external jugular vein and check for pulsation.
  (4) If vein pulsation ascends higher than 5 centimeters above the manubrium, positive neck vein distention is noted.
  (5) May indicate right heart failure.

f. Skin turgor. Skin tenting indicates intravascular volume depletion.

g. Mucous membranes. Dry mucous membranes indicate volume deficit.

h. Evaluate data from hemodynamic monitoring devices.

i. Review serum sodium levels for indications of hemoconcentration or hemodilution.

4. Dialysis access (see Module 3, Chapter 3, Vascular Access, for further detail on assessment).
  a. Bruit.
  b. Thrill.
  c. Catheter.
    (1) Exit site and dressing.
    (2) Patency of lumens.

5. Skin. Assess for changes in integrity or suppleness.
  a. Dry skin can result from the effect of the uremic state on secretion of oil and accelerate process of skin breakdown.
  b. Patients with diabetes are at risk of development of wounds as a result of the following.
    (1) Decreased blood flow to the peripheral circulation.
    (2) Decreased nerve stimulus to skin for oil production.
    (3) Nerve damage, peripheral neuropathy, can result in numbness or insensitivity to pain or temperature. Assessment and care of skin and pressure points are necessary in preventing injury (NDIC, 2013).
  c. Patients on kidney replacement therapy are at increased risk for calcific uremic arteriolopathy, also known as calciphylaxis.

6. Cardiovascular.
  a. Heart rate.
    (1) Patients with a rate < 50 or > 120 beats/min should be placed on a cardiac monitor during dialysis. Notify the physician/APRN/PA if bradycardia or tachycardia is a new onset.
    (2) Rapid heart rate may be a result of anemia, hypotension, hypovolemia, or atrial fibrillation.

(3) Monitored bradycardia or auscultated heart rate < 50 beats/min may indicate digitalis toxicity or hyperkalemia requiring an adjustment in dialysate potassium to prevent arrhythmias and medication review for other medications, such as beta blockers, that can slow the heart rate (Mohanial et al., 2013; Noble & Isles, 2006).

b. Heart rhythm. Arrhythmias (see Figure 3.1). may be due to:
   (1) Electrolyte and pH changes.
   (2) Heart failure.
   (3) Severe anemia.
   (4) Underlying ischemic and/or hypertensive cardiovascular disease.
   (5) Pericarditis.
   (6) Conduction system calcification.

c. Heart sounds (Heart Sounds, 2014).
   (1) Friction rub indicates the development of pericarditis or may indicate recent myocardial infarction. Report this finding to the nephrologist/APRN/PA prior to heparinizing the patient (University of Washington, n.d.).
   (2) Gallop may indicate myocardial infarction, valvular disease, ventricular hypertrophy, hypertension, cardiomyopathy, volume overload, or ischemia.
   (3) Muffled or distant heart sounds may indicate fluid volume excess. Report to the nephrologist/APRN/PA if this is a new onset.
   (4) Murmurs can be the result of an increase in the rate and velocity of blood flow, abnormal flow across stenosed or incompetent valves, or abnormal passages between chambers (Michigan Heart Sound and Murmur Library, n.d.).
   (5) Muffled or diminished heart sounds during inspiration may indicate pericardial effusion or cardiac tamponade.
       (a) Checking for a paradoxical pulse is indicated with these signs.
       (b) Paradoxical pulse of 10 mmHg or more is considered a hallmark of cardiac compression, pericardial effusion, and/or cardiac tamponade (see Table 3.2).
       (c) Presence of pericardial effusion and cardiac tamponade are medical emergencies.

d. Noninvasive hemodynamic monitoring: bioimpedance or impedance cardiography (ICG).
   (1) Provides hemodynamic monitoring by electrodes that are placed on the neck and lower thorax (see Figure 3.2).

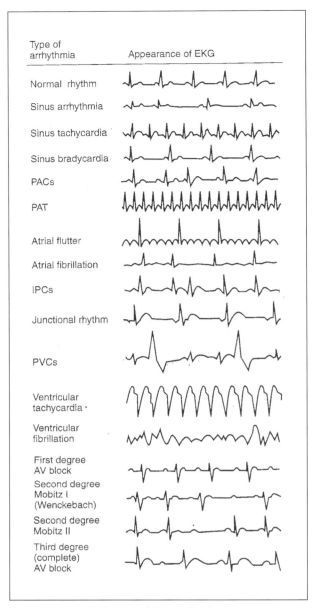

Figure 3.1. Normal EKG and types of arrhythmias.

Source: Monahan, L. (2002). *A practical guide to health assessment.* Philadelphia: W.B. Saunders Company. Used with permission.

   (2) Waveforms are reflective of the volume and velocity of aortic blood flow rather than blood pressure.
   (3) Parameters measured are stroke volume (SV), cardiac output (CO), indices of myocardial contractility, and afterload.

e. Pulmonary artery (PA)/Swan-Ganz catheter (see Figure 3.3).
   (1) Multi-lumen catheter with an inflatable balloon at the tip.
   (2) Provides hemodynamic monitoring.
   (3) Provides information about the left and right heart, differentiation of pressures, structures, and function.

Table 3.2

Measuring Paradoxical Pulse

1. After placing BP cuff on patient, inflate it above the known systolic BP. Instruct patient to breathe normally.

2. While slowly deflating the cuff, auscultate BP.

3. Listen for the Korotkoff's sounds, which will occur during expiration with cardiac tamponade.

4. Note the manometer reading when the first sound occurs, and continue to deflate the cuff slowly until Korotkoff's sounds are audible throughout inspiration and expiration.

5. Record the differences in millimeters of mercury between the first and second sounds. This is the pulsus paradoxus.

Source: Lokhandwala, K.A. (2002). Clinical signs in medicine: Pulsus paradoxus. *Clinical Signs, 48*(1), 46-49. Used with permission.

(4) The ports include proximal port for measuring central venous pressure (CVP)/pulmonary artery pressure (PAP); cardiac output port/thermistor connector; PA distal infusion port, and balloon inflation port (refer to Figure 3.3).

(5) The PA catheter is inserted through central venous approach in the external jugular or subclavian vein into the right side of the heart and into the pulmonary artery (see Figure 3.4).

(6) The PA catheter measures pressures within the right and left sides of the heart through a transducer creating a waveform on the monitor screen (see Figure 3.5).

(7) The PA catheter provides an accurate picture of the patient's fluid volume status through measurements of PAP, including pulmonary artery systolic (PAS) and pulmonary artery diastolic (PAD) (see Figure 3.6), pulmonary artery wedge pressure (PAWP), CO (see Figure 3.7), and CVP (see Table 3.3). These pressure measurements provide information about how the left side of the heart is functioning, including its pumping ability, filling pressures, and vascular volume (see Table 3.4 and Table 3.5).

f. Central venous pressure (CVP) monitoring.

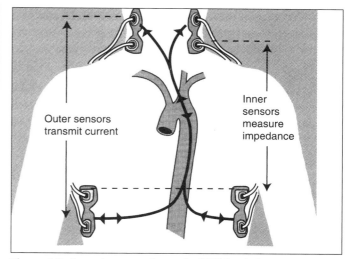

Figure 3.2. Impedance cardiography (ICG) lead placement.

Source: Hodges, R.K., Garrett, K.M., Chernecky, C., & Schumacher, L. (2005). *Real world nursing survival guide: Hemodynamic monitoring,* p. 39. St. Louis: Elsevier Saunders. Used with permission.

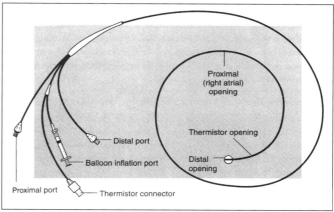

Figure 3.3. Swan-Ganz catheter ports.

Source: Hodges, R.K., Garrett, K.M., Chernecky, C., & Schumacher, L. (2005). *Real world nursing survival guide: Hemodynamic monitoring,* p. 39. St. Louis: Elsevier Saunders. Used with permission.

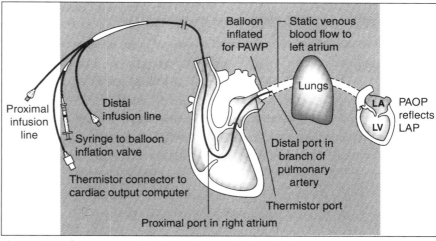

Figure 3.4. Advancement of the Swan-Ganz catheter into the heart.

Source: Hodges, R.K., Garrett, K.M., Chernecky, C., & Schumacher, L. (2005). *Real world nursing survival guide: Hemodynamic monitoring,* p. 115. St. Louis: Elsevier Saunders. Used with permission.

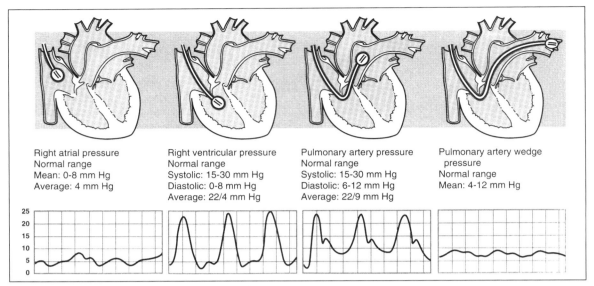

Figure 3.5. Catheter locations and pressure readings.

Source: Hodges, R.K., Garrett, K.M., Chernecky, C., & Schumacher, L. (2005). *Real world nursing survival guide: Hemodynamic monitoring*, p. 31. St. Louis: Elsevier Saunders. Used with permission.

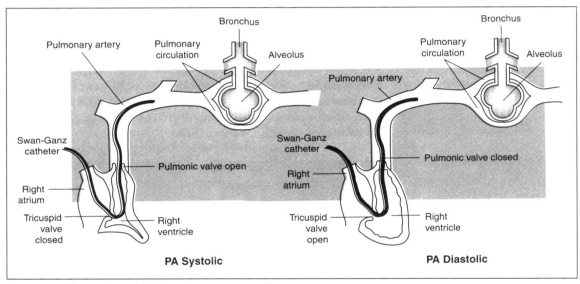

Figure 3.6. PA systolic and PA diastolic pressure readings.

Source: Hodges, R.K., Garrett, K.M., Chernecky, C., & Schumacher, L. (2005). *Real world nursing survival guide: Hemodynamic monitoring*, p. 107. St. Louis: Elsevier Saunders. Used with permission.

(1) Can be measured from a triple lumen catheter or through a PA/Swan-Ganz catheter (refer to Figure 3.6).

(2) Catheters are usually placed in the internal jugular vein (IJ) or subclavian vein.

(3) Measures the pressure of the blood in the central venous circulation returning to the left side of the heart.

(4) Useful data for indication of the patient's intravascular fluid status.

7. Pulmonary.
   a. Oxygenation (see Table 3.6).
      (1) Assess oxygenation by checking oxygenation saturation using spot or continuous pulse oximeter.

      (2) Assess FiO_2 (fraction of inspired oxygen).

      (3) Review patient's arterial blood gas trend and current values.

      (4) Review chest x-ray.

      (5) Assess patient for signs and symptoms of cyanosis.
         (a) Central cyanosis is a blue coloration of the mucous membranes, ears, lips, and nose.
         (b) Peripheral cyanosis is a blue coloration to the upper and lower extremities.

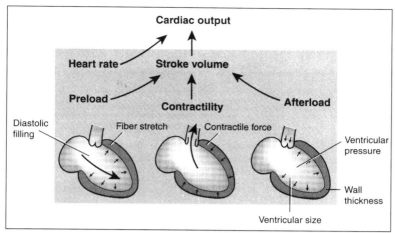

Figure 3.7. Cardiac output.

Source: Hodges, R.K., Garrett, K.M., Chernecky, C., & Schumacher, L. (2005). *Real world nursing survival guide: Hemodynamic monitoring,* p. 22. St. Louis: Elsevier Saunders. Used with permission.

Table 3.3

Hemodynamic Monitoring Definitions

Measurement		Definition	Normal Range
	Preload	Amount of blood filling the ventricle at the end of diastole.	
	Afterload	Amount of resistance against which the ventricle pumps.	
MAP	Mean arterial pressure	The average pressure in the peripheral arterial system during systole and diastole.	80–100 mmHg
PAP	Pulmonary artery pressure	Measurement of right side of heart pressures.	average: 22/9
PAS	Pulmonary artery systolic	Pressure needed to open the pulmonic valve and send blood to the pulmonary circulation.	15–30 mmHg
PAD	Pulmonary artery diastolic	Amount of resistance in the lungs between heartbeats.	6–12 mmHg
CVP/RAP	Central venous pressure/Right atrial pressure	Measurement of pressure from the right atrium. CVP taken from superior or inferior vena cava; RAP from the right atrium.	2–8 mmHg
PAWP PAOP PCWP	Pulmonary artery wedge Pulmonary artery occlusion Pulmonary capillary wedge	An indirect measurement of pulmonary venous pressure. Also reflects left atrial pressure and left ventricular end diastolic pressure. Measurement of preload.	6–12 mmHg
CO	Cardiac output	Amount of blood ejected from the heart in one minute. Determined by heart rate and stroke volume.	4–8 L/min
CI	Cardiac index	Cardiac output that is corrected for body size (body surface area).	2.5–4 L/min
SV	Stroke volume	Volume of blood ejected from the left ventricle during systole. Affected by preload, afterload, and contractility.	60–130 mL
EF	Ejection fraction	The percentage of the total volume in the left ventricle that is ejected during systole. Used as a major indicator of LV function.	60%–75%
SVR	Systemic vascular resistance	The resistance to blood flow within the peripheral blood vessels (arterioles) in the systemic circulation. LV afterload.	800–1200 dynes/sec/cm^{-5}
PVR	Pulmonary vascular resistance	The resistance to blood flow within the pulmonary blood vessels (arterioles) in the pulmonary circulation. RV afterload.	< 250 dynes/sec/cm^{-5}
SaO$_2$	Arterial oxygen saturation	Relationship between the partial pressure of oxygen (PaO$_2$) and how well saturated with O$_2$ the hemoglobin is in the arterial system.	95%–100%
SVO$_2$	Mixed venous oxygen saturation	The amount of O$_2$ in Hgb in venous blood that has returned to the RV and the PA. Helps determine balance between oxygen supply and demand in the body.	60%–80%

Adapted from Hodges, R.K., Garrett, K.M., Chernecky, C., & Schumacher, L. (2005). *Real world nursing survival guide: Hemodynamic monitoring.* St. Louis: Elsevier Saunders. Used with permission.

Table 3.4

Typical Hemodynamic Profiles in Various Acute Conditions

Condition	HR	MAP	CO/CI	CVP/RAP	PAP/PAWP	Notes
Left ventricular failure	↑	↓	↓	↑	↑	
Pulmonary edema (cardiogenic)	↑	N,↓	↓	↑	↑ PAWP > 25 mmHg	
Massive pulmonary embolism	↑	↓,V	↓	↑	↑ PAD > PAWP by > 5 mmHg	↑ PVR
Acute ventricular septal defect	↑	↓	↓	↑	↑ giant "v" wave on PAWP trace	O₂ step up noted in SvO₂
Acute mitral valve regurgitation	↑	↓	↓	↑	↑ giant "v" wave on PAWP trace	No O₂ step up noted in SvO₂
Cardiac tamponade	↑	↓	↓	↑	↑ CVP, PAD & PAW equalized	↓ RVEDVI
Right ventricular failure	↑,V	↓,V	↓	↑	PAP ↑ PAWP N,↓	↑ RVEDVI
Hypovolemic shock	↑	↓	↓	↓	↓	↑ O₂ extraction ↑ SVR
Cardiogenic shock	↑	↓	↓	↑	↑	↑ O₂ extraction ↑ SVR
Septic shock	↑	↓	↑,↓	↓,↑	↓,↑	SVR changes, ↓ O₂ extraction ↓ SVR

Key: ↑ = increased, ↓ = decreased, N = normal, V = varies

Nail bed coloration can provide an assessment of peripheral cyanosis.
b. Respiratory rate, rhythm, and pattern.
   (1) Respiratory distress/failure can develop from any condition that increases the work of breathing and/or decreases the respiratory drive (see Table 3.7).
   (2) Respiratory distress may respond to ultrafiltration of fluid with dialysis depending on the etiology.
   (3) When the lungs cannot adequately maintain tissue oxygenation or eliminate carbon dioxide, acute respiratory arrest and cardiac arrest can result.
   (4) If respiratory rate is elevated > 30 breaths per minute and the oxygen saturation is < 90%, the patient is in severe distress and immediate intervention is necessary.
   (5) Note labored respirations and use of accessory muscles.
   (6) Check equal expansion of the chest bilaterally.
c. Breath sounds.
   (1) Rales (crackles): sounds like the crinkling of cellophane.
      (a) Causes include sudden opening of alveoli in the presence of fluid, and air passing through small airways in the presence of fluid, mucus, or pus.
      (b) Consider pulmonary edema with evaluation of fluid intake and output.
   (2) Rhonchi (gurgles/sonorous wheeze): deep-rumbling sounds heard during exhalation.
      (a) May be caused by passage of air through narrowed airway.

Table 3.5 — How Selected Drugs Affect Cardiac Pressures and Function

Drug	Actions	Dose Range	HR	MAP	CO	PAWP (preload)	SVR (afterload)	PVR	Notes
Amrinone (Inocor®)	Phosphodiecrease inhibitor with strong vasodilation properties	IV loading dose: 0.75 mg/kg over 3–5 min followed by a continuous infusion of 5–10 mcg/kg/min. The bolus may be repeated in 30 minutes if required. The total daily dose should not exceed 10 mcg/kg.	O/↑	O/↑	↑	↓	↓	↓	ACLS Guideline state requires hemodynamic monitoring.
Atropine Sulfate	Antiarrythmic, which directly blocks vagal effects on SA node	0.5 to 1 mg IV push. Repeat every 3–5 minutes. Maximum dose 0.03 to 0.04 mg/kg.	↑	↑	↑	O	O	O	
Digoxin	Cardiatonic glycoside. Increases conductance by promoting extracellular calcium to move to intracellular cytoplasm. Inhibits adenosine triphosphatase. Decrease conductivity through AV mode.	Loading dose 0.5 to 1 mg IV or in divided doses PO over 14 hours. Maintenance dose 0.125 to 0.5 mg IV or PO daily 0.25 mg.	O/↓	O/↑	↑	O/↓	O	O	
Dobutamine	Directly stimulates beta 1 receptors. Moderate stimulation of beta 2 receptors. Minimal stimulation of alpha receptors.	5–15 mcg/kg/min	O/↑	↑	↑	↓	↓	↓	Potential for arrythmias and ↑O2 consumption
Dopamine	Dopaminergic effects: Renal, mesenteric vasodilation. Beta effects: Increased inotrophism Alpha effects: Vasoconstriction	0.5–3 mcg/kg/min 5.0–10 mcg/kg/min > 10.0 mcg/kg/min	↑	↑	↑	↓	↑	O	Potential for arrythmias, ↑O2 consumption, peripheral ischemia
Epinephrine	Low doses = Beta effect High doses = Alpha effect	0.005–0.02 mcg/kg/min 1 mg or > IV push; 1–4 mcg/min infusion	↑	↑	↑	↑	↑	↑	Potential for arrythmias and ↑O2 consumption, peripheral ischemia
Esmolol	Beta blocker	Loading dose 0.5 mg/kg over 1 minute followed by infusion titrate to desired effect range 50–300 mcg/kg/min	↓	↓	O/↓	O/↑	↑	↑	
Phenylephrine (Neo-synephrine®)	Alpha stimulator	0.10–0.18 mg/min until BP stable, then 0.04 0.06 mg/min	O	↓			↑	↑	peripheral ischemia
Nitroglycerin	Vasodilator with stronger effects on peripheral venous bed and coronary arteries than peripheral arterial bed	Start infusion @ 10 mcg/min and increase in increments of 10 mcg/min as needed to achieve desired effect	O	↓	O/↑	↓	↓	↓	HA & hypotension
Norepinephrine (Levophed®)	Low doses = Beta stimulation High doses = Alpha stimulation	Start at 0.05–0.01 mcg/kg/min and titrate up to 2.0–4.0 mcg/kg/min	↑	↑	↑	↑	↑	↑	peripheral ischemia
Morphine	Dilate pulmonary vascular system					↓	↑		
Furosemide (Lasix®)	Diuresis					↓	↓		

Alpha 1 receptors, vasoconstrict arterioles and coronary arteries
Beta 1 receptors, increase contractility, of myocardial cells and increase conductivity to SA /AV Nodes
Beta 2 receptors, vasodilation of coronary arterioles and bronchodilation of bronchioles
Dopamine 1 and Dopamine 2 receptors vasoconstrict and vasodilate

Source: Lichtenthal, P.R. (1998). *Quick guide to cardiopulmonary care.* Irvine, CA: Edwards Lifesciences. Used with permission.

Key   ↓ = decrease   ↑ = increase   O = unknown

Table 3.6

Oxygen Guideline for Estimating FiO$_2$ (varies with rate and depth of ventilation)

Method of Delivery	Oxygen Flow Rate	Estimated FIO$_2$ (fractionated inhaled oxygenation)
Nasal cannula • Oxygen delivery is extremely variable depending on tidal volume and ventilator pattern	1 L/min 2 L/min 3 L/min 4 L/min 5 L/min	24% 28% 32% 36% 40%
Simple mask • Need minimal flow of 5 L/min to flush out CO$_2$ • Oxygen delivery varies with changes in tidal volume, ventilator pattern, inspiratory flow rate, and whether the mask is loose or tight fitting	5–10 L/min	35% to 50%
Partial nonrebreathing mask • Mask with reservoir bag, still considered a low flow oxygen delivery system • Reservoir bag must not collapse during inspiration and must remain at least one third to one half full on inspiration	6–10 L/min	40% to 70%
Nonrebreathing mask • Is similar to the partial rebreathing mask except it has a one-way valve between the bag and the mask to prevent exhaled air from returning to the bag • Ideal method of delivering high O$_2$ concentration for short-term purposes	Minimum of 10 L/min	60% to 80%

Source: Kallstrom, T.J. (2002). American Association of Respiratory Care clinical practice guideline: Oxygen therapy for adults in the acute care facility 2002 revision & update. *Respiratory Care, 47*(6), 717-720. Used with permission.

(b) Consider asthma and bronchitis, and accumulation of secretions.
(3) Wheezes (sibilant): high-pitched musical sounds heard during exhalation.
  (a) May be caused by passage of air through narrowed airways.
  (b) Consider asthma and bronchitis.
(4) Pleural friction rub: a dry, crackling, grating, low-pitched sound heard during inspiration or exhalation.
  (a) Caused by inflamed pleural surfaces rubbing against one another.
  (b) May indicate pleurisy.
(5) Absent or diminished sounds.
  (a) Indicates presence of fluid or pus in the lung fields, muscular weakness, or splinting from pain.
  (b) If unilateral, consider mucus plug, or hemo/pneumothorax that is spontaneous or may correspond to central line placement.

(6) Mediastinal crepitus.
  (a) Indicates air in the pericardium, mediastinum, or both.
  (b) Often associated with pericardial friction rub.
8. Gastrointestinal.
  a. Presence of bowel sounds.
  b. Include stool in output.
  c. Hold anticoagulation for suspected GI bleed.
9. Genitourinary.
  a. Primary etiology of AKI or CKD.
  b. Avoid nephrotoxins (see Chapter 2, Acute Kidney Injury).
10. Endocrine: presence of diabetes and stability of serum glucose.
  a. Evaluation by HgbA1C lab value.
  b. Systemic insulin in the ICU.
    (1) Hyperglycemia; diabetic ketoacidosis.
    (2) Clearance during HD.
    (3) Considerations for dosing during HD.
    (4) Monitoring during HD.

Table 3.7

Etiology of Respiratory Distress and Failure

Pulmonary	Extrapulmonary
Acute respiratory distress syndrome (ARDS)	Acidosis
Airway obstruction	Anesthesia
Aspiration	Brain or spinal cord injury
Asthma	Cardiopulmonary bypass
Bronchitis	Disseminated intravascular coagulation (DIC)
Chronic obstructive pulmonary disease (COPD)	Drug overdose
Cystic fibrosis (CF)	Multiple sclerosis
Inhalation injury	Muscular dystrophy
Pneumonia	Myasthenia gravis
Pneumo/hemothorax	Neuromuscular blocking agents
Pulmonary emboli	Sepsis
Pulmonary edema	Severe obesity
Oxygen toxicity	Sleep apnea
Lung cancer	Shock
Radiation	Systemic inflammatory response syndrome (SIRS)
Surgical resection	Transfustion related acute lung injury (TRALI)

Courtesy of Maureen Craig, University of California Davis Medical Center, Sacramento, CA. Used with permission.

11. Neurologic.
  a. Level of consciousness/mental status.
    (1) Altered concentration.
    (2) Change in alertness.
    (3) Change in orientation to person, place, or time.
  b. Identify risk factors for patients on HD.
    (1) Disequilibrium syndrome (DDS).
    (2) Intracranial bleed and anticoagulation.
  c. Brain injury.
    (1) Intracranial pressure (ICP) monitoring.
    (2) ICP can be monitored from a burr hole through the skull via a small catheter inserted into the white matter.
      (a) Licox® monitor can also provide a reading of brain tissue oxygenation and brain temperature in addition to the ICP reading.
      (b) Ventriculostomy catheter can drain the excess spinal fluid in addition to providing an ICP reading. Consider effects of fluid removal on ICP and brain oxygenation results.
    (3) When dialyzing a patient with ICP monitoring.
      (a) Anticoagulation should not be used due to the risk of bleeding.
      (b) Precautions should be taken to prevent further brain swelling or DDS.

F. Laboratory assessment.
  1. Blood chemistry (see III. G: Dialysis solution, for further discussion of electrolytes present in dialysis solution and their physiologic importance).
    a. Sodium. Normal serum sodium is 136 to 146 mEq/L.
      (1) Low serum sodium may indicate excess fluid; dilutional value.
      (2) Elevated serum sodium may correlate with hypertension.
    b. Potassium. Normal serum potassium is 3.5 to 5 mEq/L. Elevated serum potassium may be related to diet, medications, blood transfusions, or inadequate dialysis treatment.
    c. Serum CO_2. Normal CO_2 is 24 to 32mEq/L and reflects acid/base balance. Serum carbon dioxide should be evaluated along with an arterial blood gas (ABG) to determine respiratory or metabolic acid base disturbances.
    d. Blood urea nitrogen (BUN).
      (1) The BUN is elevated in patients needing kidney replacement therapy.
      (2) A low predialysis serum level may indicate malnutrition.
      (3) BUN will increase with a GI bleed or steroid administration.
      (4) BUN is used to assess treatment adequacy

using either the urea reduction ratio (URR) or the Kt/V urea.

(5) Solutes that are easily cleared from the plasma water during a hemodialysis treatment may rebound after the treatment ends. Urea is often the marker used to assess this rebound effect.

e. Creatinine.
   (1) Creatinine is a waste product from muscle cell metabolism.
   (2) Creatinine is used to determine creatinine clearance and estimate the patient's GFR when the patient's kidney function is stable.
   (3) Creatinine levels are impacted by dialysis treatments and changing kidney function, so assessing trends in creatinine levels in light of these events is more meaningful than a single creatinine level.

f. Glucose. Normal range is 65 to 100 mg/dL.
   (1) Glucose levels may be altered in patients with diabetes.
   (2) Hypoglycemic episodes during HD may occur based upon timing of the patient taking diabetes-related medication in relation to the timing of food intake. Presence of dextrose (100 mg/dL) in the dialysate may not prevent hypoglycemia from occurring during or after HD.

g. Albumin. Normal range is 4 to 5.2 g/dL.
   (1) Low albumin levels are associated with inflammation and/or inadequate dietary protein intake.
   (2) Hypoalbuminemia is associated with increased morbidity and mortality in chronic HD patients.

h. Calcium. Normal range is 8.4 to 10 mg/dL.
   (1) Phosphorus binders may be a significant source of calcium intake.
   (2) Patients with excess calcium may be at increased risk for vascular calcifications and associated coronary events.
   (3) Calcium functions on a reciprocal basis with phosphorus.
   (4) Patients dependent on HD may experience calcium reabsorption from bone related to a state of chronic metabolic acidosis and experience loss of bone density.

i. Phosphorus levels. Normal range is 2.6 to 4.2 mg/L.
   (1) Phosphorus dietary intake is typically limited to 600 to 1200 mg/day. However, phosphorus is found in many foods, especially processed foods, dairy products, and drinks (including colas), and therefore can be a challenge for the patient to avoid.
   (2) Phosphorus binders are often prescribed to facilitate phosphorus excretion through the GI tract.

j. Calcium phosphorus product (mg/dL) = calcium x phosphorus.
   (1) The calcium/phosphorus product should be < 55 mg/dL.
   (2) A higher product can lead to the deposition of calcium phosphate crystals in the body (e.g., heart valves, lungs, joints, soft tissue, and skin).

k. Magnesium levels. Normal range is 1.8 to 2.3 mg/dL. Patients dependent on hemodialysis should avoid magnesium-containing laxatives or antacids.

l. Lipoproteins.
   (1) Cholesterol. Normal is < 150 mg/dL and elevated cholesterol may increase a patient's risk for coronary events. Total cholesterol is a combination of the following.
      (a) LDL – level below 100 mg/dL.
      (b) HDL – level above 60 mg/dL.
   (2) Triglycerides. Normal is < 150 mg/dL. Elevated triglycerides may increase a patient's risk for vascular related events.

m. Transaminase. Normal level is 8 to 40 U/L. Elevated transaminase levels may indicate liver injury or possible hepatitis.

n. Ferritin. Normal range is 9 to 200 ng/mL. Ferritin reflects the patient's iron stores.
   (1) Low levels reflect iron deficiency.
   (2) Elevated levels result from frequent blood transfusions.
   (3) Infection/inflammation can result in elevated levels of ferritin (Kalantar-Zadeh et al., 2004; Kell & Pretorius, 2014).
   (4) Further information regarding ferritin can be found at http://pubs.rsc.org/en/content/articlelanding/2014/mt/c3mt00347g#!divAbstract

o. Iron. Normal range is 40 to 175 µ/dL. Measure the amount of iron in the blood serum that is being carried by transferrin in the blood plasma.
   (1) Iron losses occur over time from red blood cell losses with the process of HD and lab draws, and bleeding from vascular access stick sites.
   (2) Patients with kidney failure are at risk for GI bleeding due to elevated level of urea.
   (3) Gastrointestinal bleeding pathogenesis is unclear. Contributing factors may include the effects of uremia on the gastrointestinal mucosa, the effects of uremia on platelet adhesiveness, and the effect of heparinization during dialysis (Shirazian & Radhakrishnan, 2010).

p. Total iron-binding capacity (TIBC).

(1) Normal level is 225 to 410 μ/dL.
(2) Measures the amount of iron that the blood would carry if the transferrin were fully saturated.

q. Transferrin saturation (%) (TSAT) measures the percentage of transferrin that is bound to iron.
   (1) Calculation: Divide the serum iron level by the TIBC.
   (2) If the TSAT is less than 20%, the patient is iron deficient and may benefit from iron repletion.

2. Hematology.
   a. White blood cell (WBC) count. Normal 4,500 to 10,000/mm^3.
      (1) Suspect infection if WBC count is elevated.
      (2) WBCs in the patient with kidney failure have decreased ability to respond to infection due to less effective phagocytosis. Phagocytosis is the process used by WBCs of engulfing and ingesting particles (e.g., bacteria) and dead cell debris (Biology Online, 2008).
   b. Hemoglobin (Hgb) and hematocrit (Hct) related to anemia.
      (1) Hgb level for transfusion is determined by the physician evaluating the state of the patient for signs and symptoms of anemia (NKF, 2007).
      (2) It is beneficial to administer the packed red blood cells (PRBC) during HD to remove the excess volume and potassium.
      (3) Potassium content in PRBCs increases as the unit of blood approaches its expiration date due to cell lysis (Malament et al., 1975). When blood is stored, intracellular potassium slowly leaks from the red blood cells into the extracellular solution which carries the packed RBCs. This results in transfusion of a solution containing increased extracellular potassium along with the infusion of the packed RBCs which could be hazardous for a patient who is already hyperkalemic (Olson et al., 2013).
   c. Platelet count. Normal range is 150,000 to 350,000/μL of blood (George, 2011).
      (1) Platelet count is related to clotting ability. Platelets have the ability to adhere to subendothelial tissue and subsequent aggregation, attracting other clotting factors such as fibrin to form clots (George, 2011).
      (2) Decrease in platelet count > 50% from baseline (prior to heparin exposure) may indicate heparin-induced thrombocytopenia (HIT).

(a) Antibodies are specific for heparin bound to platelet factor 4.
(b) Platelet activation increases the risk of thrombosis while paradoxically increasing the risk for bleeding from the decreasing platelet count.

3. Coagulation.
   a. Prothrombin time (PT), partial thromboplastin time (PTT), and international normalized ratio (INR) are used to evaluate coagulation.
   b. D-dimer is used to evaluate for disseminated intravascular coagulation (DIC) or deep vein thrombosis (DVT).
   c. Heparin-induced thrombocytopenia (HIT) antibody is used to assess for safe heparin exposure. When HIT is suspected clinically, all formulations of heparin, including heparin flushes for catheters, are discontinued (Ahmed et al., 2007). Studies have suggested alternative locking solutions to include sodium citrate 4% (Grudzinski et al., 2007; Lok et al., 2006) and tissue plasminogen activator (Firwana et al., 2011).
   d. Transfusion of blood products that treat bleeding disorders.
      (1) Fresh-frozen plasma (FFP) can be administered during HD, allowing for removal of fluid volume.
      (2) Platelets may be administered during or after HD, as specified by nephrologist/APRN/PA.
      (3) Infused platelets may be captured in the dialyzer if given during HD. Anticoagulation needs to be evaluated and adjusted per provider order as platelet counts change.
      (4) If ordered to be given during HD, administer platelets using an infusion pump via venous chamber during the last 30 minutes of treatment.
         (a) An intravenous (IV) infusion pump that is administering an infusion into the venous chamber may need its pressure parameters adjusted to administer the infusion against a positive pressure in the venous chamber.
         (b) The positive pressure present in the venous chamber is typically higher than that in a vein. An infusion pump may interpret this higher positive pressure inaccurately as a downstream occlusion.

4. Other possible laboratory data for analysis.
   a. Digoxin.
      (1) Provide guidance for adjustment of potassium in dialysate.

(2) Evaluate the patient's adherence to taking digoxin as prescribed.

b. Therapeutic antibiotic levels. Determine re-dosing prescriptions.

(1) Collection of lab for trough (lowest concentration in the patient's bloodstream) and peak levels (highest concentration of a drug in the patient's bloodstream) is used to evaluate the appropriate dosage levels of many drugs.

(2) Optimal time to draw samples can be found looking at guidelines for the drug and procedures of the institution.

c. Beta-type natriuretic peptide (BNP) levels during congestive heart failure episodes.

III. The HD treatment plan.

A. In the acute setting, the dialysis prescription by the nephrologist/APRN/PA will vary according to the patient's clinical presentation and lab results.

1. The role of the acute dialysis nurse is unique and requires experience and critical thinking skills.

2. This role is autonomous, yet consultative, with communication of patient information as needed by the nephrology nurse and intermittent onsite contact with the nephrologist/APRN/PA.

3. The treatment plan is determined by an accurate patient assessment, application of treatment protocols, and collaboration with the nephrologist.

4. See Appendix 3.2: Acute Hemodialysis Order Form.

B. Dialysis adequacy.

1. The effectiveness of the dialysis treatment is dependent on the session length, the blood flow rate, and the dialysis solution flow rate.

2. In the acute setting, dialysis adequacy is complicated by the following.

a. Increased use of venous catheters for dialysis access that may deliver a substantially lower blood flow rate.

b. Increased recirculation in venous catheters, especially those placed in the femoral vein.

c. Decreased treatment time due to intradialytic patient complications.

d. Increased sequestration of urea in muscles due to use of vasopressors, resulting in decreased blood flow to muscles and skin.

e. Interruptions to the prescribed dialysis treatment plan.

(1) The patient's primary reason for hospitalization with its subsequent procedures, therapies, surgeries, and tests may take precedence over a single planned hemodialysis treatment.

(2) It is the duty of the nephrologist and the acute care nephrology team to assess the patient's kidney replacement therapy needs and to provide adequate dialysis.

C. Dialysis disequilibrium syndrome (DDS).

1. Etiology. DDS is a set of neurologic and systemic symptoms related to an acute increase in brain water content.

a. DDS is most likely to occur when a patient is first dialyzed, or has missed dialysis treatment, or at a time when the dialysis treatment aggressively lowers solutes in the patient's plasma.

b. Occurs when blood urea nitrogen (BUN) values are very high > 175 mg/dL.

c. When plasma solute levels are rapidly lowered during a dialysis treatment, the solute concentration in brain cells and cerebral spinal fluid is much higher than that of plasma due to the difference in permeability of the blood-brain barrier. Water shifts from plasma into the brain tissue causing cerebral edema.

d. Acute changes in pH of the cerebral spinal fluid during hemodialysis are caused by a more rapid diffusion of carbon dioxide than bicarbonate across the blood/brain barrier.

e. Patients who are very young, elderly, small body size, or who have primary CNS disease (seizure disorders, stroke, brain aneurysms) are more susceptible to DDS.

f. Patients on chronic HDs who are under-dialyzed are also susceptible due to elevated BUN.

2. Review predialysis labs and patient history to identify those at risk for DSS.

3. Support the osmolality of the blood during dialysis.

a. Urea, sodium, and glucose are all important osmolar molecules.

b. Each represents an important role (see Table 3.8).

4. The use of prophylactic anticonvulsants in patients predisposed to seizures should be considered until uremia is controlled.

5. Signs and symptoms (see Table 3.9).

a. Headache.

b. Nausea and vomiting.

c. Restlessness.

d. Hypertension.

e. Increased pulse pressure.

f. Decreased sensorium.

g. Convulsions.

h. Coma.

6. Prevention (see Table 3.10).

a. Short, inefficient dialysis treatments with slow solute removal.

Table 3.8

Osmolar Molecule Table

Urea	Na⁺	Glucose
Depending on the body weight of the patient, only a 30% reduction in plasma urea nitrogen is desired on the initial treatment. Low blood flow rates (BFR) 150–250 mL/min or a BFR that is about three times the body weight in kg is recommended and gradually increased with consecutive treatment. Shortened length of treatment (2 hours) is recommended (and gradually increased with consecutive treatment).	A dialysate sodium level of at least 140 mEq per L helps maintain serum osmolality during hemodialysis. Use of sodium gradient dialysis with dialysate sodium level > 145 mEq/L reduces incidence of DDS. In patients who are already hypernatremic, it is safer to set the dialysate sodium level to a value close to the patients plasma sodium level, not lower. In these cases, sodium modeling may not be appropriate.	A dialysate solution that contains at least 200 mg/dL of dextrose should be used.

Courtesy of DCI Acute Program, Omaha, Nebraska. Used with permission.

(1) Small dialyzer.
(2) Slow dialysate flow rate.
(3) Slow blood flow rate.
  b. Administration of a suitable osmotic agent, such as mannitol, to counteract the rapid fall in plasma osmolality that occurs with clearance of BUN molecules from the blood plasma.
7. When DDS occurs, the hemodialysis treatment may need to be terminated, or at the very least efficiency of diffusion reduced.
8. After the initial HD session, the patient should be reevaluated.
  a. Patient is usually dialyzed again the following day.
  b. Gradually increase the length of treatment and the BFR over a series of treatments.
  c. Dialysate flow rates are slowly raised toward 500 to 800 mL/min as prescribed by the nephrologist/APRN/PA.
9. If a longer dialysis session is required for purposes of fluid removal, isolated ultrafiltration (UF or PUF) can be performed in which dialysate flow bypasses the dialyzer resulting in a decreased effect on osmolality.

D. The prescription for time on dialysis is based upon evaluation of the patient's clinical presentation and may range from short sessions for patients at risk for DDS to longer sessions such as with drug overdose situations or a patient's response to ultrafiltration rates.

E. Determining dialysate flow rates (DFR).
  1. Generally, for acute HD, the DFR is 500 to 600 mL/min.
  2. The rate may be higher for the hypercatabolic patient if DDS is not a risk.

3. With the advancement in technology, some dialysis machines have the capability of automatically adjusting the DFR to 1.5 times the BFR for efficiency of treatment.

F. Dialyzer.
  1. Biocompatible synthetic membranes obtain the best patient outcomes in the acute setting.
  2. Copolymer of polyacrylonitrile and sodium methallyl sulfonate membranes have caused an

Table 3.9

DDS Signs and Symptoms

Mild To Early Disequilibrium
Nausea/vomiting
Blurred vision
Restlessness
Headache
Hypertension
Increased pulse pressure
Muscle cramps
Dizziness not related to BP
Asterixis

Severe Disequilibrium
Confusion
Disorientation
Muscle twitching/tremors
Seizures
Arrhythmias
Coma (improved within 24 hours)
Death

Courtesy of DCI Acute Program, Omaha, Nebraska. Used with permission.

Table 3.10

Sample DDS Prevention Protocol

Treatment Day 1

1. The prescribed BFR for the 1st treatment is calculated by taking the patient's approximate dry weight multiplied by 3 = _____ mL/min.
   Examples:
   50 kg patient x 3 = 150 mL/min BFR
   70 kg patient x 3 = 210 mL/min BFR
   90 kg patient x 3 = 270 mL/min BFR, not to exceed 300 mL/min

2. Treatment time: 2 hours

3. DFR = 500 mL/min

4. Heparin free until BUN < 100 mg/dL
   Tight low total heparin if BUN ≤ 100 mg/dL

5. Hyperosmolar agents to prevent DDS
   a. 25% mannitol, 6.5 to 12.5 g mannitol administered IVP hourly; do not administer last 30 minutes of treatment. Mannitol will be used on all patients with preexisting seizure conditions, and patients exhibiting mild or moderate to severe CNS symptoms from dialysis disequilibrium.
   b. Exponential sodium modeling of 150

6. Weight loss according to fluid assessment

Treatment Day 2

1. If BUN > 100 mg/dL predialysis, use the same protocol as 1st treatment except increase treatment time to 2.5 hours.

2. If BUN < 100 mg/dL, increase BFR by 50 mL/min from last treatment.

3. DFR = 500 mL/min

4. Heparin free until BUN < 100 mg/dL
   Tight low total heparin if BUN ≤ 100 mg/dL

5. Hyperosmolar agents to prevent DDS
   a. 25% Mannitol, 6.5 to 12.5 g mannitol administered IVP hourly, do not administer last 30 minutes of treatment. Mannitol will be used on all patients with preexisting seizure conditions, and patients exhibiting mild or moderate to severe CNS symptoms from dialysis disequilibrium.
   b. Exponential sodium modeling of 150

6. F160 NR dialyzer or equivalent _____.

7. Weight loss according to fluid assessment.

Treatment Day 3

1. 3-hour treatment

2. DFR = 500 mL/min

3. Maximum BFR as tolerates

4. Tight low total heparin

5. Sodium modeling as indicated

6. F160 NR dialyzer or equivalent _____.

7. Weight loss according to fluid assessment.
   If BUN is still > 100 mg/dL on day 3, access is functioning adequately and/or patient is in a catabolic state, call nephrologist for treatment order clarification. If access is a potential problem associated with clearance, notify nephrologist.

Adapted from Creighton Nephrology, Creighton University, Omaha, Nebraska. Used with permission.

increased risk of anaphylactic reactions in patients taking angiotensin-converting enzyme (ACE) inhibitors and should be avoided in this group of patients.

3. Prepare the dialyzer for use by first rinsing with normal saline following manufacturer's recommendations to remove residual sterilant and other manufacturing materials.

4. Dialyzer membrane reaction.
   a. Signs and symptoms.
      (1) Dyspnea.
      (2) Feeling of warmth at the exit site or throughout the body.
      (3) Sense of impending doom.
      (4) Chest pain.
      (5) Back pain.
      (6) Anaphylaxis.
      (7) Cardiac arrest.
      (8) Death.
   b. Treatment.
      (1) Stop dialysis treatment without returning the patient's blood.
      (2) Provide supplemental oxygen to the patient.
      (3) Monitor patient's vital signs. Notify nephrologist/APRN/PA of the reaction and results of patient assessment.
      (4) Treatment of anaphylaxis follows hospital protocols, generally with IV antihistamines (diphenhydramine), steroids, and epinephrine until patient stabilizes.

5. Refer to Module 3, Chapter 2, Hemodialysis, for information on various dialyzer filters and membrane types, sizes, and specific attributes.

G. Dialysis solution.
   1. Dialysis solution composition should be tailored according to the patient's clinical presentation and laboratory values according to the nephrologist/APRN/PA's orders.
   2. "Standard" dialysate composition prescribed for outpatient HD may not be appropriate in an acute care setting while the patient is experiencing an acute illness.
   3. Plasma bicarbonate levels are normally 24 mEq/L.
      a. In the absence of kidney function, patients may present with metabolic acidosis, as the generated acids are not excreted.
      b. These acids may be buffered by available bicarbonate in the blood and the patient will then present with a lower bicarbonate level.
      c. Bicarbonate in the dialysate diffuses to the patient's blood during a dialysis treatment when the dialysis solution bicarbonate concentration is higher than the bicarbonate concentration in the patient's plasma.
      d. The dialysis solution bicarbonate concentration is selected in collaboration with the nephrologist/APRN/PA to achieve the desired changes in the patient's plasma bicarbonate level.

4. Dialysis solution sodium.
   a. The normal range for serum sodium is 135 to 145 mEq/L.
   b. Sodium and water are closely related in the body. The normal range of serum sodium reflects the relationship between sodium and volume status.
   c. To learn the definitions and signs and symptoms of hyponatremia and hypernatremia clinical presentations, see the following tables.
      Table 3.11. Hyponatremia and Hypovolemic/Hyponatremia.
      Table 3.12. Hypervolemic/Hyponatremia.
      Table 3.13. Isovolemic/Hyponatremia.
      Table 3.14. Hypernatremia.
      Table 3.15. Hypervolemic/Hypernatremia.
      Table 3.16. Hypovolemic/Hypernatremia.
   d. Sodium correction with hemodialysis.
      (1) The goal is to achieve an euvolemic status and normal body sodium at the end of the dialysis treatment.
      (2) This can be achieved by using osmotic agents, ultrafiltration, and a dialysis solution with the desired sodium content.
      (3) Review serum sodium levels predialysis.
      (4) Assess patient for volume overload or volume depletion.
         (a) Assess the patient's fluid balance to determine if sodium imbalance is due to hemodilution or hemoconcentration.
         (b) If predialysis serum sodium levels are < 130 mEq/L, it is dangerous to achieve normonatremia quickly (Simon et al., 2014; Wendland & Kaplan, 2012).
            i. Rapid correction may cause osmotic demyelination syndrome (ODS) Wendland & Kaplan, 2012), characterized clinically by an acute progressive dysarthria, dysphagia, or weakness progressing to quadriplegia, and alterations of consciousness.
            ii. Patients at greatest risk of the syndrome include those with chronic alcoholism, malnutrition, prolonged diuretic use, liver failure, extensive burns, or a history of an organ transplant.
         (c) If predialysis serum sodium levels are > 145 mEq/L, it is dangerous to attempt to correct hypernatremia by

Table 3.11

Hyponatremia and Hypovolemic/Hyponatremia

Electrolyte Imbalance	Cause	Signs and Symptoms
Hyponatremia Serum sodium level < 135 mEq. Critically low levels may be < 125 mEq.	1) Sodium deficiency in relation to body water; body fluids are diluted and cells swell from decreased extracellular fluid osmolality.	1) Signs and symptoms vary depending on how quickly the sodium level drops. If the level drops quickly, the patient will be more symptomatic.
Hypovolemic/hyponatremia	1) Is defined as deficits of both total body water and sodium, but sodium loss is greater than water loss (true hyponatremia). 　a) Renal Causes 　　i) Osmotic diuresis 　　ii) Salt-losing nephrites 　　iii) Adrenal insufficiency 　　iv) Diuretic use (primarily thiazides) 　b) Nonrenal causes 　　i) Vomiting 　　ii) Diuresis 　　iii) GI fistulas 　　iv) Gastric suctioning 　　v) Excessive sweating 　　vi) Cystic fibrosis 　　vii) Burns 　　viii) Wound drainage	1) Signs and symptoms include: 　a) Apprehension 　b) Dizziness 　c) Postural hypotension 　d) Cold, clammy skin 　e) Decreased skin turgor 　f) Tachycardia 　g) Oliguria 　h) Decreased CVP, PAP, PAW 　i) Elevated HCT

Courtesy of DCI Acute Program, Omaha, Nebraska. Used with permission.

Table 3.12

Hypervolemic/Hyponatremia

Electrolyte Imbalance	Cause	Signs and Symptoms
Hypervolemic/Hyponatremia	1) Both water and sodium levels increase in the extracellular area, but the water gain is more impressive. Serum sodium levels are diluted. 　a) Heart failure 　b) Liver failure 　c) Nephrotic syndrome 　d) Excessive administration of hypotonic IV fluids 　e) Hypoaldosteronism 　f) Severe hyperglycemia in diabetic dialysis patients. For every increase of 100 mg/dL in serum glucose, there is a corresponding initial decrease of 1.3 mEq/L in the serum sodium concentration due to osmotic shift of water from the intercellular to the extracellular compartment. Because osmotic diuresis does not occur, the excess plasma water is not excreted. Insulin administration reverses the water shift and corrects the hyponatremia.	1) Signs and symptoms include: 　a) Disorientation 　b) Muscle twitching 　c) Nausea/vomiting 　d) Abdominal cramps 　e) Headache 　f) Seizures 　g) Edema 　h) Hypertension 　i) Weight gain 　j) Rapid bounding pulse 　k) CVP and PAP elevated

Courtesy of DCI Acute Program, Omaha, Nebraska. Used with permission.

Table 3.13

Isovolemic/Hyponatremia

Electrolyte Imbalance	Cause	Signs and Symptoms

Isovolemic/Hyponatremia	1) Extracellular fluid is equal to intracellular fluid volume.
	  a) Glucocorticoid deficiency (inadequate fluid filtration by the kidneys)
	  b) Hypothyroidism (limited water excretion)
	  c) Kidney failure
	  d) Syndrome of inappropriate antidiuretic hormone (SIADH) secretion
	    i) Concerns especially of duodenum, pancreas and oat-cell (small-cell) carcinoma of the lung
	    ii) CNS disorders, trauma, tumors, and stroke
	    iii) Pulmonary disorder, tumors, asthma, and COPD
	    iv) Medications, oral antidiabetic drugs, chemotherapeutic drugs, psychoactive drugs, diuretics, synthetic hormones, and barbituates
		1) No physical signs and symptoms of volume excess.

Courtesy of DCI Acute Program, Omaha, Nebraska. Used with permission.

Table 3.14

Hypernatremia

Electrolyte Imbalance	Cause	Signs and Symptoms
Hypernatremia Serum sodium level > 145 mEq/L	An excess of sodium relative to body water occurs when there is an increase in sodium or loss of free water. Can occur with decreased, normal, or increased body water.	Body fluids become hypertonic; more concentrated fluid moves by osmosis from inside the cell to outside the cell to balance the concentration in the two compartments. As fluid leaves them, the cells become dehydrated, especially those of the CNS. Patients may show signs of fluid overload from increased extracellular fluid volume in the blood vessels. Symptoms are more severe if high sodium level develops rapidly instead of over time. Neurologic symptoms include: 1) Restlessness/agitation 2) Weakness 3) Lethargy 4) Stupor 5) Confusion 6) Seizures/coma 7) Neuromuscular irritability (twitching) 8) Low grade fever/flushed skin

Courtesy of DCI Acute Program, Omaha, Nebraska. Used with permission.

Table 3.15

Hypervolemic/Hypernatremia

Electrolyte Imbalance	Cause	Signs and Symptoms

Hypervolemic/Hypernatremia	1) Excessive sodium gain
	2) Food and medication (kayexalate)
	3) Excessive IV administration of sodium solutions (sodium bicarbonate, hypertonic saline solutions)
	4) Excessive adrenocortical hormones
	   a) Cushing's syndrome
	   b) Hyperaldosteronism
		1) Signs and symptoms include:
		   a) Increased BP
		   b) Bounding pulse
		   c) Dyspnea

Courtesy of DCI Acute Program, Omaha, Nebraska. Used with permission.

Table 3.16

Hypovolemic/Hypernatremia

Electrolyte Imbalance	Cause	Signs and Symptoms

Hypovolemic/Hypernatremia	1) Loss of a small amount of sodium and a large amount of water, with a greater emphasis on loss of body water.
	   a) Impaired thirst regulation (hypothalamic disorders)
	   b) People who can't drink voluntarily (infants, confused elderly, immobile or unconscious patients)
	   c) Fever, heat stroke
	   d) Pulmonary infections/hyperventilation
	   e) Excessive burns
	   f) Diarrhea/GI losses
	   g) Hyperglycemia/osmotic diuresis
		1) Signs and symptoms include:
		   a) Dry mucous membranes
		   b) Oliguria
		   c) Orthostatic hypotension

Courtesy of DCI Acute Program, Omaha, Nebraska. Used with permission.

dialyzing against a low-sodium dialysis solution.
- i. May cause cerebral edema, hypotension, and muscle cramping.
- ii. In this case, the dialysate sodium level should be set close (within 5 mEq/L) to that of the pretreatment plasma level.
5. Dialysis solution potassium.
   - a. Potassium is the major cation (positive charge) in the intracellular fluid and plays a critical role in many metabolic cell functions. Normal range for a serum potassium is 3.5 to 5 mEq/L.
     - (1) Only 2% of the body's potassium is found in the extracellular fluid.
     - (2) 98% is in the intracelluluar fluid.
     - (3) Small, untreated alterations in serum potassium levels can seriously affect

neuromuscular and cardiac functioning.
   - b. Normal kidney function is needed to maintain the potassium balance.
     - (1) 80% of the daily excretion of potassium is done by the kidneys.
     - (2) 20% is lost via the bowel and sweat glands.
   - c. The sodium/potassium pump is an active transport mechanism that moves ions across the cell membrane against a concentration gradient. The pump moves sodium from the cell into the extracellular fluid and maintains high intracellular potassium levels by pumping potassium into the cell.
   - d. Magnesium helps sodium and potassium ions move across the cell membrane, affecting sodium and potassium levels both inside and outside the cell.
   - e. A change in pH may affect serum potassium

levels because hydrogen ions move into the cells and push potassium into the extracellular fluid.

(1) Acidosis and/or hyperglycemia can cause hyperkalemia as potassium moves out of the cell to maintain balance (ADA, 2014).

(2) Alkalosis and/or insulin can lower serum potassium levels as potassium moves into the cell to maintain balance.

(3) To learn the potential causes and signs and symptoms of hypokalemia and hyperkalemia, see Tables 3.17 and 3.18.

f. Potassium imbalance is corrected with HD to achieve a serum potassium level within safe range of 3.5 mEq/L to 5.0 mEq/L.

(1) Hypokalemia.

(a) Review serum potassium levels predialysis to determine the correction needed.

(b) Assess patient for clinical evidence of hypokalemia.

(2) Hyperkalemia.

(a) Review serum potassium levels predialysis to determine the severity of the hyperkalemia and how much correction is needed.

(b) Make sure the results are current and accurate.

(c) A hemolyzed lab sample will cause a false high serum potassium level.

(d) Mild hyperkalemia.

i. Patients with some kidney function may be treated with a loop diuretic to increase potassium removal by the kidneys.

ii. Educate patient and restrict PO and IV potassium intake.

iii. Screen medications and nutritional supplements for potassium.

iv. Treat underlying disorders leading to the high potassium: hyperglycemia, hypomagnesemia, and acidosis.

(e) Moderate to severe symptomatic hyperkalemia usually requires HD. While arrangements for HD are being made, the patient may need to be treated medically.

i. Assess cardiac rhythm changes associated with potassium (see Figure 3.8).

ii. Kayexalate 30 grams in 50 mL of sorbitol by mouth or 50 grams of Kayexalate without sorbitol if given as a retention enema, as sorbitol can cause intestinal necrosis if given as an enema.

[a] Onset 1 to 2 hours with duration of action 4 to 6 hours.

[b] As the medication coats the intestines, sodium moves across the bowel wall into the blood and potassium moves out of the blood into the intestines.

[c] Loose stools remove potassium from the body.

[d] Monitor for development of congestive heart failure due to sodium retention.

iii. 10% calcium gluconate (10 mL IV over 3 min). *Note*: This is not a treatment for hyperkalemia; it is only used to protect the myocardium from the effects of hyperkalemia. Calcium antagonizes the effects of hyperkalemia at the cellular level by shifting the threshold potential to a less negative value, returning myocyte excitability back to normal, increasing the electrochemical gradient across the myocyte, and reversing the myocyte depression seen with severe hyperkalemia (Noble, 2006; Parkham et al., 2006).

[a] Onset is 1 to 3 minutes and the effects last 1 to 3 hours.

[b] AVOID if digitalis toxicity is suspected, since calcium and digitalis have similar effects on the heart and can result in undesired bradycardia, even to the point of cardiac arrest.

iv. Sodium bicarbonate 50 mEq IV over 5 min: Effects last 1 to 3 hours.

[a] Decreases serum potassium level by temporarily shifting potassium into the cells in a patient with acidosis. Treatment with medications such as insulin, glucose, and sodium bicarbonate are temporizing measures that move potassium into cells, while definitive loss of excess potassium must be achieved with cation exchange resins, dialysis, or by increasing renal excretion (Lederer, Alsauskas, Mackelaite, et al., 2014).

[b] This is a hypertonic solution and may exacerbate fluid overload and hypernatremia.

[c] Bicarbonate administration is no longer indicated once dialysis is

Table 3.17

Hyperkalemia Imbalances

Electrolyte	Cause	Signs and Symptoms

Hyperkalemia Serum potassium level rises above 5.5 mEq/L	1) Pseudohyperkalemia
	  a) Hemolysis
	  b) Improper phlebotomy techniques
	    i) Prolonged tight tourniquet prior to lab draw
	    ii) Fist clenching and unclenching prior to drawing specimen may increasing serum K^+ levels by as much as 2.5 mEq/L
	    iii) Use of small gauge needle or finger sticks to obtain blood sample
	  c) Thrombocytosis (chemotherapy)
	  d) Leukocytosis (chemotherapy)
	2) Decreased renal excretion – acute or chronic oliguric renal failure
	  a) Decreased renal perfusion (CHF, sepsis)
	  b) Adrenal insufficiency (hypoaldosteronism/Addison's)
	  c) HIV
	  d) Drugs: ACE inhibitor/angiotension receptor blockers, heparin, cyclosporine and K^+ sparing diuretics
	3) Transcellular shift (intracellular to extracellular)
	  a) Metabolic acidosis (moves K^+ out of the cells as hydrogen ions shift into the cell). For each 0.1 decrease in pH typically there is an increase in K^+ of 0.5–0.8 mEq/L.
	  b) Drugs: beta blockers, angiotension receptor blockers, succinylcholine, digitalis (in large doses poisons the NA^{++}/K^+ ATPase pump resulting in K^+ release from the cells)
	  c) Tissue destruction: rhabdomyolysis, crush injuries, lungs, severe infections
	  d) Tumor lysis, hemolysis
	  e) Cardiac surgery
	  f) Diabetes – insulin deficiency (elevated blood sugar causes K^+ to rise)
	4) Factors due to increased intake
	  a) PRBC transfusions close to expiration date
	  b) Oral supplement, salt substitutes, IV potassium, tube feedings
	  c) GI bleeding related to gut reabsorption of hemolyzed RBCs
		1) Muscle weakness is usually the first sign, spreads from the legs to the trunk eventually involving the respiratory muscles. Paralysis seen with serum $K^+ > 8.0$, patients often report falling due to leg weakness
		2) Smooth muscle hyperactivity causing nausea, cramps, and diarrhea
		3) Paresthesias of face, tongue, feet, and hands (stimulation of pain receptors)
		4) EKG changes occur in the following progression as K^+ rises (see Figure 3.8, EKG changes with hypo/hyperkalemia)
		  a) Tall, peaked t-wave
		  b) Prolonged P-R internal (greater than 2.0 sec.)
		  c) Loss of P wave
		  d) Slight widening of QRS complex
		  e) Very wide QRS complex
		  f) Bradycardia
		  g) Sine wave pattern (QRS complex merges with T-wave)
		  h) Ventricular fibrillation or standstill

Courtesy of DCI Acute Program, Omaha, Nebraska. Used with permission.

initiated, as hemodialysis provides bicarbonate to the patient via diffusion from the dialysate to the blood.
  v. Beta2 adrenergic agonist-nebulized albuterol 10 mg (Parham et al., 2006).
    [a] Onset in 30 minutes with a duration of 2 to 4 hours.
    [b] This option moves potassium intracellularly but does not reduce total body potassium.
  g. Dialysis solution potassium may affect the stability of a HD treatment.

(1) Obtain the most recent serum potassium level.
(2) Use a serum potassium level drawn just prior to dialysis if changes are suspected.
(3) Dialysis solution potassium concentrations are prescribed to correct potassium imbalance at a safe rate while avoiding patient complications of hyperkalemia or hypokalemia.
(4) For patients having the serum potassium level drawn by the dialysis nurse, collaborate with the nephrologist/APRN/PA regarding initiating treatment with a 2K^+

Table 3.18

Hypokalemia Imbalances

Electrolyte	Cause	Signs and Symptoms

Hypokalemia Serum potassium level < 3.5 mEq/L	1) Gastrointestinal losses
	 a) Diarrhea
	 b) Prolonged gastric suctioning/vomiting
	 c) Secretory tumors (villous adenoma)
	 d) Intestinal drainage (fistulas, surgical drains)
	 e) Recent ileostomy
	2) Renal losses: not uncommon in patients with nonoliguric acute kidney failure
	 a) Drugs: diuretics, high dose corticosteroids, insulin, high dose penicillins, drugs causing hypomagnesemia (amphotericin B, aminoglycosides, cisplatin), beta agonists (including pressors and broncho dilators such as albuterol), and insulin overdose
	 b) Magnesium depletion (magnesium is needed for sodium and potassium ions to cross the cell membrane)
	  i) See drugs causing hypomagnesemia
	  ii) Hyperalimentation (causes hypomagnesemia due to shifting of magnesium into cells during anabolism)
	 c) Renal tubular acidosis
	 d) Cushing's syndrome
	 e) Increased GFR (osmotic diuresis with hyperglycemia, newly functioning transplanted kidney)
	3) Severe diaphoresis
	4) Poor dietary intake (anorexia, alcoholism, debilitation)
	5) Transcellular shift (extracellular to intracellular)
	 a) Alkalosis (potassium moves into the cell as hydrogen ions move out)
	 b) Elevated beta-adrenergic activity related to stress, coronary ischemia, or delerium tremens
	 c) Drugs (Beta agonists and insulin overdose)
	 d) Hypothermia
	 e) Hyperalimentation
		Hypokalemia: symptoms are rare if serum K^+ is > 3.0 mEq/L
		1) Skeletal muscle weakness, especially in the legs
		2) Paresthesia, leg cramps, restless legs, and decreased or absent deep tendon reflexes
		3) Ascending paralysis with respiratory compromise
		4) Rarely, prolonged hypokalemia can cause rhabdomyolysis, a condition where there is breakdown of muscle fibers leading to myoglobin in the urine, eventually leading to hyperkalemia
		5) Anorexia, nausea and vomiting, decreased bowel sounds, constipation, and/or ileus
		6) Cardiac problems
		 a) Weak, irregular pulse
		 b) Orthostatic hypotension
		 c) EKG changes
		  i) Flattened T-wave
		  ii) Depressed ST segment
		  iii) Enlarging U-wave superimposed on T wave to give appearance of prolonged Q-T
		  iv) Increased potential for bradycardic response to digitalis glycoside toxicity, as potassium is needed to balance the level of digoxin in the blood and cells
		  v) Cardiac arrest
		  vi) Frequent PVCs unresponsive to lidocaine
		  vii) Tachyarrhythmias if patient is volume depleted
		 d) Worsens the effects of digoxin toxicity, as potassium is needed to balance the level of digoxin in the blood

Courtesy of DCI Acute Program, Omaha, Nebraska. Used with permission.

or 3K$^+$ dialysate and adjust the dialysate if required when the serum level is available.

(5) Increased ectopy during a treatment may be resolved by increasing the potassium in the bath.

h. When determining the potassium dialysate bath to be used during acute HD, consider the following options: two potassium dialysate protocols are provided (see Tables 3.19 and 3.20).

6. Dialysis solution calcium.

a. Calcium is a positively charged cation found in both the extracellular fluid and the intracellular fluid.

(1) The normal range for the total serum calcium is 8.4 to 10.0 mg/dL.

(2) 99% of all calcium is concentrated in the skeletal system (OSU, 2014). Calcium, along with phosphorus, is responsible for bone and teeth formation.

(3) Only 1% of all calcium is found in the serum and soft tissue (OSU, 2014).

(4) Nearly half of all serum calcium is bound to albumin. Changes in serum albumin correlate with changes in serum calcium (see Figure 3.9).

(a) Evaluate the patient's albumin and calcium level together.

(b) Calculate the corrected calcium. (Pharmacology Weekly, 2014). Corrected calcium (mg/dL) = measured total calcium (mg/dL) + 0.8(4 – serum albumin [g/dL]), where 4.0 represents the average albumin level.

(c) Example: Serum calcium of 9 (mg/dL), albumin of 3 (g/dL).

(d) 9(mg/dL)+ 0.8(4-3[g/dL]) = 9.8 (mg/dL) corrected calcium level.

(5) Ionized calcium is the physiologically active form of calcium (4.65 to 5.25 mg/dL), most directly influencing physiologic functioning of nerves and muscles (Crawford & Harris, 2012). The range of ionized calcium reference values vary between male/female and age (Mayo Clinic, 2014), and its interpretation is in conjunction with the total serum calcium measurement (Goldberg, 2012). Several systemic functions are dependent on ionized calcium levels.

(a) Cell membrane permeability and nerve impulse transmission.

(b) Contraction of skeletal, smooth, and cardiac muscle.

(c) Blood clot formation.

b. Calcium is absorbed in the small intestine and excreted in the urine and feces. Several factors influence calcium levels in the body.

(1) Serum pH has an inverse relationship with the ionized calcium level.

(a) If the serum pH rises (the blood becomes alkaline), more calcium binds with protein and the ionized calcium level drops.

(b) Conversely, when pH falls (acidosis), less calcium binds with protein, raising the ionized calcium level (Crawford & Harris, 2012).

(c) The patient with alkalosis is usually hypocalcemic, and the

Table 3.19

Potassium Dialysate Protocol – Option A

Standard Dialysate Bath Adjustments	
Serum potassium	**Dialysate potassium**
> 5.0 mEq/L	2.0 mEq/L
4.0–5.0 mEq/L	3.0 mEq/L
3.5–3.9 mEq/L	3.5 mEq/L
< 3.5 mEq/L	4.0 mEq/L
Notify nephrologist of serum K+ < 3.5 mEq/L	
Consider higher than usual bath for patients at high risk for arrhythmias, cardiomyopathy, s/p CABG, metabolic acidosis anticipated to be corrected by dialysis, or other cardiac compromise.	

Source: Courtesy of Dr. Geraldine Corrigan, Medical Director. Western Nephrology Acute Dialysis, Denver, Colorado. Used with permission.

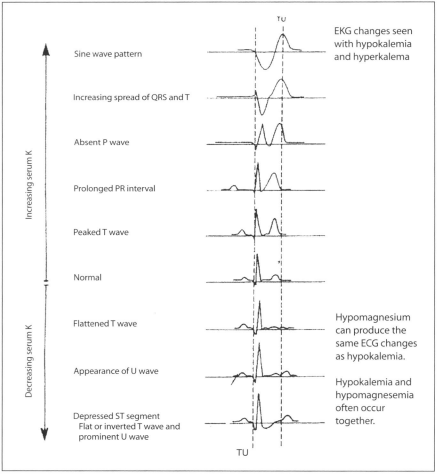

Figure 3.8. EKG changes with hypo/hyperkalemia.
Courtesy of DCI Acute Program, Omaha, Nebraska. Used with permission.

Table 3.20

Potassium Dialysate Protocol – Option B

Potassium dialysate bath considerations play an important role in achieving the goal of safe and effective hemodialysis treatment stability for the acutely ill patient with AKI.

1. The K^+ bath should be collaboratively verified with the orders of the nephrologist/APRN/PA on the following patients:
   a. Patients with impaired kidney function receiving digitalis medications, who are exhibiting signs and symptoms of digitalis toxicity.
   b. Patients with kidney failure ordered to receive blood transfusions.
   c. Patients with kidney failure ordered to receive isolative UF on a routine dialysis day.
   d. Patients with impaired kidney function presenting with hyperglycemia and hyperkalemia.
   e. Patients with impaired kidney function recently experiencing a cardiac condition or cardiac surgery.

2. If serum K^+ is < 4.0 mEq/L, use $4K^+$ mEq/L dialysate bath.

3. If serum K^+ is 4.1 to 4.5 mEq/L, use $3K^+$ mEq/L dialysate bath.

4. If serum K^+ is 4.6 to 5.5 mEq/L, use $2K^+$ mEq/L dialysate bath.

5. If serum K^+ is 5.6 to 6.5 mEq/L, use $1K^+$ mEq/L dialysate bath.

6. If serum K^+ is > 6.5 mEq/L, obtain direct K^+ bath orders from nephrologist/APRN/PA.
   a. In patients exhibiting cardiac arrhythmias, draw a serum K+ level at baseline and hourly. Monitor patient closely for arrhythmias, refer to Table 3.15: EKG changes related to high or low potassium.
   b. A 0 K^+ bath is always contraindicated. The steep gradient between the serum potassium and the dialysis solution potassium may result in additional arrhythmias.
   c. Reducing the gradient between the serum potassium and the dialysis solution potassium will reduce this risk of arrhythmia (e.g., for a serum potassium of 10 mEq/L, select a dialysis potassium of 2 mEq/L). The dialysis treatment may need to be lengthened to achieve the desired removal of potassium from the patient.
   d. The potassium content in the dialysis solution may also be stair-stepped down each hour to achieve the final desired serum potassium for the patient.

7. The potassium (K^+) dialysate protocol Option B listed, is a guideline only and does not replace communication with the ordering nephrologists, critical nursing assessment, and evaluation of the patient with AKI or kidney failure.

Source: Creighton Nephrology, Creighton University, Omaha, Nebraska. Used with permission.

patient with acidosis is usually hypercalcemic.
   (2) For the definition, etiology, signs, and symptoms of hypocalcemia and hypercalcemia, see Table 3.21 and Table 3.22. Assess the patient for clinical evidence of hypocalcemia if total calcium level is < 8.7 mg/dL or ionized calcium is < 1.1 mmol/L.
   c. Calcium is present in dialysis solution to prevent precipitous loss of calcium during treatment and resulting hypocalcemia.
   (1) KDOQI guidelines recommend that in patients receiving calcium-based phosphate binders, the dialysate calcium concentration should be targeted to physiologic levels of 2.5 mEq/L. In patients not receiving calcium-containing phosphate binders, the dialysate calcium should be targeted to 2.5 to 3.0 mEq/L based on serum calcium levels and the need for therapy with active vitamin D sterols (NKF, 2005).
   (2) The dialysis solution calcium directly affects the serum-ionized calcium during a hemodialysis treatment.
      (a) A dialysis solution calcium level of 2.5 mEq/L is equivalent to a 1.25 mmol/L.
      (b) The normal range for serum-ionized calcium is 1.2–1.4 mmol/L.
   (3) Some authorities do not support using a dialysate solution containing 2.5 mEq/L of calcium in the critically ill patient. Changes in ionized calcium levels have a pivotal role

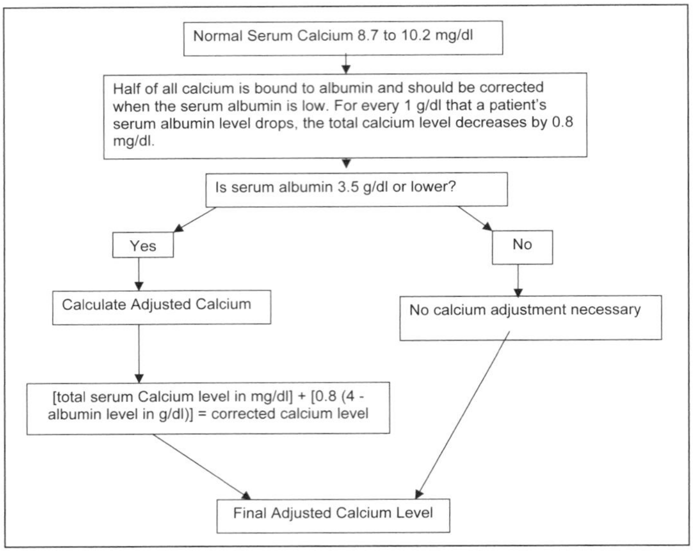

Figure 3.9. Calcium's relationship to albumin.

Courtesy of DCI Acute Program, Omaha, Nebraska. Algorithm compiled from: Springhouse Corporation. (1997). *Fluid and electrolytes made incredibly easy* (p. 135). Philadelphia: Lippincott, Williams & Wilkins. Used with permission.

Table 3.21

Hypocalcemic Imbalances

Electrolyte	Cause	Signs and Symptoms

Hypocalcemia Serum calcium levels drop below 8.7 mg/dL	1) Decreased intake or absorption
	  a) Insufficient dietary intake
	  b) Protein malnutrition (decreased albumin)
	  c) Alcoholism
	  d) Hypoparathyroidism/parathyroidectomy
	  e) Radical neck surgery
	  f) Hypomagnesemia (PTH is magnesium dependent)
	  g) Acute & chronic renal failure (the kidney is unable to activate vitamin D)
	  h) Liver disease
	  i) Steroids/Cushings
	  j) Sepsis
	  k) Anticonvulsants (phenobarb and dilantin interfere with calcium absorption)
	2) Increased excretion
	  a) Diuretics
	  b) Chronic diarrhea
	  c) High phosphorus levels
	  d) Diuretic phase of AKI
	  e) Pancreatic insufficiency/acute pancreatitis cause malabsorption of calcium
	  f) Burns (distressed tissues trap calcium ions from extracellular fluid)
	3) Increased calcium binding
	  a) Citrate containing blood products
	  b) Alkalosis (causes increased protein bonding)
	  c) Drugs
	    i) Anticonvulsants (phenytoin and phenobarbital)
	    ii) Calcitonin
	    iii) Drugs that lower serum magnesium levels (cisplatin & gentamycin)
	    iv) Edetate disodium (disodium EDTA)
	    v) Loop diuretics
	    vi) Mithramycin
		1) Neurologic
		  a) Anxiety
		  b) Confusion
		  c) Irritability
		  d) Seizures (usually generalized)
		2) Neuromuscular
		  a) Paresthesia of the toes, fingers, or face (especially around the mouth)
		  b) Twitching/tremors
		  c) Muscle cramps (laryngeal & abdominal muscles are particularly prone to spasm)
		  d) Tetany (positive Trousseau or Chvostek's signs)
		  e) Hyperactive deep tendon reflexes
		3) Cardiac response
		  a) Diminished response to digoxin
		  b) Decreased cardiac output
		  c) Prolonged ST segment
		  d) Lengthened QT interval (risk for ventricular tachycardia)
		  e) Hypotension

Courtesy of DCI Acute Program, Omaha, Nebraska. Used with permission.

Table 3.22

Hypercalcemic Imbalances

Electrolyte	Cause	Signs and Symptoms

Hypercalcemia Adjusted serum calcium levels above 10.2 mg/dL	1) Increased calcium intake
	  a) Excessive intake of supplement or calcium antacids
	2) Increased absorption
	  a) Low phosphorus levels
	  b) Vitamin A & D overdose/toxicity
	3) Increased mobilization of calcium from bone
	  a) Hyperparathyroidism
	  b) Malignancy (especially breast, lung, lymphoma, multiple myeloma) causes bone destruction
	  c) Multiple fractures
	  d) Prolonged immobilization
	4) Decreased calcium excretion
	  a) Lithium & thiazide diuretics
	  b Renal tubular acidosis
	5) Acidosis (increases calcium ionization)
	6) Children have higher serum calcium levels than adults and may be markedly increased during bone growth (especially adolescence)
		Caused by the effects of excess calcium in the cells, which causes a decrease in cell membrane excitability.
		1) Effects on skeletal muscle
		  a) Muscle weakness – flaccidity
		  b) Hyporeflexia
		  c) Decreased muscle tone
		2) Effects on heart muscle
		  a) Bradycardia/cardiac arrest
		  b) Shortened QT interval
		  c) Shortened ST segment
		  d) Increased PR interval
		  e) Evidence of digoxin toxicity
		  f) Hypertension
		3) Effects on nervous system
		  a) Confusion
		  b) Personality changes/psychosis
		  c) Lethargy/coma
		4) Decrease in GI motility causing: anorexia, nausea, vomiting, decreased bowel sounds, constipation, paralytic ileus
		5) Bone pain due to pathologic fractures
		6) Flank pain due to development of kidney stones

Courtesy of DCI Acute Program, Omaha, Nebraska. Used with permission.

in myocardial contractility, which could influence blood pressure stability during hemodialysis (Toussaint & Cooney, 2006; van der Sande et al., 1998).

(a) For an adjusted serum calcium > 10.2 mg/dL, use a dialysis solution with 2.5 mEq/L of calcium.

(b) For an adjusted serum calcium < 10.2 mg/dL, use a dialysis solution with 3 to 3.5 mEq/L of calcium.

(c) Patients receiving large volumes of blood products may need to use a dialysis solution calcium of 3.0 to 3.5 mEq/L to counteract the effect of the citrate anticoagulant present in most blood products.

  i. Citrate binds to available calcium and is metabolized by the liver to bicarbonate.

  ii. Once the citrate has been metabolized, the calcium is then released back into the serum.

d. Alternate methods to correct serum calcium.

(1) For hypocalcemia, administer 1 gram of calcium gluconate IV push over 10 minutes.

(2) Calcium gluconate is preferable to calcium chloride, as calcium chloride must always be infused into a central line as it may cause sloughing and necrosis of tissue if a peripheral IV site infiltrates.

(3) Gram for gram, calcium chloride contains three times the available calcium as calcium gluconate; if given too rapidly, calcium chloride may cause bradycardia and even cardiac arrest.

(4) Correction of hypomagnesemia (< 1.5 mEq/L), hyperphosphotemia (> 4.5 mg/dL), and alkalosis is imperative for IV calcium to be effective (see Figure 3.10). Hypomagnesemia is commonly associated with other electrolyte abnormalitites including hypokalemia and hypocalcemia. Intravenous calcium infusions should not be given with severe hyperphosphatemia due to the risk of precipitation. Alkalosis causes an increase in the binding of calcium to albumin (Moe, 2008).

(5) If a patient is receiving IV calcium, watch for arrhythmias, especially if the patient is also taking digoxin.

(a) Calcium and digoxin have similar effects on the heart.

(b) Place patient on cardiac monitor and evaluate for changes in rate and rhythm.

H. Ultrafiltration.
　1. Ultrafiltration is the removal of water from the plasma through the semipermeable membrane of the dialyzer by hydrostatic pressure or osmotic force.
　2. Fluid assessment and calculations.
　　a. Use the information obtained during the predialysis patient assessment to anticipate the patient's volume status and available fluid for ultrafiltration.
　　　(1) Calculate the fluid balance since the last hemodialysis treatment or hospital admission for patient new to hemodialysis, using I/O and weight measurements.

　　　(a) For established ambulatory or wheelchair bound patients, the ultrafiltration goal can be calculated by the difference in weight since the last HD treatment.
　　　(b) Fluid removal based on weight gain should include correlation with intake and output measurements since different scales can produce different results.
　　(2) Assess patient's intravascular fluid status using BP, CVP, PAWP, hematocrit, and serum sodium levels. Excess fluid in this space responds well to ultrafiltration.
　　(3) Assess the patient for edema, ascites, changes in skin turgor, and mucous membranes. Excess fluid in the form of

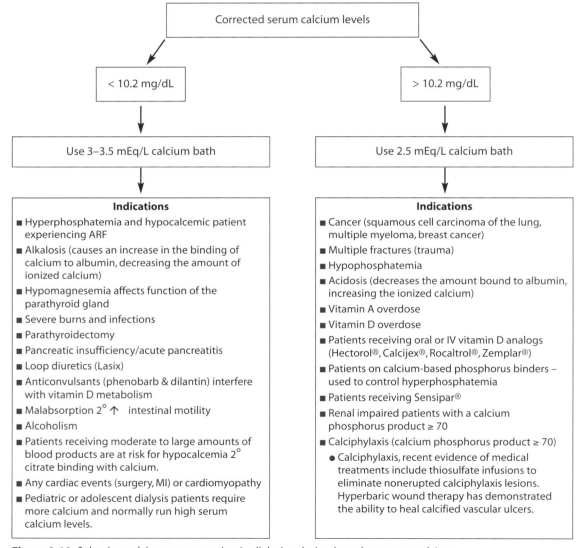

Figure 3.10. Selecting calcium concentration in dialysis solution based on serum calcium.

Adapted from Creighton Nephrology, Creighton University, Omaha, Nebraska. Algorithm compiled using references from Santos, P.W., Hartle, J.E., II, & Quarles, L.P. (2006) & Daugirdas, J.T., Blake, P.G., & Ing, T.S. (2001). Used with permission.

edema and ascites is more resistant to removal with ultrafiltration than excess fluid in the intravascular space.
 b. Calculate anticipated intake during the hemodialysis treatment.
  (1) Saline for prime and rinseback.
  (2) Saline flushes.
  (3) Volume from anticoagulant (e.g., citrate and calcium).
  (4) Volume from blood products administration.
  (5) Other PO or IV intake.
3. Review the prescribed ultrafiltration goal with the nephrologist as needed. Discrepancies may exist between the UF goal prescribed earlier and the current patient assessment of fluid excess.
4. Interventions that may assist with ultrafiltration.
 a. Third spacing, poor cardiac function, and/or intravascular hypovolemia may necessitate the use of osmotic agents to facilitate shifting the fluid back into the intravascular compartment for removal with dialysis.
 b. Anticipate the need for osmotic agents and collaborate with the nephrologist/APRN/PA to select and make these agents available (see Table 3.23).
  (1) Osmotic pressure is exerted by solutes across a selectively permeable membrane. The capillary membrane is selectively permeable, and fluid will move across the capillary membrane to the higher concentration of particles (Klabunde, 2014a). For example, administration of

25% mannitol injection or 50% dextrose during dialysis would increase the intravascular concentration of solutes (osmolality), promoting fluid shift into the intravascular compartment available for ultrafiltration on hemodialysis
  (2) Oncotic pressure is exerted by large protein molecules (i.e., albumin generates about 70% of the oncotic pressure within the capillary, drawing water back into the capillaries) (Klabunde, 2014a).
  (3) Normal capillary permeability can be altered by the presence of proinflammatory mediators (e.g., histamine, bradykinin) and/or injury to the structural integrity of capillaries as in tissue trauma, burns, severe inflammation (Klabunde, 2014b).
 c. Blood products act like osmotic agents to pull fluid into the vascular space.
 d. Lower the dialysate temperature (35° to 36° C) to improve vascular tone.
 e. UF profiling. A continuously decreasing linear pattern of UF is well tolerated and is associated with fewer hypotensive episodes.
 f. Conductivity profiling, also known as sodium modeling (Oliver et al., 2001).
  (1) Use cautiously to avoid leaving the patient with elevated serum sodium level that will drive rapid fluid gain posthemodialysis.
  (2) Most effective when used in conjunction with UF profiling.
 g. Sequential (isolated) ultrafiltration.
  (1) Isolated ultrafiltration removes iso-osmolar

Table 3.23

Osmotic Agents

Medication	Administration	Special Considerations
25% albumin	50 mL administered IV via the arterial chamber. The mechanism of action causes approximately 175 mL of additional fluid shift into circulation within 15 minutes. Administer up to 2 times during HD session, 30 minutes apart, not in last hour of treatment.	Is expensive and sometimes in shortage in certain geographic areas. Is an effective osmotic agent. Is not an effective agent for fluid shifting when the serum albumin level is normal.
25% mannitol (12.5 g)	10–20 mL IVP into venous dialysis tubing. Mechanism of action, promotes osmotic fluid shift. Administer up to 3 times during HD session, 30 minutes apart, not in last hour of treatment.	
50% dextrose	10–25 mL IV via venous chamber port over 3–5 minutes. The mechanism of action is an immediate increase in plasma osmolarity contributing to a fluid shift. Administer up to 3 times during HD session, 30 minutes apart, not in last hour of treatment.	For use in the nondiabetic patient.

Adapted from DCI Acute Program, Omaha, Nebraska. Used with permission.

fluid from the intravascular compartment, removing excess fluid without significantly changing the blood solute concentrations. The iso-osmolar fluid contains mainly water and nonprotein bound low-molecular weight solutes (i.e., electrolytes, urea, creatinine), which are removed at about the same concentration as found in the plasma levels (Robbins, 2006).

   (2) Better cardiovascular stability with isolated ultrafiltration may be accounted for by avoiding the decrease in plasma osmolality that occurs during hemodialysis process. A rise in plasma oncotic pressure due to rise in plasma protein level facilitates refilling of the vascular space by fluid from the interstitial space. Total peripheral resistance may result from a lower core body temperature, promoting peripheral vasoconstriction (White et al., 2008).

   (3) Because the solute removal is essentially isotonic, evaluation for conventional dialysis to correct solute concentrations is performed (Mulloy, 2002).

   h. Online blood volume monitoring (BVM). BVM devices measure blood plasma refill via a relative hematocrit (Katzarski, 1996; Sinha et al., 2009).

   i. Position patient with feet elevated; lower head of bed as needed.
      (1) Make certain positioning patient does not compromise the patient's condition.
      (2) Keep the patient's head of bed at ≥ 30 degrees for patients with elevated intracranial pressure (ICP) to minimize intracranial pressure.
      (3) Patients who are ventilator dependent or receiving a tube feeding are at risk for aspiration of secretions or feeding and should not be left flat.

   j. Thrombo-embolic-deterrent (TED) hose or sequential lower leg compression device.

I. Anticoagulation.
   1. Use the information obtained during the predialysis patient assessment to determine the patient's bleeding risk and response to anticoagulation. Bleeding risk may be elevated by any of the following.
      a. BUN > 100 mg/dL may cause uremic platelet dysfunction.
      b. Low platelet count (including causes such as TTP, HIT).
      c. Impaired liver function.
      d. Medications that may affect blood clotting such as ibuprofen, naproxen (NSAIDs), warfarin,

aspirin, platelet inhibitors such as clopidogrel (Plavix®), anticoagulants such as enoxaparin (Lovenox®), dalteparin (Fragmin®), danapariod (Orgaran®), factor Xa inhibitors rivaroxaban (Xarelto®) and fondaparinux (Arixtra®), and thrombin inhibitor such as desirudin (Iprivask®) (Drugs.com, 2015, http://www.drugs.com/condition/deep-vein-thrombosis-prophylaxis.html).

      e. Chemotherapeutic agents causing thrombocytopenia.
      f. Antibiotics affecting platelet function (cephalosporins, erythromycin, amphotericin B, and most aminoglycosides).

   2. Patients with minimal bleeding risk.
      a. These patients may receive "tight" or "low" total heparinization to minimize patient bleeding risk.
      b. The goal is to prolong the patient's clotting time to avoid thrombus formation in the extracorporeal circuit.
      c. Anticoagulation is achieved with an initial heparin bolus followed by a heparin infusion or boluses at a prescribed rate during the hemodialysis treatment.
      d. The nephrologist/APRN/PA may adjust the heparin dose based on the patient's and/or extra corporeal circuit's response in previous hemodialysis treatments.
      e. PTTs may be used to titrate intradialytic heparin administration.
      f. Goal PTT may be 45 to 65 seconds.
      g. Heparin adjustment in the acute care setting is under the direction of a registered nurse in collabration with the nephrologist/APRN/PA and established protocols.
      h. Patient response to heparin varies. Heparin half-life is patient dependent and ranges from 30 minutes to 2 hours.

   3. Patients with high bleeding risk.
      a. Patients who are actively bleeding, who are at high risk of bleeding, or in whom the use of heparin is contraindicated should have hemodialysis without heparin.
      b. Indications for heparin-free dialysis include:
         (1) Pericardial effusion/pericarditis.
         (2) Recent surgery with bleeding complications or risk (especially vascular, cardiac, eye, kidney transplant, and brain).
         (3) Known coagulopathy/thrombocytopenia.
         (4) Heparin allergy (HIT).
         (5) Active bleeding.
         (6) Severe uremia (especially during the first three dialysis treatments).
         (7) Patients receiving dialysis immediately before or after an operation or

interventional procedure (e.g., kidney biopsy, cardiac cath).
  (8) Patients at risk for GI bleed (esophageal varices, ulcer disease).
  (9) Recent stroke, trauma, or burn.
  c. Heparin-free dialysis may include the following techniques.
    (1) Heparin rinse of the extracorporeal circuit with heparinized saline (3000 units/L) during the priming procedure, followed by a normal saline flush prior to initiating dialysis so the heparin in the circuit is not given to the patient. CAUTION: NOT APPROPRIATE FOR PATIENTS WITH HIT.
    (2) The blood flow is set as high as tolerated during dialysis (at least 250 mL/min). CAUTION: NOT APPROPRIATE FOR PATIENTS AT RISK FOR DDS.
    (3) A 25 to 200 mL rapid saline rinse of the dialyzer is performed every 30 to 60 minutes throughout the dialysis treatment. The rinsing allows inspection of the extracorporeal circuit and may assist in avoiding circuit clotting. The ultrafiltration calculations are adjusted to remove the fluid given as flushes.
  d. Alternative anticoagulation options.
    (1) Regional citrate anticoagulation using anticoagulant citrate dextrose formula A (ACD-A) or 4% trisodium citrate.
    (2) Hemodialysis using dialysate containing citric acid.
    (3) Other systemic anticoagulants may also be used.

IV. Intradialytic assessment and interventions.

A. The goal of intradialytic patient care is to assess, apply interventions, and evaluate the patient's response to the interventions, providing a safe, effective, and comfortable hemodialysis treatment.

B. Both the hemodialysis system and the water treatment system must be monitored throughout the hemodialysis treatment and findings documented.

C. Patient assessment and documentation of findings.
  1. The intradialytic assessment will include the hemodialysis system BFR, arterial pressure (AP), venous pressure (VP), transmembrane pressure (TMP), and ultrafiltration rate (UFR), as well as the patient's vital signs, pain level, I/O, vascular access, anticoagulation received, lab results, and any patient complaints or changes in patient behavior.

  2. The patient on intermittent hemodialysis must be monitored continuously by the patient care provider.
    a. The patient's vascular access must be visible throughout the entire treatment.
    b. Changes in the patient's condition or vascular access can happen quickly, and it is critical that the patient care provider be present to quickly resolve any treatment complication (e.g., hypotension, catheter disconnection, or needle dislodgement).
  3. Documentation should occur every 15 minutes in critical care settings and in patients receiving HD for the first time.
  4. Documentation may occur every 30 minutes in general acute care settings.
  5. During unstable patient situations, documentation occurs as often as interventions are occurring and patient responses are being evaluated.

D. Patient parameters.
  1. Vital signs.
    a. Blood pressure and pulse are indicative of the patient's tolerance to fluid removal. Hypotension and increased pulse rate often signal intravascular hypovolemia.
    b. Assess both the apical and radial heart rate for signs of atrial fibrillation or other arrhythmias intermittently and when hypotension occurs.
    c. Respirations.
      (1) Increased respirations initially can indicate decreasing blood pressure or acidosis.
      (2) Decreased respirations can indicate severe hypotension or alkalosis.
    d. Temperature as warranted by changes in patient condition (e.g., shaking chills, or during the administration of blood products).
  2. Fluid removal and blood pressure monitoring.
    a. Most patients who require kidney replacement therapy have some UF needs.
    b. The total volume ultrafiltrated, as well as rapid removal of fluid volume (high ultrafiltration rate), contribute to hypotension.
      (1) Hypotension is the most common complication during HD occurring in up to as many as 30% of treatments (Kotanko & Henrich, 2014).
      (2) Defined by the following qualities.
        (a) Systolic blood pressure (SBP) < 100 mmHg.
        (b) Diastolic blood pressure (DBP) < 40 mmHg.
        (c) Drop in SBP > 40 mmHg.
        (d) Mean arterial pressure (MAP) < 65.
      (3) Hypotension is related to intravascular volume, cardiac output, and systemic vascular resistance.

(4) 20% to 25% decrease in cardiac output = decrease of > 20 mmHg in SBP or DBP upon standing.
c. Contributing factors to intradialytic hypotension.
  (1) Solute gradient changes.
  (2) Eating a large meal immediately before or during the hemodialysis treatment has been known to cause severe hypotension as well as nausea and vomiting.
    (a) To promote healing, every effort should be made to help the patient maintain nutritional intake in the hospital setting.
    (b) One option is to be sure the patient's meal is delivered early so he/she can eat 1 hour prior to the planned treatment.
    (c) A nutritional supplement can be prescribed and offered in small amounts to the patient during treatment to maintain caloric intake and avoid hypotension.
    (d) The bedside nurse should be instructed to hold the patient's tray until the patient's hemodialysis treatment is complete, even when the patient is receiving the hemodialysis in the dialysis treatment room. With eating a meal, arterioles in the splanchnic bed dilate, resulting in increased blood flow in the superior mesenteric artery with postprandial hemodynamic changes maximal at 30 minutes (Alagiakrishnan, 2007).
  (3) Decreased compensatory mechanisms.
  (4) Oxygen saturation level.
    (a) Oxyhemoglobin is oxygen bound to hemoglobin molecules in red blood cells (RBCs) and a measurement is SaO_2.
    (b) A normal oxyhemoglobin saturation should be greater than 95% (Pruitt & Jacobs, 2003, 2004).
    (c) A drop in arterial saturation could be due to a low inspired oxygen and/or a decrease in cardiac output.
    (d) SvO_2 (mixed venous saturation) monitoring reflects oxygen consumption and under normal conditions is 75%, indicating tissues extract 25% of the oxygen delivered.
    (e) A decrease in SvO_2 can reflect a change in hemoglobin, cardiac output, arterial saturation, or tissue oxygen requirements (Morgan, 2012; Reyer, 2013).
    (f) Decrease in saturation can be induced by ultrafiltration depleting the intravascular blood volume.
    (g) During HD the PO_2 may drop 5 to 23 mmHg, creating a problem in patients with severe preexisting pulmonary or cardiac disease, especially in the elderly (Diroll, 2014).
  (5) Autonomic dysfunction.
  (6) Medications (e.g., antihypertensive medications).
  (7) Laboratory values (e.g., low blood glucose, hypocalcemia, or low hematocrit).
d. Prevention of hypotension and promotion of safe ultrafiltration with plasma refill occurs by following the interventions that may assist with UF.
e. Treating intradialytic hypotension. Each step should be taken and blood pressure reassessed until hypotension resolves.
  (1) Decrease ultrafiltration rate to minimum.
  (2) Recline the patient if this position is not contraindicated.
  (3) Bolus with normal saline (volume dependent on the patient size and condition) and/or titrate vasopressors if available.
  (4) Additionally, apply the interventions that may assist with UF as indicated (see III.H.4 in this chapter).
3. Vascular access monitoring.
  a. Monitor the hemodialysis system arterial pressure (AP) and the venous pressure (VP).
  b. Directly observe the catheter, fistula, or graft. Observe and verify the security of needle placement and/or bloodline connections.
  c. The patient's vascular access must be visible throughout the entire treatment (Axley et al., 2013).
4. Response to treatment. The patient should be encouraged to report complaints of dizziness, cramping, and restlessness as these symptoms may indicate hypotension or volume depletion.
5. Observe and document the patient's level of consciousness.

E. Equipment parameters.
1. Integrity of the extracorporeal circuit.
  a. Verify that all lines are open and that connections are intact and secure every 30 minutes. More frequent observations could be indicated if the patient is restless, confused, etc.
  b. Keep connections visible at all times.
2. Observe color of blood in dialyzer and bloodlines.
  a. Dark color can precede filter clotting.
  b. Cherry soda-pop appearance indicates hemolysis.
3. Monitor pressure readings.

a. Venous pressure (VP) measures the resistance encountered when blood is being returned to the patient through the venous access.
   (1) Should not exceed 250 mmHg.
   (2) High VP pressure may indicate clotting in venous chamber, bloodline, or venous needle.
   (3) Low VP may indicate venous access disconnection.

b. Arterial pressure (AP) measures the negative pressure applied by the blood pump between the needle site and the blood pump.
   (1) Should not exceed negative 250 mmHg.
   (2) Low AP indicates hypotension, excessive suction on wall of access, or a clotted arterial needle or access port.
   (3) Sudden drop in AP may indicate needle migration or infiltration.
   (4) High AP may indicate clotting of dialyzer or system.

c. Transmembrane pressure (TMP) is a calculated pressure derived from the venous pressure minus the dialysate pressure in mmHg.
   (1) The TMP is influenced by the porosity of the dialyzer membrane.
   (2) High-flux dialyzers will have a lower TMP.
   (3) TMP rises slowly throughout a hemodialysis treatment in response to ultrafiltration with resultant increased blood viscosity.
   (4) TMP must be monitored to detect rapid large shifts in pressure, which may indicate excess ultrafiltration, a dialysate leak, or system clotting.

4. Anticoagulant delivery and effectiveness.
   a. The anticoagulant pump should be observed to make certain the anticoagulant is being infused as prescribed.
   b. Monitor patient and system response to anticoagulant by direct observation or blood specimen testing.
   c. Discontinue anticoagulant as indicated in treatment order, typically 30 to 60 minutes prior to treatment termination for patients who need to achieve hemostasis after needle removal from their graft or fistula.
   d. For patient bleeding, discontinue anticoagulation and consult the nephrologist/APRN/PA for additional laboratory and/or medication orders.

5. Blood and dialysate flow rates ensure that prescribed rates are being delivered to achieve desired patient solute clearance. Dialysis time may need to be increased if the prescribed rates are not achievable.

6. Ultrafiltration rate (UFR) should be set and adjusted based on patient response to treatment.

7. Conductivity. Dialysate conductivity monitoring ensures the delivery of a dialysis solution with an electrolyte concentration that will not harm red blood cells by causing hemolysis or crenation.

F. Intradialytic patient education.
   1. An acute nephrology nurse should assess the patient receiving hemodialysis for knowledge deficits, readiness to learn, and preferred method of learning.
   2. Patient education should meet the identified knowledge deficits using a method that meets the patient's needs (e.g., audio, visual, or kinesthetic).
   3. The 1:1 bedside education helps to allay concerns about the dialysis process and offers an opportunity to educate and answer questions related to kidney health, whether the patient is experiencing AKI or CKD. See Appendix 1.1, Patient Education Brochure, in Chapter 1 of this module.
   4. Education should be provided for the CKD patient approaching stage 5. This education should include exposure to all treatment options that are available to the patient (e.g., in-center hemodialysis, home hemodialysis, continuous ambulatory peritoneal dialysis, automated peritoneal dialysis, living donor kidney transplant, deceased donor kidney transplant, and conservative care). Refer to Module 2, Chapter 3, The Individual with Kidney Disease.
   5. Vascular access.
      a. Educate the patient about the care and maintenance of his/her existing access.
      b. Educate the patient about vascular access options and the steps the patient will take to achieve a successful fistula or graft if needed.
      c. Educate the patient about care of a catheter vascular access. See Appendix 3.3: Catheter Instructions for the Patient and Appendix 3.4: Patient Catheter Release Form.
   6. Most important, education of patients with CKD and/or family should include the information that kidney replacement therapy may be integrated into their lives, helping them feel better so they can fully live.

V. Posthemodialysis assessment and evaluation.

A. The purpose of the posthemodialysis assessment and evaluation is to evaluate the patient, his/her response to treatment, changes in the overall condition, and the achievement of treatment goals.
   1. Any unexpected changes in patient condition or failure to achieve the expected treatment goals should be reported to the charge nurse and/or provider. Changes to the patient's care should be anticipated.

2. The posthemodialysis patient assessment should be performed as indicated below and verbally reported to the receiving bedside nurse. The report should include the following.
   a. Blood glucose monitoring and laboratory tests drawn, predialysis, intradialysis, or postdialysis.
   b. Amount and type of anticoagulation administered.
   c. All medications administered (oral, intravenous, and parenteral).
   d. Amount and type of blood products administered.
   e. Before and after vital signs.
   f. Net fluid balance.
   g. Condition of vascular access.
      (1) Fistula or graft: patent with bruit and thrill and type of dressing.
      (2) Catheter: exit-site condition and dressing change.
   h. Response or complications experienced throughout treatment.
   i. Clarify any orders to be carried out after dialysis to avoid an assumption that they may have already been completed, such as administration of antibiotics.
3. If the hemodialysis treatment occurred in a dialysis treatment room, the patient's condition and mode of departure should be documented on the hemodialysis treatment record as well.

B. The patient and extracorporeal circuit are evaluated after the treatment is discontinued and the assessment documented on the hemodialysis treatment flowsheet.
   1. Vital signs.
      a. BP: lying, sitting or standing, as patient condition permits. Consider a sitting and standing BP prior to removing needles so that additional saline may be infused if hypotensive.
      b. Standing BP is taken to assess for orthostatic hypotension; if patient is unable to stand, consider elevating the head of the bed 80 to 90 degrees.
      c. Assess the pulse rate and rhythm by apical auscultation and radial pulse comparison.
         (1) Increased rate may indicate fluid volume depletion or atrial fibrillation in response to volume depletion.
         (2) A change in heart rate to > 120 or < 50 beats/min should be reported to the nephrologist/APRN/PA.
      d. Temperature.
         (1) Compare to predialysis temperature.
         (2) Elevation may indicate access infection or infection related to other illness manifestations.
      e. Respiration.
         (1) Rate and quality: labored or rapid.
         (2) Auscultate breath sounds.
         (3) Oxygen saturation rate.
   2. Weight.
      a. Compare to predialysis weight to determine amount of fluid removed during dialysis.
      b. Compare to dry weight to determine if fluid removal achieved euvolemia.
   3. Vascular access (whether newly placed or established) condition.
      a. Estimate blood loss, length of time bleeding, type of dressing applied, and patency of access at time the patient is returned to the care of the bedside nurse.
      b. Observe vascular access for signs and symptoms of infection (e.g., redness, warmth, swelling, and drainage). Obtain culture as needed.
   4. Sense of well-being.
      a. Record the patient's response to treatment (e.g., "tolerated treatment well without complications").
      b. Level of consciousness (LOC).
         (1) Note changes in patient's LOC prior to return to general care.
         (2) Include description such as alert, oriented, disoriented, agitated, confused, obtunded, unconscious, combative, depressed, etc.
   5. Dialyzer and extracorporeal circuit condition.
      a. Residual blood loss.
         (1) Estimate and document after the rinseback of blood from the dialyzer.
            (a) Small = 25% clotted/streaked fibers noted.
            (b) Moderate = 25 to 50% clotted/streaked fibers noted.
            (c) Large = 50 to 100% clotted/streaked fibers noted.
         (2) Estimate the amount of surfaced area clotted in the chambers, correlating the total amount of anticoagulant administered during treatment.
      b. A large amount of clotting and streaking would be an indicator of inadequate anticoagulation, and adjustments should be anticipated on subsequent hemodialysis treatments.

C. Obtain postdialysis laboratory tests.
   1. BUN for Kt/Vurea or URR, blood cultures, serum drug levels.
   2. Ensure that blood chemistries are drawn no sooner than 1 to 2 hours after treatment, to allow the patient's body to re-equilibrate serum electrolyte levels and avoid treating an electrolyte level in the midst of equilibration (e.g., giving IV potassium for a low serum potassium level).

D. Provide patient education.
   1. The approximate date of next dialysis treatment.
   2. Access care.
   3. Diet.
   4. Fluid restrictions.
   5. Medications.
   6. Instruction and reinforcement in any areas needed.
   7. For the ARF patient undergoing hemodialysis for the first time, use ARF patient educational material. Refer to Appendix 1.1 in Chapter 1 of this module for a Patient Education Brochure to provide patient and family education relative to ARF and the hemodialysis treatment.

References

Ahmed, I. Majeed, A., & Power, R. (2007). *Heparin induced thrombocytopenis: Diagnosis and management update.* Retrieved from http://.ncbi.nlm.nih.gov/pmc/articles/PMC2600013/

Alagiakrishnan, K. (2007). Postural and postprandial hypotension: *Approach to management.* Retrieved from http://www.medscape.com/viewarticle/559578_5

Albers, G.W., & Amarenco, P. (2001). *Combination therapy with clopidogrel and aspirin: Can the CURE results be extrapolated to cerebrovascular patients?* Retrieved from http://stroke.ahajournals.org/content/32/12/2948.full.pdf+html

Amato, R.L., Klebovy, D., King, B., & Salai, P.B. (2008). Hemodialysis. In C.S. Counts (Ed.), *Core curriculum for nephrology nursing* (5th ed., pp. 690-692). Pitman, NJ: American Nephrology Nurses' Association.

American Heart Association (AHA). (2005). *New AHA recommendations for blood pressure measurement.* Retrieved from http://www.aafp.org/afp/2005/1001/p1391.html

American Diabetes Association (ADA). (2004). *Hyperglycemic Crises in diabetes.* Retrieved from http://care.diabetesjournals.org/content/27/suppl_1/s94.full

American Diabetes Association (ADA). (2014). Clinical practice recommendations. *Diabetes Care, 37*(1), 558.

American Stroke Association (ASA). *Anti-clotting agents explained.* Retrieved from http://www.strokeassociation.org/STROKEORG/

Aurigemma, G.P., Konkle, B.A., & Gaasch, W.H. (2014). *Antithrombotic therapy in patients with prosthetic heart valves.* Retrieved from http://www.uptodate.com/contents/antithrombotic-therapy-in-patients-with-prosthetic-heart-valves

Axley, B., Speranza-Reid, J., & Williams, H.F. (2013). Venous needle dislodgement in patients on hemodialysis. *Nephrology Nursing Journal, 39*(6), 435-445.

Bagshaw, S.M., & Bellomo, G.C. (2008). *Early acute kidney and sepsis: A multicentre evaluation.* Retrieved from http://www.ncbi.nlm.nih.gov/pubmed/18402655

Baskin, J.L., Puj, C., Reiss, U., Wilimas, J.A., Metzger, M.L., Ribeiro, R.C., & Howard, S. C. (2009). Management of occlusion and thrombosis associated with long-term indwelling central venous catheters. Retrieved from http://www.ncbi.nlm.nih.gov/pmc/articles/PMC2814365/

Biology Online. (2008). *Phagocytosis.* Retrieved from http://www.biology-online.org/dictionary/Phagocytosis

Bristol-Myers Squibb. (2013). *Coumadin (warfarin sodium) and you.* Retrieved from http://www.coumadin.com/html/index.htm

Burns, M.J., Friedman, S.L., & Larson, A.M. (2014). *Acetaminophen (paracetamol) poisoning in adults: Pathophysiology, presentation and diagnosis.* Retrieved from http://www.uptodate.com/contents/acetaminophen-paracetamol-poisoning-in-adults-pathophysiology-presentation-and-diagnosis?topicKey=EM%2F340&elapsedTimeMs=5&view=print&displayedView=full

Centers for Disease Control and Prevention (CDC). (2007). Nephrogenic fibrosing dermopathy associated with exposure to gadolinium-containing contrast agents – St. Louis, Missouri, 2002-2006. *Morbidity and Mortality Weekly Report, 56*(7), 137-141. Retrieved from http://www.cdc.gov/mmwr/preview/mmwrhtml/mm5607a1.htm

Centers for Disease Control and Prevention (CDC). (2010) *Glossary; antibiotic/antimicrobial resistance A–Z index.* Retrieved from http://www.cdc.gov/drugresistance/about.html

Centers for Disease Control and Prevention (CDC). (2012). *Meningococcal disease: Epidemiology and prevention of vaccine-preventable disease.* Retrieved from http://www.cdc.gov/vaccines/pubs/pinkbook/mening.html

Centers for Disease Control and Prevention (CDC). (2013). *Colorectal cancer screening tests.* Retrieved from http://www.cdc.gov/cancer/colorectal/basic_info/screening/

Centers for Disease Control and Prevention (CDC). (2014). *Infection prevention and control recommendations for hospitalized patients with known or suspected Ebola virus disease in U.S. hospitals.* Retrieved http://www.cdc.gov/vhf/ebola/healthcare-us/hospitals/infection-control.html

Crawford, A. & Harris, H. (2012). Fluid and electrolyte series balancing act calcium & phosphorus. Retrieved from http://www.nursingcenter.com/skincarenetwork/JournalArticle?Article_ID=1281585&Journal_ID=54016&Issue_ID=1281516&expiredce=1

Chan, K.E., Edelman, E.R., Wenger, J.B., Thadhani, R. I., & Maddux, F.W. (2015). Dabigatran and rivaroxaban use in atrial fibrillation patients on hemodialysis. Retrieved from http://circ.ahajournals.org/content/early/2015/01/16/CIRCULATIONAHA.114.014113.full.pdf+html

Chan, K.E., Mazarus, M., & Hakim, R.M. (2010). *Digoxin associates with mortality in ESRD.* Retrieved from http://jasn.asnjournals.org/content/early/2010/06/24/ASN.2009101047.full.pdf+html

Cincotta, E., & Schonder, K.S. (2008). Pharmacologic aspects of chronic kidney disease. In C.S. Counts (Ed.), *Core curriculum for nephrology nursing* (5th ed., pp. 579-595). Pitman, NJ: American Nephrology Nurses' Association.

Cleveland Clinic. (2013). *Disease & conditions: Orthostatic hypotension.* Retrieved from http://my.clevelandclinic.org/health/diseases_conditions/hic_orthostatic_hypotension

Craig, M. (2008). Slow extended daily dialysis and continuous renal replacement therapies. In C.S. Counts (Ed.), *Core curriculum for nephrology nursing* (5th ed., pp. 237-238). Pitman, NJ: American Nephrology Nurses' Association.

Craig, R.C., & Hunter, J.M. (2008). *Recent developments in the perioperative management of adult patients with chronic kidney disease.* Retrieved from http://bja.oxfordjournals.org/content/101/3/296.full

Davenport, A. (2009). *Review article: Low-molecular weight heparin as an alternative anticoagulant to unfractionated heparin for routine outpatient hemodialysis treatment.* Retrieved from http://onlinelibrary.wiley.com/doi/10.1111/j.1440-1797.2009.01135.x/pdf

DeAbreu, K.L., Silva, G.B., Jr., Barreto, A.G.C., Melo, F.M., Oliveria, B.B., Mota, R.M., ... Daher, E.F. (2010). *Acute kidney injury after trauma: prevalence, clinical characteristics and RIFLE classification.* Retrieved from http://www.ncbi.nlm.nih.gov/pmc/articles/PMC3021827

Diroll, A. (2014). *The importance of oxygen during hemodialysis.*

Retrieved from http://www.rsnhope.org/health-library/article-index/the-importance-of-oxygen-during-hemodialysis/

Drugs.com (2014a). *Curarization definition.* Retrieved from http://www.drugs.com/dict/curarization.html

Drugs.com (2014b). *Myoneural junction definition.* Retrieved from http://www.drugs.com/dict/myoneural.html

Drugs.com (2014c). *Neuromuscular blocking agents.* Retrieved from http://www.drugs.com/dict/neuromuscular-blocking-agents.html

Drugs.com (2015). *Deep vein thrombosis, prophylaxis medications.* Retrieved from http://www.drugs.com/condition/deep-vein-thrombosis-prophylaxis.html

Ejaz, A.A., & Mohandas, R. (2014). *Are diuretics harmful in the management of acute kidney injury?* Retrieved from http://www.ncbi.nlm.nih.gov/pubmed/24389731

Firwana, B.M., Hasan, R., Ferwana, M., Varon, J., Stem, A., & Gidwani, U. (2011). *Tissue plasminogen activator versus heparin for locking dialysis catheters: A systematic review.* Retrieved from http://www.ncbi.nlm.nih.gov/pmc/articles/PMC3507063/

Garg, S., Singhal, S., Sharma, P., & Jah, A.A. (2012). *Inotropes and vasopressors review of physiology and clinical use.* Retrieved from http://omicsonline.org/inotropes-and-vasopressors-review-of-physiology-and-clinical-use-2161-105X.1000128.pdf

George, J.N. (2011). *Platelets.* Retrieved from http://www.ouhsc.edu/platelets/Platelets/platelets%20intro.html

GlobalRPh. (2012). *Mean arterial pressure (MAP) Calculator.* Retrieved from http://www.globalrph.com/map.htm

Goldberg, D. (2012). *Calcium, ionized.* Retrieved from http://emedicine.medscape.com/article/2087469-overview

Grams, M.E., Estrella, M.M., Coresh, J., Brower, R.G., & Liu, K.D. (2011). *Fluid balance diuretic uses, and mortality in acute kidney injury.* Retrieved from http://www.ncbi.nlm.nih.gov/pubmed/21393482

Grudzinski, L., Quinan, P., Kwok, S., & Pierratos, A. (2007). Sodium citrate 4% locking solution for central venous dialysis catheters – An effective, more cost-efficient alternative to heparin. *Nephrology Dialysis Transplantation, 22*(2), 471-476. Retrieved from http://ndt.oxfordjournals.org/content/22/2/471.full

Heart Sounds. (2014). Retrieved from http://www.easyauscultation.com/heart-sounds

Himmelfarb, J., Joannidis, M., Molitoris, B., Schietz, M., Okusa, M.D., Warnock, D., … Kellum, J.A. (2008). *Evaluation and initial management of acute kidney injury.* Retrieved from http://cjasn.asnjournals.org/content/3/4/962.full

Kalantar-Zadeh, K., Rodriguez, R.A., & Humphresy, M.H. (2004). Association between serum ferritin and measures of inflammation, nutrition and iron in haemodialysis patients. *Nephrology Dialysis Transplantation, 19*, 141-149.

Katzarski, K.S. (1996) *Monitoring blood volume during haemodialysis treatment of acute renal and multiple organ failures.* Retrieved from http://ndt.oxfordjournals.org/content/11/supp8/20.full.pdf

Kidney Disease: Improving Global Outcomes (KDIGO). (2012). *KDIGO clinical practice guidelines for acute kidney injury.* Retrieved from http://www.kdigo.org/clinical_practice_guidelines/pdf/KDIGO%20AKI%20Guideline.pdf

Kell, D.B., & Pretorius, R. (2014). *Serum ferritin is an important inflammatory disease marker, as it is mainly a leakage product from damaged cells.* Retrieved from http://pubs.rsc.org/en/content/articlelanding/2014/mt/c3mt00347g#!divAbstract

Klabunde, R.E. (2014a). *Cardiovascular physiology concepts: Hydrostatic and oncotic pressures.* Retrieved from http://www.cvphysiology.com/Microcirculation/M012.htm

Klabunde, R. E. (2014b). *Cardiovascular physiology concepts: Tissue edema and general principles of transcapillary fluid exchange.* Retrieved from http://www.cvphysiology.com/Microcirculation/M010.htm Kotanko, P., & Henrick, W.L. (2014). *Intradialytic*

hypotension in an otherwise stable patient. Retrieved from http://www.uptodate.com/contents/intradialytic-hypotension-in-an-otherwise-stable-patient

Kyle, T. (2008). *Essentials of pediatric nursing: Performing a physical examination; measurement of vital signs.* Retrieved from http://books.google.com/books?id=qdmBXAtC3lMC&pg=PA263&lpg=PA263&dq=placement+of+blood+pressure+cuff+in+children&source=bl&ots=pChASYWziG&sig=Px8qYTwTpduR3jNpF58imS5VJws&hl=en&sa=X&ei=SLJzVLe3B4itogTdo4CoAg&ved=0CCwQ6AEwBA#v=onepage&q=placement%20of%20blood%20pressure%20cuff%20in%20children&f=false

Lederer, E., Alsauskas, Z.C., Mackelaite, L., & Nayak, V. (2014). *Hyperkalemia treatment and management.* Retrieved from http://emedicine.medscape.com/article/240903-treatment#aw2aab6b6b2

Lentino, J.R., & Leehey, D.J. (1994). Special problems in the dialysis patient. Chapter 28: Infections. In J.T. Daugirdas & S.I. Todd (Eds.). *Handbook of dialysis* (2nd ed., pp. 479). New York: Little, Brown.

Lewis, S.L. (1992). *Fever: Thermal regulation and alterations in end stage renal disease patients.* Retrieved from http://www.ncbi.nlm.nih.gov/pubmed/1546884

Lok, C.E., Appleton, D., Bhola, C., Khoo, B., & Richardson, R.M.A. (2006). *Trisodium citrate 4% – An alternative to heparin capping of haemodialysis catheters.* Retrieved from http://ndt.oxfordjournals.org/content/22/2/477.full

Malament, I.B., Uhlman, W., & Eisinger, R.P. (1975). P*otassium load from blood transfusion in dialysis patients.* Retrieved from http://rd.springer.com/article/10.1007%2FBF02082677#page-1

Mao, H., Katz, N., Ariyanon, W., Blanca-Martos, L., Adybelli, Z., Giuliani, A., … Ronco, C. (2013). Cardiac surgery-associated acute kidney injury. *Cardiodrenal Medicine, 3*(3), 178-199. Retrieved from http://www.karger.com/Article/FullText/353134 doi:10.1159/000353134

Mayo Clinic. (2013a). *Deep vein thrombosis.* Updated July 3, 2014. Retrieved from http://www.mayoclinic.com/health/deep-vein-thrombosis/DS01005/METHOD=print&DSECTION=all

Mayo Clinic. (2013b) *Secondary-hypertension.* Updated March 15, 2013. Retrieved from http://www.mayoclinic.com/health/secondary-hypertension/DS01114/METHOD=print

Mayo Clinic. (2014). *Interpretive handbook: Test 8378: Calcium, ionized, serum clinical information.* Mayo Medical Laboratories: Reference Laboratory Services for Health Care Organizations. Retrieved from http://www.mayomedicallaboratories.com/interpretive-guide/?alpha=C&unit_code=8378

McGhee, B.H., & Bridges, M.E..J. (2002). *Monitoring the arterial blood pressure: what you may not know.* Retrieved from http://ccn.aacnjournals.org/content/22/2/60.full.pdf+html

McNeely, J., Parikh, S., Valentine, C., Haddad, N., Ganesh, S., Rovin, B., Hebert, L., & Agarwal. A. (2012). *Bath salts: A newly recognized cause of acute kidney injury.* Retrieved from http://www.hindawi.com/journals/crin/2012/560854/

Merck Sharp & Dohme Corporation. (2014). *Edema.* Retrieved from http://www.merckmanuals.com/professional/cardiovascular_disorders/symptoms_of_cardiovascular_disorders/edema.html

Moe, S.M. (2008). *Disorders involving calcium, phosphorus, and magnesium.* Retrieved from http://www.ncbi.nlm.nih.gov/pmc/articles/PMC2486454/

Mohanial, V. Haririan, A., & Weinman, E.J. (2013). *Bradycardia without "classical" EKG changes in hyperkalemic hemodialysis patients.* Retrieved from http://www.ncbi.nlm.nih.gov/pubmed/22784561

Morgan, B. (2012). *SvO$_2$ (mixed venous oxygen saturation) or SCVO$_2$ (central venous oxygen saturation).* Retrieved from http://www.lhsc.on.ca/Health_Professionals/CCTC/edubriefs/svo2.htm

National Diabetes Information Clearinghouse (NDIC). (2013). *Diabetic neuropathies: The nerve damage of diabetes.* Retrieved from http://diabetes.niddk.nih.gov/dm/pubs/neuropathies/

National Institutes of Health, U.S. National Library of Medicine. (2013). *Rhabdomyolysis.* Retrieved from http://www.nlm.nih.gov/medlineplus/ency/article/000473.htm

National Kidney Foundation (NKF). (2002). *KDOQI clinical practice guideline on hypertension and antihypertensisve agents in chronic kidney disease: Guideline 12: Use of diuretics in CKD.* Retrieved from http://www2.kidney.org/professionals/KDOQI/guidelines_bp/guide_12htm

National Kidney Foundation (NKF). (2005). *KDOQI clinical practice guidelines for bone metabolism and disease in children with chronic kidney disease. Guideline 10. Dialysate Calcium Concentrations.* Retrieved from http://www2.kidney.org/professionals/KDOQI/guidelines_pedbone/guide10.htm

National Kidney Foundation (NKF). (2006). *KDOQI clinical practice guidelines and clinical practice recommendations for anemia in chronic kidney disease.* (2006). Retrieved from https://www.kidney.org/sites/default/files/docs/anemiainckd.pdf

National Kidney Foundation (NKF). (2006). *KDOQI clinical practice guidelines and clinical practice recommendations for anemia in chronic kidney disease in adults. SPR 3.4: Transfusion therapy.* Retrieved from http://www2.kidney.org/professionals/KDOQI/guidelines_anemia/cpr34.htm

National Kidney Foundation (NKF). (2012). *KDOQI clinical practice guidelines for diabetes and CKD: 2012 update.* Retrieved from https://www.kidney.org/sites/default/files/docs/diabetes-ckd-update-2012.pdf

Noble, K., & Isles, C. (2006). *Hyperkaleamia causing profound bradycardia.* Retrieved from http://www.ncbi.nlm.nih.gov/pmc/articles/PMC1861116/

Ochiai, Y., McCarthy, P.M., Smedira, N.G., Banbury, M.K., Navia, J.L., Feng, J., … Fukamachi, K. (2002). *Predictors of severe right ventricular failure after implantable left ventricular assist device insertion: Analysis of 245 patients.* Retrieved from http://www.ncbi.nlm.nih.gov/pubmed/12354733

Ogbru, O. (2014). *Warfarin, coumadin, Jantoven.* Retrieved from http://www.medicinenet.com/wararin/article.htm

Oliver, M.J., Edwards, L.J., & Churchill, D.N. (2001). *Impact of sodium and ultrafiltration profiling on hemodialysis-related symptoms.* Retrieved from http://jasn.asnjournals.org/content/12/1/151.full

Olson, J., Talekar, M., Sachdev, M., Castellani, W., De la Cruz, N., Davis, J., … George, M. (2013). *Potassium changes associated with blood transfusion in pediatric patients.* Retrieved from http://ajcp.ascpjournals.org/content/139/6/800.full.pdf+html

Oregon State University (OSU). (2014). *Calcium.* Retrieved from http://lpi.oregonstate.edu/infocenter/minerals/calcium/index.html#summary

Overgaard, D.B., & Dzavik, V. (2008). *Inotropes and vasopressors: review of physiology and clinical use in cardiovascular disease.* Retrieved from http://circ.ahajournals.org/content/118/10/1047.full

Parham, W.A. Mehdirad, A.A., Biermann, K.M., & Fredman, C.S. (2006). *Hyperkalemia revisited.* Retrieved from http://www.ncbi.nlm.nih.gov/pmc/articles/PMC1413606/

Park, B.J., Peck, A.J., Keuhnert, M.J., Newbern, C. Smerker, C., & Comer, F.A. (2004). Lack of SARs transmission among healthcare workers, United States. Retrieved from http://www.ncbi.nlm.nih.gov/pmc/articles/PMC3322937/

Patel, A.M., Adeseun, G.A., Ahmed, I., Mitter, N., Rame, J.E., & Rudnick, M.R. (2013). Published online 2012. *Renal failure in patients with left ventricular assist devices.* Retrieved from

http://cjasn.asnjournals.org/content/early/2012/10/10/CJN.06210612.full

Pearson Education. (2007). *Grading pitting edema.* Retrieved from http://wps.prenhall.com/wps/media/objects/2791/2858109/toolbox/Figure18_24.pdf

Pergola, P.E., Habiba, N.M., & Johnson, J.M. (2004). *Body temperature regulation during hemodialysis in long-term patients: Is it time to change dialysate temperature prescription?* Retrieved from http://www.ncbi.nlm.nih.gov/pubmed/15211448

Pharmacology Weekly. (2014). *Calcium correction for hypoalbuminemia medical calculator.* Retrieved from http://www.pharmacologyweekly.com/app/medical-calculators/calcium-correction-albumin-calculator

Phelps, K.R. (1990). *Edema.* Retrieved from http://www.ncbi.nlm.nih.gov/books/NBK348/

Preidt, R. (2014). *Prescribe blood thinner Pradaxa with caution, study warns.* Retrieved from http://www.webmd.com/heart-disease/news/20141103/prescribe-blood-thinner-pradaxa-with-caution-study-warns

Pruitt, W.C. & Jacobs, M. (2003). *Breathing lessons: Basics of oxygen therapy.* Retrieved from http://www.shulmanusa.com/Nursingpdf/Pruitt%20and%20Jacobs%20-%20Basics%20of%20Oxygen%20Therapy.pd

Pruitt, W.C. & Jacobs, M. (2004). *Interpreting arterial blood gases: Easy as ABC.* Retrieved from http://www.acu.edu.au/__data/assets/pdf_file/0020/54443/Arterial_blood_gases.pdf

Reyer, E. (2013). *The hemodynamic and physiological relevance of continuous central venous oxygenation monitoring: It's not just for sepsis.* Retrieved from http://www.icumed.com/media/402627/M1-1430%20Reyer%20-%20SCVO2%20Oximetry%20White%20Paper%20Rev.01-Web.pdf

Rice, E.K., Isbel, N.M., Becker, G.J., Atkins, R.C., & McMahon, L.P. (2000). *Heroin overdose and myoglobiniric acute renal failure.* Retrieved from http://www.ncbi.nlm.nih.gov/pubmed/11140805

Robbins, K.C. (2006). Hemodialysis: Prevention and management of treatment complications. In A. Molzahn & E. Butera (Eds.), *Contemporary nephrology nursing: Principles and practice.* Pitman, NJ: American Nephrology Nurses' Association.

RxList. (2014). *Lanoxin (Digoxin tablets) drug information: Clinical pharmacology.* Retrieved from http://www.rxlist.com/lanoxin-tablets-drug/clinical-pharmacology.htm

Santos, P.W., Hartle, J.E., & Quarles, L.D. (2014). *Calciphylaxis (calcific uremic arteriolopathy).* Retrieved from http://www.uptodate.com/contents/calciphylaxis-calcific-uremic-arteriolopathy

Shen, J.I., & Winkelmayer, W.C. (2012). *Use and safety of unfractionated heparin for anticoagulation during maintenance hemodialysis.* Retrieved from http://www.ncbi.nlm.nih.gov/pubmed/22560830

Shirazian, S., & Radhakrishnan, J. (2010). Gastrointestinal disorders and renal failure: Exploring the connection: Gastrointestinal bleeding. *Nature Reviews Nephrology, 6,* 480-492. doi:10.1038/nrneph.2010.84

Siegel, J.D., Rhinehart, E., Jackson, M., Chiarello, L., & the Healthcare Infection Control Practices Advisory Committee. (2007). *2007 guideline for isolation precautions: Preventing transmission of infectious agents in healthcare settings.* Retrieved from http://www.cdc.gov/hicpac/2007IP/2007isolationPrecautions.html

Simon, E.E., Hamrahian, S.M., & Teran, F.J. (2014). *Hyponatremia clinical presentation.* Retrieved from http://emedicine.medscape.com/article/242166-clinical

Sinha, A.D., Light, R.P., & Agarwal, R. (2010). *Relative plasma volume monitoring during hemodialysis aids the assessment of dry weight.* Retrieved from http://www.ncbi.nlm.nih.gov/pmc/articles/PMC2819307

Texas Heart Institute. (2012a). *Beta-blockers*. Retrieved from http://www.texasheartinstitute.org/HIC/Topics/Meds/betameds.cfm

Texas Heart Institute. (2012b). *Calcium channel blockers*. Retrieved from http://www.texasheartinstitute.org/HIC/Topics/Meds/calcmeds.cfm

Texas Heart Institute. (2013a). *Antiplatelet therapy*. Retrieved from http://www.texasheart.org/HIC/Topics/Meds/antiplatelet.cfm

Texas Heart Institute. (2013b). *Digitalis medicines*. Retrieved from http://www.texasheart.org/HIC/Topics/Meds/digimeds.cfm

The VA/NIH Acute Renal Failure Trial Network. (2008). Intensity of renal support in critically ill patients with acute kidney injury. *New England Journal of Medicine, 359*(1), 7–20. Retrieved from http://www.ncbi.nlm.nih.gov/pmc/articles/PMC2574780/

Toussaint, N., Cooney, P., & Kerr, P.G. (2006). Review of dialysate calcium concentration in hemodialysis. *Hemodialysis International, 10*, 326–337. doi: 10.1111/j.1542-4758.2006.00125.x Retrieved from http://jasn.asnjournals.org/content/12/1/151.full

University of Michigan Heart Sound and Murmur Library. (n.d.). Retrieved from http://www.med.umich.edu/lrc/psb/heartsounds/

University of Washington Department of Medicine. (n.d.). *Demonstrations: Heart sounds and murmurs*. Retrieved from http://depts.washington.edu/physdx/heart/demo.html

van der Sande, F.M., Cheriex, E.C., van Kuijk, W.H., & Leunissen, K.M. (1998). *Effect of dialysate calcium concentrations on intradialytic blood pressure course in cardiac-compromised patients*. Retrieved from http://www.ncbi.nlm.nih.gov/pubmed/9669433

Warkentin, T.D., Levine, M.N., Hirsh, J., Horsewood, P., Roberts, R.S., Gent, M., & Kelton, J.G. (1995). Heparin-induced thrombocytopenia in patients treated with low-molecular-weight heparin or unfractionated heparin. *The New England Journal of Medicine, 332*, 1330-1336.

Wendland, E.M., & Kaplan, A.A. (2012). *A proposed approach to the dialysis prescription in severely hyponatremic patients with end-stage renal disease*. Retrieved from http://www.ncbi.nlm.nih.gov/pubmed/21906168

White, J.J., Mulloy, L.L., Caruana, R.J., & Ing R.S. (2008). Isolated ultrafiltration. In A.R. Nissenson & R.N. Fine (Eds.), *Handbook of dialysis therapy*. Philadelphia: Saunders Elsevier.

Appendix 3.1. Sample Acute Hemodialysis Flowsheet

Source: Western Nephrology Acute Dialysis, Denver, CO. Used with permission.

WESTERN ACUTE DIALYSIS, P.C.
HEMODIALYSIS RECORD

DATE _____ # of Setups _____
LOCATION: Dialysis Rm ____ Pt Rm ____
PT ROOM # _____ OP Unit ____
# of Pt's Run: 1 ____ 2 ____ 3 ____
HOSPITAL: _____
PATIENT NAME: _____

HEMODIALYSIS ORDERS:
Dialyzer: _____ Total Tx Time: _____ Time On: _____
BFR: _____ Ultrafiltration: _____ Time Off: _____
Dialysate: K⁺ ____ CA⁺⁺ ____ HCO₃ ____ **Dialysate △s:**
Programmable Sodium: _____ K⁺ ____ Ca⁺ ____
Heparin: Temp: _____ HCO₃ ____
Bolus: _____ **LABS TO DRAW:** **LAB RESULTS**
Continuous: _____ Chem Screen CA⁺⁺ Mg⁺⁺
Off At: _____ CBC PO₄
Total: _____ Coag Albumin

Fluid To Remove:
Prime/RB _____
IV Fluids _____
Replacement Fluid _____
PO Fluids _____
PRBC _____
Machine Set To Remove: _____
Total Fluids Given During Tx _____
Liters Processed _____
Consent Signed ____ Yes ____ No

PATIENT ASSESSMENT: Diagnosis: _____

Pulmonary	**Cardiovascular**	**Edema**	**Access**
Breath Sounds	Rhythm	None Ext	Type: R L
Rate/Rhythm	Comments	Slight Sacral	IJ SC
O₂ Mode/Rate	Neuro AAO x	Moderate Abd	Fem
SPO₂	Responds to Sound	Pitting Orbital	Fistula
FIO₂	Pain No Response		

Bruit _____ Insertion Date _____
Redness _____ Dr. _____
Edema _____ Drsg. Chg'd Y N
Bruising _____ Catheter Volume
Drainage _____ A ___ ml V ___ ml

	BP	APICAL	TEMP
PRE		bpm	
POST		bpm	

MACHINE CHECKLIST
Bleach ____ Neg. ____ Pos.
Chloramines ____
Alarm Test ____
Pressure Test ____
Conductivity ____ pH ____

EDUCATION
Modality Training ☐
Family/Patient Education ☐
Printed Instructions ☐
Verbal Instructions ☐

IV Medications/Amt _____

EPO _____
Total Hourly _____

I+O
INTAKE (Since last Rx) ____ kg
OUTPUT (Since last Rx) ____ kg
Cartridge # _____

Dialysis Mach # _____
GAIN ____ kg DRY WT ____ kg
LOSS ____ kg LAST TX POST WT ____ kg

RO Mach # _____
° PRE/WT
° POST/WT

NURSING NOTES
Verified correct patient, procedure, site and equipment Initial _____ Timeout Performed _____

TIME	BP	PULSE	BLOOD FLOW	FLUIDS GIVEN	UFR	ACT	PRESSURES Art/Neg	VEN	TMP

Staff Signature/Initials _____

Appendix 3.2. Sample Acute Hemodialysis Order

Source: Western Acute Dialysis in Denver, Colorado. Used with permission.

☐ **STAT**

Hemodialysis Orders
Meditech category: Hospitalist/Internal Medicine
Meditech Name:

Ⓜ

Important: Pharmacy must receive a copy of all medication orders (new & change orders). Please scan to Pharmacy As Soon As Possible.

A Therapeutic or generic equivalent drug approved by the Pharmacy may be substituted.

Orders	Progress Notes

Rev: 07/07   **PPO.955**
HEMODIALYSIS ORDERS
Treatment Date: _____ Allergies: _____
Dialyzer: ☐ F160NR   ☐ PF 14OH   ☐ Other: _____
 	
Tx time: _____ BFR: _____ ml/min DFR _____ ml/min UFR: _____kg
PUF for _____time_____kg
☐ Calculate Kt/V   EDW _____ kg
 	
Dialysate:
Temp: Normal (37C) or _____C
☐   Potassium _____ and adjust per protocol
☐   Potassium_____ do not adjust per protocol
     Serum Potassium   Dialysate Potassium
     > 5   mmol/L   2 mEq/L
     4 – 5   mmol/L   3 mEq/L
     3.5 – 3.9   mmol/L   3.5 mEq/L
     < 3.5   mmol/L   4 mEq/L
 	
☐   Calcium _____ Notify MD of Calcium levels > 11 mg/dL or < 7.5 mg/dL
☐   Bicarb mEq per liter_____   Na_____
☐   Programmable Sodium   150_____ 145_____ 140_____
 	
☐ Profile 1: UF Custom step ▦   Na Progr Curve 150-140 ⌐
☐ Profile 2: UF Constant   Na Progr Curve 148-138 ⌐
☐ Profile 3: UF Step 1.5 / 1 / 0.5 ⌐   Na Constant _____
☐ Profile 4: UF Progressive Curve ⌐   Na Constant _____
☐ Profile 5: UF Step 1.5 / 1 / 0.5 ⌐   Na Step 14.8 / 14.5 / 13.8 ⌐
☐ Profile 6: UF Progressive Curve ⌐   Na Progr Curve 148-138 ⌐
 	
Anticoagulation (for hemodialysis treatment only):
☐   Heparin bolus_____units; hourly_____units; off at _____min
☐   None
☐   Other; Specify: _____
☐   Review anticoagulation orders with MD if patient already on anti coag meds (Such as: Aggrastat, Alteplase, Aspirin, Coumadin, Fragmin, Heparin IV or Sub-Q, Hirudin, Lovenox, Plavix, ReoPro, Xigris)
 	
Weights:
☐   Daily   ☐ Dialysis days only   ☐ Pre and post dialysis treatment
 	
Labs:
☐   No labs
☐   Draw early to be on chart by 6am_____ OR dialysis staff to draw pre-treatment_____
☐   Basic Metabolic/Chem Panel ☐ Comprehensive Metabolic/Chem Panel
☐   Renal   ☐ CBC   ☐ Albumin   ☐ Calcium   ☐ Phosphorus
☐   Magnesium   ☐ Vanco Random   ☐ Pt/PTT
☐   T& C for _____units Leuko poor RBC's   ☐ Give PRBC's_____# units
 	
Signed: _____MD Date/Time: _____
	Medications:
	☐ **HYPOTENSION:**
	   ☐ NS Bolus_____ml PRN to maximum of _____ml
	   ☐ Albumin 25%_____gm for SBP less than ____ max of ____gm
	   ☐ Hypertonic Saline IV per protocol
	   ☐ Pressors: _____
	   ☐ Other: _____
	☐ Mannitol _____gms Instructions: _____
	☐ Epogen _____units IV/Sub-Q M, W, F / T, T, S / Q dialysis day
	                       / weekly on _____
	
	Access:
	☐ Fistula ☐ Graft
	     Special Instructions: _____
	☐ Catheter pack with:☐ Heparin ☐ TPA ☐ 4% Sodium Citrate
	     Volume = A _____ ml V _____ ml
	
	Signed: _____MD Date/Time: _____
	
	Progress Notes

FORM BARCODE LABEL HERE	**PATIENT BARCODE LABEL MUST BE PLACED IN THIS SPACE**

Appendix 3.3. Catheter Instructions for the Patient

Source: Creighton Nephrology, Creighton University, Omaha, Nebraska. Used with permission.

Catheter Instructions for the Patient

Name:_____Date:_____

Catheter Type:_____Placement Date:_____

Catheter Placed by: Dr._____

Central Venous Access Devices (Catheters) may be:
   A. Temporary
   B. Permanent (Perm Cath)

A. Temporary
   1. Description: A device used on a temporary basis for vascular cannulation and circulatory access for hemodialysis until a permanent method can be prepared, or until a different mode of dialysis therapy can be instituted. These devices are currently made of carbothane, Teflon, polyurethane or silicone, all biocompatible materials.
   2. A hemodialysis catheter is needed when:
      a) Immediate access to the venous circulation is needed for in-patients experiencing acute kidney failure
      b) While waiting for a graft or AV fistula to mature
      c) After removal of permanent access because of an infection
      d) Before initiation of peritoneal dialysis or during episodes of peritonitis

   3. Types (usually based on location of placement)
      a) Subclavian vein catheter (SVC)
      b) Jugular vein catheter (IJC)
      c) Femoral vein catheter (FVC)

B. Permanent Catheter
   1. Description: Operative placement of dual or single lumen catheter in the internal jugular or subclavian is tunneled subcutaneously to exit site on chest wall. The biocompatible cuff is designed to inhibit infection in tunnel and provide catheter immobilization in the chest, keeping it in place for months.

POSSIBLE COMPLICATIONS OF CATHETER PLACEMENT

   1. Immediate postinsertion complications as traumatic hemo or pneumothorax (air or blood in the chest cavity); inadvertent subclavian artery puncture; brachial plexus injury; air embolism (air entering the blood circulation). A chest x-ray is done postinsertion, before the catheter is used, to assure proper placement/position of a catheter.
   2. Other complications include the following:
      a) Bleeding at insertion site during hemodialysis or after catheter removal.
      b) Hematoma (bruise) at insertion site.
      c) Thrombosis or clotting creating resultant poor blood flow.

Continued on next page

Appendix 3.3. Catheter Instructions for the Patient (continued)

Source: Creighton Nephrology, Creighton University, Omaha, Nebraska. Used with permission.

d) Emboli (air or dislodged blood clots)

e) Cardiac arrhythmias (abnormal heart irregularity).

f) Infection and Sepsis (an infection in the blood). Commonly infection of insertion site especially when catheter left in place for longer periods of time.

g) Other complications may arise as kinked catheter, anchor suture removal, accidental removal of entire catheter, accidental unclamping, or uncapping of catheter.

CARE OF YOUR CATHETER

1. The catheter dressing is changed at each dialysis treatment by a Registered Nurse or a Licensed Practical Nurse under strict aseptic technique. It may be done at the start, during or after dialysis treatment. As a patient, you are not allowed to change the catheter dressing or to manipulate your catheter in any way. However, if there is a dire need to change dressing or manipulate catheter, please call the nurse for assessment of situation and to receive instructions. Never use scissors in handling catheters and dressings.

2. Keep your catheter exit site or dressing clean, sterile, and dry. Do not get dressing wet when showering or bathing. If dressing accidentally gets wet, call clinic nurse.

3. Report immediately to the nurse (either by phone or during your clinic visit) the following signs or symptoms:
   a) Dressing soaked with any type of discharge from exit site
   b) Any foul smell from catheter site
   c) Blood soaked dressing
   d) Uncapped or unclamped catheter
   e) Fever of any cause and/or unknown cause
   f) Pain, redness, swelling around catheter site

EMERGENCY SITUATIONS

1. When bleeding from unclamped and uncapped catheter, press with thumb and forefinger the two clamps until you hear it click or feel it snap. If you find it difficult to do pinching action, bend or kink catheter just below the caps, or if this is not possible for you to do, cover open ports with fingers. Call the clinic or physician office immediately. If blood loss from uncapped/unclamped catheter is great and/or you feel dizzy, lightheaded, shortness of breath, or chest pain, call emergency 911, lie down, and limit ambulation.

2. When bleeding from accidental removal/yanking of catheter, immediately apply direct firm pressure over catheter site, lie down and limit movements and ambulation. If site continues to bleed for more than 15 minutes and/or you feel dizziness, lightheaded, shortness of breath, or chest pain, call emergency 911. Continue to apply direct pressure until help arrives.

3. When there is continuous bleeding from the catheter exit or the dressing site a few days after catheter placement, call the physician office or dialysis unit for instruction. If site continues to bleed for more than 15 minutes and/or you feel dizziness, lightheaded shortness of breath, or chest pain, call emergency 911. Continue to apply direct firm pressure until help arrives.

4. When accidental removal of a new catheter dressing occurs, call the clinic.

Appendix 3.4. Patient Catheter Release Form

Source: Creighton Nephrology, Creighton University, Omaha, Nebraska. Used with permission.

Patient Catheter Release Form

I, _____, having a temporary/permanent catheter as a vascular access for hemodialysis, have been advised and educated on the importance of catheter care and emergency procedures.

I have been shown and have returned demonstration on how to handle threatening situations involving catheters such as bleeding or leaking from exit site, bleeding from uncapped or unclamped catheter, and/or accidental removal of my catheter.

I have also been given a Catheter Instruction Sheet that I can take home and review or use as a referral when the need arises.

Outside the clinical setting, I agree to assume full responsibility for any actions I would take in case of catheter emergency and will not hold Dialysis Clinic, Inc. responsible for any outcomes of such actions.

Addendum: If the patient is unable to understand and/or perform the catheter procedures, a family member must be instructed on the above emergency care.

Nurse's Comments:

_____

_____

_____   _____
Date   Patient/Legal Representative Signature

_____   _____
Date   Clinic Representative – Name and Title

Water Treatment in the Acute Care Setting

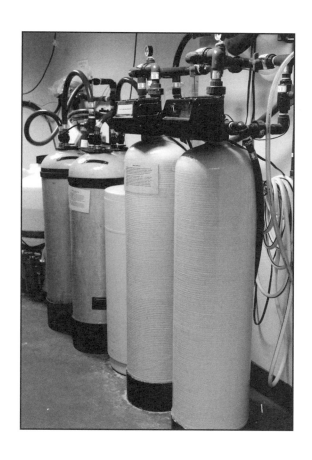

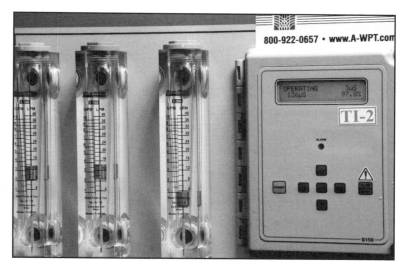

Chapter Editor
Helen F. Williams, MSN, BSN, RN, CNN

Author
Glenda M. Payne, MS, RN, CNN

CHAPTER **4**

Water Treatment in the Acute Care Setting

This offering for **1.4 contact hours** is provided by the American Nephrology Nurses' Association (ANNA).

American Nephrology Nurses' Association is accredited as a provider of continuing nursing education by the American Nurses Credentialing Center Commission on Accreditation.

ANNA is a provider approved by the California Board of Registered Nursing, provider number CEP 00910.

This CNE offering meets the continuing nursing education requirements for certification and recertification by the Nephrology Nursing Certification Commission (NNCC).

To be awarded contact hours for this activity, read this chapter in its entirety. Then complete the CNE evaluation found at **www.annanurse.org/corecne** and submit it; or print it, complete it, and mail it in. Contact hours are not awarded until the evaluation for the activity is complete.

Example of reference for Chapter 4 in APA format. One author for entire chapter.

Payne, G. . (2015). Water treatment in the acute care setting. In C.S. Counts (Ed.), *Core curriculum for nephrology nursing: Module 4. Acute kidney injury* (6th ed., pp. 107-118). Pitman, NJ: American Nephrology Nurses' Association.

Interpreted: Chapter author. (Date). Title of chapter. In …

Cover photos by Counts/Morganello.

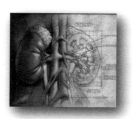

CHAPTER 4

Water Treatment in the Acute Care Setting

Purpose

To provide basic information regarding water treatment for nurses who provide acute hemodialysis.

Objectives

Upon completion of this chapter, the learner will be able to:
1. Discuss the responsibilities of the acute hemodialysis nurse in ensuring safe water and dialysate.
2. Describe two ways the quality of the water used for hemodialysis is measured.
3. List minimum treatment components necessary to produce water for dialysis.

I. **Water for acute hemodialysis (HD) may be prepared using a central water treatment system or individual water treatment systems that may be portable.**

A. Central water treatment systems (systems that deliver water to three or more machines) are described in detail in the chronic HD section of the *Core Curriculum* (see Module 3, Chapter 2, Section B, Ensuring Water and Dialysate Safety and Quality for Chronic Hemodialysis).
   1. In the description of the central water treatment system, references are made to requirements of the Centers for Medicare and Medicaid Services (CMS) for end-stage renal disease (ESRD) facilities providing outpatient dialysis.
   2. Although CMS regulations for outpatient dialysis facilities do not apply to acute dialysis services, those requirements are based on the Association for the Advancement of Medical Instrumentation (AAMI) recommendations.
   3. State surveyors and surveyors from accreditation agencies such as The Joint Commission (TJC) would view the AAMI recommendations as describing the minimum standard for safe practice.

B. Individual water treatment systems will be described in this chapter.

II. **Ensuring the water used for HD is safe.**

A. The most important water treatment "component" is the human element.
   1. Selecting and training personnel to recognize the risks to patients from water and dialysate is a critical management responsibility.
   2. Staff assigned to operate or monitor the water treatment system should complete a training program specific to the water treatment system in use that describes the individual's responsibilities for the maintenance and operation of that system.
   3. Audits of the practices related to water treatment and dialysate preparation should be conducted routinely to verify assigned staff members follow expected procedures and perform as expected.
   4. Education of all responsible staff members should include the "whys" for each step in the water treatment and dialysate preparation, with emphasis on the reasons that safe water is critical to patient safety. Understanding "why" decreases the risks of staff members altering expected practice or taking shortcuts.

B. Responsibility for safe water and safe dialysate.
   1. Each person operating an individual water treatment system is responsible for ensuring that system is safe for use.
   2. The operator of the equipment is responsible to

follow facility procedures and to notify the nurse in charge and the responsible biomedical personnel if there is any question or problem with the system.

3. The registered nurse (RN) in charge is responsible for the following.
   a. Knowing the basics of water and dialysate safety.
   b. Monitoring those working with the system to ensure that tests are performed accurately and results are recorded correctly.
   c. Notifying the responsible physician immediately if problems cannot be resolved quickly.
   d. Ensuring the responsible physician is aware of any issue with the water and dialysate systems.
4. The nurse manager is responsible for ensuring all staff assigned any responsibility for water treatment or dialysate preparation are qualified by training and have the proper documentation of current competency.
5. The medical director or physician responsible for the acute HD unit and the governing body of the hospital are ultimately responsible for the water and dialysate systems.

C. For more about the risks of unsafe water and dialysate to patients who require hemodialysis, see Module 3, Chapter 2, Hemodialysis, Section B, Ensuring Water and Dialysate Safety and Quality for Chronic Hemodialysis.

III. Measuring the quality of HD water.

A. Chemical contaminates. See Table 4.1 for the maximum chemical contaminate levels allowed in water used for HD.

B. Microbiological contaminates. See Tables 4.2 and 4.3 for the maximum and action levels for bacteria and endotoxin allowed in water used for HD. The AAMI adopted the International Standards Organization's (ISO) documents with a deviation that allows the continued use of the previous methodology for cultures (i.e., time, temperature, and media).

IV. Regulatory requirements and standards for water used for hemodialysis.

A. The Association for the Advancement of Medical Instrumentation (AAMI) is a voluntary standard-setting body that develops recommended practices and standards for healthcare equipment, medical devices, and products.
   1. The AAMI standards program consists of more than 100 technical committees and working groups that produce standards, recommended

Table 4.1

List of Maximum Allowable Levels of Chemicals

Maximum allowable levels of toxic chemicals and dialysis fluid electrolytes in dialysis water [a]	
Contaminant	Maximum concentration mg/L [b]
Contaminants with documented toxicity in hemodialysis	
Aluminum	0.01
Total chlorine	0.1
Copper	0.1
Fluoride	0.2
Lead	0.005
Nitrate (as N)	2
Sulfate	100
Zinc	0.1
Electrolytes normally included in dialysis fluid	
Calcium	2 (0.05 mmol/L)
Magnesium	4 (0.15 mmol/L)
Potassium	8 (0.2 mmol/L)
Sodium	70 (3.0 mmol/L)

[a] The physician has the ultimate responsibility for ensuring the quality of water used for dialysis.
[b] Unless otherwise noted.

Maximum allowable levels of trace elements in dialysis water	
Contaminant	Maximum concentration mg/L
Antimony	0.006
Arsenic	0.005
Barium	0.1
Beryllium	0.0004
Cadmium	0.001
Chromium	0.014
Mercury	0.0002
Selenium	0.09
Silver	0.005
Thallium	0.002

Source: ANSI/AAMI 13959:2014, Tables 1 and 2 (ANSI/AAMI, 2014a). Used with permission.

practices, and technical information reports for medical devices (go to http://www.aami.org for more information).

2. The AAMI Standards and Recommended Practices represent a national consensus. Many of the AAMI standards have been approved by the American National Standards Institute (ANSI) as American National Standards.

3. For hemodialysis, the AAMI Renal Disease and Detoxification Committee (RDD) comprises representatives from major manufacturers of dialysis machines and supplies, outpatient and hospital providers of dialysis, professional organizations, and regulatory agencies including CMS, the Centers for Disease Control (CDC), and the Food & Drug Administration (FDA).

   a. The RDD Committee develops consensus standards in all areas related to HD (e.g., water and dialysis quality, water treatment equipment, dialysis equipment, and reprocessing of hemodialyzers).

   b. ANSI/AAMI RD:52:2004 was incorporated into the 2008 update of the ESRD Conditions for Coverage (CfC) for outpatient dialysis facilities by CMS. Many acute units choose to follow the ANSI/AAMI RD:52:2004 recommendations for water quality and safety (AAMI, 2004).

   c. In 2011, the AAMI adopted a set of international standards as replacement for ANSI/AAMI RD:52, and in 2014, adopted a United States (U.S.) deviation to those documents (see below). At the time of publication of this text, CMS had not updated the ESRD CfC to incorporate these updated standards.

   d. In the context of this document, the statement "recommended by the AAMI" means that this expectation is present as a recommended practice in both the ANSI/AAMI RD 52 document and the current AAMI documents related to water and dialysate (see Table 4.4).

B. International Standards Organization (ISO). While the AAMI is the organization that develops medical device standards in the United States, ISO serves this function internationally.

Table 4.2

Comparison of RD 52 and ANSI/AAMI Recommendations for Dialysis Water Microbiological Quality

Contaminant	AAMI Max Level	AAMI Action Level	RD 52 Max Level	RD 52 Action Level
Total viable bacteria count (TVC)	< 100 CFU/mL	50 CFU/mL	< 200 CFU/mL	50 CFU/mL
Endotoxin	< 0.25 EU/mL	0.125 EU/mL	< 2 EU/mL	1 EU/mL

Source: Adapted from ANSI/AAMI 11663:2014 (AAMI, 2014c).

Table 4.3

Comparison of RD 52 and ANSI/AAMI Recommendations for Dialysis Fluid (Dialysate) Microbiological Quality

Contaminant	AAMI Max Level	AAMI Action Level	RD 52 Max Level	RD 52 Action Level
Total viable bacteria count (TVC)	< 100 CFU/mL	50 CFU/mL	< 200 CFU/mL	50 CFU/mL
Endotoxin	< 0.5 EU/mL	0.25 EU/mL	< 2 EU/mL	1 EU/mL

Source: Adapted from ANSI/AAMI 11663:2014 (AAMI, 2014c).

1. The AAMI is a participant in the ISO process. It is advantageous for both the manufacturer and the user to have standards that are congruent across the globe.

2. In 2011, the AAMI adopted a suite of five ISO documents as the U.S. recommended practices for hemodialysis (refer to Table 4.4). In 2014, the AAMI adopted a U.S. deviation to those documents.

   a. The major differences in the AAMI documents that CMS adopted as regulation for outpatient dialysis facilities in 2008 and the five ANSI/AAMI documents that are the current AAMI recommendations are in the action and maximum allowable levels for microbiological contamination.

   (1) The ANSI/AAMI documents recommend lower maximum levels for colony forming units (CFU) for bacteria, and lower maximum and action levels for endotoxin (refer to Tables 4.2 and 4.3).

   (2) The ANSI/AAMI documents include a deviation from the ISO documents. This U.S. deviation allows the continuation of use of the culture methodology described in RD 52.

   (a) Incubation time: 48 hours.

Table 4.4

Documents Adopted by AAMI in Replacement of RD 52

Identification #	Title
ANSI/AAMI 11663:2014	Quality of dialysis fluid for hemodialysis and other related therapies
ANSI/AAMI 13958:2014	Concentrates for hemodialysis and related therapies
ANSI/AAMI 13959:2014	Water for hemodialysis and other related therapies
ANSI/AAMI 26722:2014	Water treatment equipment for hemodialysis applications and related therapies
ANSI/AAMI 23500:2014	Guidance for the preparation and quality management of fluids for hemodialysis and related therapies

(b) Incubation temperature: 35°C (95°F).
(c) Culture media: Trypticase soy agar (TSA) or standard methods agar and plate count agar (also known as TGYE).

C. CMS –Hospital Conditions of Coverage (CoP). To receive reimbursement for the care of Medicare-covered patients, hospitals must meet the CMS Hospital CoP. While the word "dialysis" appears only under the Condition of Discharge Planning, the following hospital conditions and standards include requirements applicable for acute dialysis services (CMS, 2014). (Download this entire document at http://www.cms.gov/Regulations-and-Guidance/Guidance/Manuals/Downloads/som107ap_a_hospitals.pdf).
1. §482.12 CoP: Governing Body (CMS tag: A0043).
2. §482.12 (e) Standard: Contracted services: "The governing body must be responsible for services furnished in the hospital whether or not they are furnished under contracts. The governing body must ensure that services permit the hospital to comply with all applicable conditions of participation and standards for the contracted services" (CMS tag: A0083).
3. §482.12 (e) (1) Standard: "The governing body must ensure that the services performed under a contract are provided in a safe and effective manner" (CMS tag: A0084).
4. §482.13 (c) (2) Standard under Patient Rights. "The patient has the right to receive care in a safe setting" (CMS tag: A0144).
5. §482.21 CoP: Quality Assessment and Performance Improvement Program. "The hospital must develop, implement, and maintain an effective, ongoing, hospital-wide, data-driven quality assessment and performance improvement program. The hospital's governing body must ensure that the program reflects the complexity of the hospital's organization and services, involves all hospital departments and services (including those services furnished under contract or arrangement), and focuses on indicators related to improved health outcomes and the prevention and reduction of medical errors" (CMS tag: A0263).
6. §482.23 (b) (3) Standard: "A registered nurse must supervise and evaluate the nursing care for each patient" (CMS tag: A0395).
7. §482.23 (b) (6) Standard: "Non-employee licensed nurses who are working in the hospital must adhere to the policies and procedures of the hospital" (CMS tag: A0398).
8. §482.41 CoP: Physical Environment (CMS tag: A0700).
9. §482.41(c) Standard: Facilities: "The hospital must maintain adequate facilities for its services" (CMS tag: A0722). Survey procedures for this Standard include: "Review the facility's water supply and distribution system to ensure that the water quality is acceptable for its intended use (drinking water, irrigation water, lab water, etc.). Review the facility water quality monitoring and, as appropriate, treatment system" (CMS, 2014).
10. §482.41(c) (2) Standard: "Facilities, supplies, and equipment must be maintained to ensure an acceptable level of safety and quality" (CMS tag: A0724). Survey procedures for this requirement include, "There must be a regular periodic maintenance and testing program for medical devices and equipment. A qualified individual such as a clinical or biomedical engineer or other qualified maintenance person must monitor, test,

calibrate, and maintain the equipment periodically in accordance with the manufacturer's recommendations and Federal and State laws and regulations. Equipment maintenance may be conducted using hospital staff, contracts, or through a combination of hospital staff and contracted services" (CMS, 2014).

11. §482.42 CoP: Infection Control. "There must be an active program for the prevention, control, and investigation of infections and communicable diseases" (CMS tag: A0747).

12. §482.42(b) (1) Standard: Responsibilities of Chief Executive Officer, Medical Staff, and Director of Nursing Services. (2) "Be responsible for the implementation of successful corrective action plans in affected problem areas" (CMS tag: A0756).

13. §482.43 CoP Discharge Planning. "The hospital must have in effect a discharge planning process that applies to all patients. The hospital's policies and procedures must be specified in writing." (CMS tag: A0799). Also note that many of the Standards under this CoP will also apply to acute HD services.

D. Accrediting organizations. There are four organizations that have "deemed" status for hospitals.
  (1) "Deemed status" means the surveys by these organizations are deemed to meet the requirements of CMS CoPs, and thus exempt hospitals accredited by those organizations from routine state surveys for CMS requirements.
  (2) The four accrediting organizations with deemed status are as follows.
    (a) The Joint Commission (TJC).
    (b) The American Osteopathic Association's (AOA) Healthcare Facilities Accreditation Program (HFAP).
    (c) DNV GL Healthcare (DNV GL).
    (d) Center for Improvement in Healthcare Quality (CIHQ).

E. While survey procedures and focus vary, all surveys focus on patient safety, and expect hospitals to continuously monitor the outcomes of the acute dialysis program, to analyze the monitoring data, and take action to continuously improve quality.

V. State hospital licensing requirements.

A. Most states require hospitals to be licensed. If a state licensing survey is conducted, the acute HD services would be included in that survey.

B. It is important to be aware of any specific requirements under those state licensing rules that address dialysis. For example, the state of Texas has fairly extensive rule language related to water treatment for acute HD (http://www.dshs.state.tx.us/hfp/rules.shtm#hosp_gen).

VI. Portable water treatment systems for acute dialysis.

A. Basic vs. optional components.
  1. Basic, at a minimum:
    a. A method to remove total chlorine.
    b. A purification component, i e., reverse osmosis (RO) or deionization (DI).
    c. A water quality monitor is necessary to ensure safe water for acute HD (AAMI, 2014a).
  2. Optional water treatment equipment.
    a. May include components such as water softeners or sediment filters.
    b. Dependent on need as defined through the analysis of the hospital's source water.
    c. Must follow the manufacturer's guidance for the purification component.

B. Maintenance and repair of dialysis equipment must not be done when a patient is connected to the equipment.

C. Utilities.
  1. Backflow prevention: acute water treatment systems are generally connected to the incoming city water. Local plumbing codes may require the use of a device to prevent backflow of fluid (which could be disinfectant) from the water treatment system into the city's water distribution system.
  2. Electrical supply.
    a. The manufacturer's guidance for the water treatment components and the dialysis machine should be followed. Generally a separate power source is required for each.
    b Careful maintenance of the water treatment and dialysis machines ensures electrical leakage is minimized. This equipment is frequently used in environments where life support equipment is also in use. Testing for electrical leakage should be done:
      (1) At least annually, and
      (2) After any repair to the electrical power system.
  3. Drain: Spent dialysate and the reject water from reverse osmosis (RO) should be discharged to drain in a way that does not contaminate the patient's environment.
    a. If a dedicated drain is not available, a sink may be used if it can be dedicated to this purpose

during the dialysis treatment; it should be cleaned and disinfected afterward.
   b. An air gap between the discharge hose and the drain must be maintained to prevent backflow into the equipment.

D. Pretreatment components. A portable water treatment system should not be operated without all its pretreatment components online.
   1. Softener.
      a. The manufacturer's guidance for the purification device will determine if a softener is required.
      b. Portable softeners do not include a brine tank. They must be regenerated off-line (not during patient treatment) using a brine tank and a water source.
      c. If the hospital centrally softens the potable water supply, the engineering department should be informed of potential negative impact on the dialysis equipment if the central softener is regenerated during dialysis treatments.
   2. Carbon filtration.
      a. Previous AAMI recommendations made a blanket exception for portable dialysis to the requirement for two carbon adsorption filters and a 10-minute Empty Bed Contact Time (EBCT) because of the weight the tanks added to the equipment carts.
         (1) With the advent of newer technology, both in different types of carbon filters and in portable cart design, there is less reason for this exception. If at all possible, each acute dialysis water treatment system should include redundant carbon filtration and a 10-minute EBCT.
         (2) Patients needing acute dialysis may be more susceptible to harm from exposure to chlorine breakthrough.
         (3) If it is not possible to provide redundant carbon filtration, more frequent monitoring for total chlorine during treatment should be done.
      b. EBCT: a 10 minute-EBCT refers to the volume of water in the media space (if the tank was empty of media) that would run the reverse osmosis for 10 minutes. For more information about EBCT, see Module 3, Chapter 2, Section B, Ensuring Water and Dialysate Safety and Quality for Chronic Hemodialysis.
      c. Testing should be done before each treatment to verify that the level of total chlorine is less than 0.1mg/L.
         (1) The equipment should run for at least 15 minutes before the test sample is drawn to ensure that the water tested has not been

sitting in the carbon media for longer than the EBCT.
         (2) According to the AAMI, when the water treatment system is used for longer treatments, such as continuous veno-venous hemodialysis (CVVHD), continuous venovenous hemodiafiltration (CVVHDF), or sustained low-efficiency daily dialysis (SLEDD), testing may be performed approximately every 8 hours if the EBCT of the carbon media is based on a dialysate flow rate of at least 500 mL/min, and the actual dialysate flow rate is not more than 300 mL/min (AAMI 23500, 2014a).
      d. Carbon options.
         (1) Granulated activated carbon (GAC), if used, should have a minimum iodine rating of 900 or equivalent, be virgin carbon (i.e., non-regenerated) and have a mesh size of 12 x 40 or smaller.
            (a) If possible, two tanks in series (plumbed so that the water exiting one tank goes into the second tank) with 10-minute EBCT should be used.
            (b) In acute settings, exchange carbon tanks are used. These tanks are not back-washable, and must be exchanged for tanks filled with unused carbon. Because carbon provides an excellent media for bacterial growth, the tanks should be changed out frequently, even if there has been no breakthrough of total chlorine. Follow the manufacturer's recommendation for exchange. In the absence of such guidance, replace the carbon media at least every 6 months.
         (2) Carbon block: activated carbon block technology uses a blend of fine activated carbon and a binder, mixed together, molded, and hardened. The finer mesh size of the carbon allows faster and greater adsorption capacity than the same volume of GAC. The uniform pores of the carbon block do not support "channeling," so that water flows through more open pores, increasing the contact time.
            (a) Carbon block filters are smaller and lighter in weight than GAC.
            (b) The manufacturers of carbon block technology used for dialysis water treatment must provide evidence to the user that the carbon block provides adsorption capacity equivalent to 10-minute EBCT when a single dialysis machine is connected to the portable water treatment system.

(3) Hybrid systems: the portable system for carbon adsorption may include one GAC tank, followed by one carbon block for polishing, with a testing port between.
3. Cartridge filters: a cartridge filter may be placed postcarbon to remove particles of carbon fines that could damage the purification component.

E. Water purification (treatment) components.
1. Reverse osmosis (RO).
   a. Daily monitoring of the RO should include both percent rejection and product-water conductivity. Monitoring both parameters is necessary because an increase in the feed-water contaminants could mean the product water is not suitable for use for dialysis, even though the percent rejection remains high.
   b. In the event the water quality falls below the set limits for conductivity or rejection, there should be a means to prevent the product water from reaching the patient. This could be an automatic divert to drain valve, RO shutdown, or immediate response by the operator.
   c. Maintenance should include disinfection of the RO as bacteria can grow through the membrane.
      (1) The disinfection schedule should follow the manufacturer's guidance.
      (2) More frequent disinfection should be considered if the equipment is not operated for several days or if test results above the action levels demonstrate that the recommended disinfection schedule is not sufficient.
2. Deionization (DI).
   a. AAMI recommends use of two portable mixed-bed DI tanks (i.e., tanks that contain both cation- and anion-attracting ions) in a worker-polisher configuration. If separate cation and anion tanks are used, they should be followed by a mixed-bed tank (AAMI 23500, 2014a).
   b. Must be continuously monitored for resistivity using a temperature-compensated audible and visual alarm.
   c. Must include a system to prevent product water from reaching the patient if the resistivity of the water falls to 1 MΩ·cm or less.
   d. Must be followed by an ultrafilter or endotoxin-retentive filter because DI does not remove bacteria or endotoxin and can add to the bioburden because the DI resin bed supports bacterial growth.

F. Posttreatment components. Endotoxin retentive filter. AAMI recommends that in-line dialysate filters be used in acute dialysis (AAMI 23500, 2014a).

1. Patients requiring acute HD may be more vulnerable to infection.
2. Acute dialysis equipment is often used intermittently and is subject to frequent connection and disconnection, which presents greater opportunity for microbiological contamination.

G. Distribution system.
1. Direct feed – portable water treatment systems provide water directly to the dialysis machine, without a loop or a storage tank.
2. Central system – with indirect feed provides water to several dialysis machines after circulating from a storage tank through a loop.

VII.   Ensuring safe water for patient treatment.

A. Daily monitoring.
1. Chlorine testing.
   a. Test sensitivity. The testing method must be sufficiently sensitive to identify levels of total chlorine of less than 0.1 mg/L.
   b. Timing.
      (1) Test before each patient treatment if using individual water treatment equipment.
      (2) If using a central water treatment system, test before each shift of patients or every 4 hours.
      (3) All tests should be done after the system has been running for at least 15 minutes.
   c. Location of testing port.
      (1) The chlorine test should be run on a sample of water taken from between the two carbon filters.
      (2) This allows monitoring of the function of the first tank and provides a level of safety should the first tank fail.
   d. Test results.
      (1) If the test result after the first tank is > 0.1 ppm total chlorine, notify the physician responsible and test after the second tank.
      (2) If the test after the second tank is > 0.1 ppm, stop treatment until the carbon tanks can be replaced or other equipment secured.
      (3) If the test after the first tank is > 0.1 ppm, but the test after the second tank is < 0.1 ppm, treatment can continue with more frequent monitoring after the second tank (e.g., every 30 to 60 minutes). Arrangements should be made to exchange the carbon tanks prior to using the system again.
   e. Common errors in testing include the following.
      (1) Not running the equipment for at least 15 minutes prior to taking the test sample.

(2) Using a test method that does not test to 0.1 ppm.

(3) Not following the directions for the test (e.g., test sample volume, timing, use of a blank).

(4) Errors in recording the results.

f. Audits of practice (i.e., observing actual practice) allow identification of areas for improvement, provision of education, and reinforcement of the reasons following policy protects patients.

2. Water quality.

a. Measures used on a daily basis.

(1) Resistivity of water is a measure of the ability of the water to resist an electrical current.

(2) Conductivity of water is a measure of the ability of the water to conduct an electric current.

(3) Both resistivity and conductivity are related to the amount of ionic material dissolved in the water, also called total dissolved solids (TDS).

b. RO: Feed water conductivity = the quantity of particles presented to the RO.

c. Product water conductivity = the quantity of particles remaining in the RO treated water.

d. RO rejection rate = the percent of particles presented to the RO that are rejected to the drain.

e. DI: Resistivity is the measure used to monitor the quality of water produced by DI.

(1) Because toxic levels of contaminants can be immediately released by an exhausted DI system, these systems must be more closely monitored than RO systems.

(2) This includes recording the resistivity prior to each treatment and requiring an automatic divert-to-drain valve to immediately shunt the DI product water to drain if the resistivity limit is exceeded.

f. Chemical analysis. Each portable water treatment system should be tested at least annually to verify that the system produces water that meets the AAMI chemical contaminate standards (refer to Table 4.1).

B. Protecting the water treatment and HD systems from microbiologic contamination.

1. The disinfection system and schedule for the water treatment equipment and dialysis machines should be designed to prevent bacterial proliferation and to maintain the equipment within the AAMI limits for bacterial growth. The purpose of disinfection is to prevent excessive growth that would result secondary to an inadequate disinfection program. The purpose is not to eradicate growth.

2. Standard dialysate is used in most of the United States. The maximum and action levels for microbial contamination of standard water and dialysate are listed in Tables 4.2 and 4.3 respectively.

3. Ultrapure dialysate. To lessen patient's exposure to low levels of endotoxins, which may increase the risk for some of the long-term complications of HD, European countries have long endorsed the use of ultrapure dialysate.

a. Ultrapure dialysis fluid is defined as having a total viable microbiological count of less than 0.1 CFU/mL and an endotoxin concentration less than 0.03 EU/mL.

b. Obtaining these low levels of microbial contamination requires the use of endotoxin-retentive filters.

4. Portable water treatment equipment and dialysis machines are at greater risk of contamination due to their intermittent use and frequent connection and disconnection.

a. One strategy to decrease bacterial proliferation is to run each system for 15 minutes each day, whether or not that system is being used that day.

b. Another option to decrease bacterial proliferation is to store RO systems filled with a bacteriostatic agent when they are not used for several days. Caution is required to ensure clear labeling of the status of this equipment and complete rinsing before use.

c. If a single dialysis machine is used to perform multiple treatments during the day, it should be cleaned following each treatment and disinfected at the end of the day according to the manufacturer's instructions.

d. During a treatment day, if more than 4 hours pass between uses of a single machine, that machine should be disinfected before its next use.

e. If a machine has not been disinfected each day, it should be disinfected before use.

5. Cultures and endotoxin testing.

a. All samples should be collected in the "worst case" scenario: as distant in time from the last disinfection as possible.

b. Samples for water cultures and endotoxin levels should be collected from each portable water treatment system at least monthly.

c. Samples for dialysate cultures and endotoxin levels should be collected from a sample of dialysis machines each month, using a system to ensure that every machine is tested at least annually and different machines are tested each month.

(1) If the dialysis machines are disinfected after samples are taken, and if those sample results are above the action levels, additional samples should be taken immediately.

(2) A single test result above the action levels does not require removal of that dialysis machine from service; repeated results above action levels for the same machine should result in a thorough investigation, including observation of sample collection and consultation with the physician responsible for the dialysis service.

(3) Samples above the maximum level require that the machine be taken offline, re-disinfected, and retested until it is again below the maximum level and safe to use for patient care.

6. Culture methodology.
   a. While ANSI/AAMI RD 52:2004 allowed the use of dip samplers, the current ANSI/AAMI recommendations found in ANSI/AAMI 23500 and 13959 do not allow the use of dip samplers (AAMI, 2004, 2014a, 2014b).
   b. ANSI/AAMI/ISO 13959 recommends that the culture media should be tryptone glucose extract agar (TGEA), Reasoners 2A (R2A), or other media that can be demonstrated to provide equivalent results (AAMI, 2014). Blood agar and chocolate agar must not be used. A calibrated loop must not be used. Incubation temperatures of 17°C to 23°C (62.6°F to 73.4°F) and incubation time of 7 days are recommended.
   c. In 2014, ANSI/AAMI approved a United States (U.S.) deviation to the culture methodology, based on the language in ANSI/AAMI/ISO 13959, which states that other media, incubation, times, and temperatures may be used if demonstrated that they provide equivalent results. The U.S. deviation allows the use of Trypticase soy agar (TSA) media, at an incubation temperature of 35°C (95°F), for an incubation time of 48 hours. These parameters reflect those used in RD 52.

VIII. Quality assessment and performance improvement (QAPI) for acute dialysis water treatment systems.

A. Recordkeeping.
   1. Documentation of monitoring to ensure delivery of safe water includes the following.
      a. Daily logs for each portable system.
      b. Culture and endotoxin reports.
      c. Maintenance and repair records.

2. Data should be displayed in a way that allows visual identification of trends.
   a. At least three data points are required to begin to see a trend; six points provide a fuller view.
   b. Develop a system to allow identification of commonalities. For example, was the same portable water treatment system in use for more than one incident? Which dialysis machine was used with which water treatment system?

B. Reporting: to allow action to be taken proactively.
   1. Immediately report significant problems with the water treatment systems to the unit manager or charge nurse and the medical director or the physician responsible for the acute dialysis program. Consider the following examples.
      a. If maximum culture or endotoxin levels are exceeded.
      b. If action levels for cultures or endotoxins are exceeded 2 consecutive months for the same equipment.
      c. If a patient has a pyrogen reaction during treatment.
   2. Routinely report on the water treatment systems during unit QAPI meetings.
      a. Display data in a manner to allow discovery of trends and patterns.
      b. Report results of practice audits.
      c. Develop action plans and review implementation of previous action plans.
      d. Recognize the importance of reviewing the effectiveness of each action plan at every QAPI meeting and revise plans as indicated.

References

Association for the Advancement of Medical Instrumentation (AAMI). (2004). ANSI/AAMI RD52:2004. *Dialysate for hemodialysis.* Arlington, VA: AAMI

Association for the Advancement of Medical Instrumentation (AAMI). (2014a). ANSI/AAMI 23500:2014. *Guidance for the preparation and quality management of fluids for hemodialysis and related therapies. Annex A: Special considerations for acute hemodialysis.* Arlington, VA: AAMI.

Association for the Advancement of Medical Instrumentation (AAMI). (2014b). ANSI/AAMI 13959:2014. *Water for hemodialysis and related therapies.* Arlington, VA: AAMI.

Association for the Advancement of Medical Instrumentation (AAMI). (2014c). ANSI/AAMI/ISO 11663:2014. *Quality of dialysis fluid for hemodialysis and related therapies.* Arlington, VA: Author.

Centers for Medicare and Medicaid Services (CMS). (2014). *State operations manual Appendix A: Survey protocol, regulations and interpretive guidelines for hospitals.* (Rev. 116, 6-06-14). Retrieved from http://www.cms.gov/Regulations-and-Guidance/Guidance/Manuals/Downloads/som107ap_a_hospitals.pdf

Core Curriculum for Nephrology Nursing, Sixth Edition © 2015 American Nephrology Nurses' Association

CHAPTER **5**

Peritoneal Dialysis in the Acute Care Setting

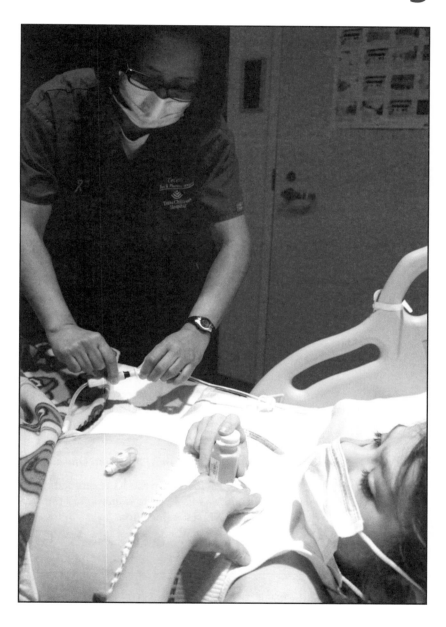

Chapter Editor
Helen F. Williams, MSN, BSN, RN, CNN
Author
Linda L. Myers, BS, RN, CNN, HP

CHAPTER **5**

Peritoneal Dialysis in the Acute Care Setting

This offering for **1.2 contact hours** is provided by the American Nephrology Nurses' Association (ANNA).

American Nephrology Nurses' Association is accredited as a provider of continuing nursing education by the American Nurses Credentialing Center Commission on Accreditation.

ANNA is a provider approved by the California Board of Registered Nursing, provider number CEP 00910.

This CNE offering meets the continuing nursing education requirements for certification and recertification by the Nephrology Nursing Certification Commission (NNCC).

To be awarded contact hours for this activity, read this chapter in its entirety. Then complete the CNE evaluation found at **www.annanurse.org/corecne** and submit it; or print it, complete it, and mail it in. Contact hours are not awarded until the evaluation for the activity is complete.

Example of reference for Chapter 5 in APA format. One author for entire chapter.

Myers, L.L. (2015). Peritoneal dialysis in the acute care setting. In C.S. Counts (Ed.), *Core curriculum for nephrology nursing: Module 4. Acute kidney injury* (6th ed., pp. 119-142). Pitman, NJ: American Nephrology Nurses' Association.

Interpreted: Chapter author. (Date). Title of chapter. In …

Cover photo by Robin Davis, BS, CCLS, Child Life Specialist, Texas Children's Hospital.

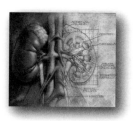

CHAPTER 5

Peritoneal Dialysis in the Acute Care Setting

Purpose

The purpose of this chapter is to describe the care of patients undergoing peritoneal dialysis (PD) in the acute care setting.

Objectives

Upon completion of this chapter, the learner will be able to:
1. Describe the nephrology nurse's role in coordinating and facilitating the care of the patient on PD in the acute care setting.
2. Outline the steps to initiate and manage the admission, discharge, and handoff of care of the patient on PD in the acute care setting.
3. Discuss the assessment of potential complications of PD in the acute care setting.

I. Nursing management of the patient on PD in the acute care setting.

A. The patient on PD may be admitted to the medical/surgical unit for the following reasons.
1. PD catheter insertion or catheter-related complications.
2. Infectious or noninfectious dialysis complications.
3. Transferred from a critical care setting.
4. Admitted for elective, nonemergent reasons.
   a. Elective and nonemergent surgery.
   b. Elective diagnostic procedures.
      (1) Invasive cardiac studies.
      (2) Complicated endoscopy and/or colonoscopy.
      (3) Arthroscopy.
   c. Medical indications.
      (1) Cardiac ischemia.
      (2) Pulmonary problems.
         (a) Pneumonia.
         (b) Asthma.
         (c) Chronic obstructive pulmonary disease (COPD).
         (d) Evaluation of sleep apnea.
         (e) Gastroparesis.
      (3) Gastrointestinal issues.
         (a) Hiatal hernia.
         (b) Severe reflux disease.
         (c) Gastrointestinal bleeding.
         (d) Pancreatitis.
      (4) Metabolic and endocrine disorders.
      (5) Orthopedic procedures.
      (6) Diabetes and complications.
      (7) Neurologic disorders.
      (8) Peripheral vascular disease.
      (9) Localized and systemic infections.
      (10) Psychiatric disorders.

B. Preparations for an elective admission.
1. The home training or acute care PD nurse may be active in the coordination of the patient's admission.
2. Preparation will vary with each institution and may include the following.
   a. Determine if the hospital unit can safely perform PD therapy.
   b. Establish a channel of communication between the hospital unit and the outpatient PD nurses.
   c. Identify the hospital PD resources for the staff nurse on the unit.
   d. Provide in-service educational programs for the hospital staff.
   e. Provide written educational information and tools for the hospital staff.
   f. Provide the patient's chronic kidney disease (CKD) and dialysis history following Health Insurance Portability and Accountability Act (HIPAA) guidelines.
   g. Share information concerning the patient's learning style and coping mechanisms.
   h. Identify and/or provide a PD catheter, PD solution, drain bags, and other PD equipment which may include a cycler.

i. Identify the PD nurse as an advocate for both the patient and for PD.
j. Provide liaison service for hospital staff and the PD healthcare team (Blake, 2006; Czajkowski et al., 2013; Piraino, 2006).

C. Specific issues that may need to be addressed during the hospitalization of a patient on peritoneal dialysis (see Appendix 5.1).
1. Staff may lack experience with PD and need frequent support and educational offerings.
2. Staff may need review of policies and procedures (Bernardini et al., 2006; Farina, 2008).
3. PD orders/prescriptions may need clarification.
4. Ordering adequate supplies.
5. Protocols for adjustment of intraperitoneal PD solution volume for invasive procedures. These adjustments will vary according to the healthcare provider's (physician/APRN/PA) preference and experience as well as the hospital's policies and procedures.
   a. A patient on PD who is having a cardiac catheterization, for example, may need a temporary reduction in fill volume during the procedure to provide patient comfort and to diminish the possibility of respiratory complications.
   b. A patient on PD needing a colonoscopy, a procedure that may lead to transient bacteremia resulting in peritonitis, may need additional care, including:
      (1) Draining the PD fluid prior to the procedure.
      (2) Administering antibiotic prophylaxis. The International Society for Peritoneal Dialysis (ISPD) recommends ampicillin 1 gm IV before the procedure with single dose of aminoglycoside with or without metronidazole (Guest, 2014; Piraino et al., 2011; Yip et al., 2007).
6. Changes to the patient's PD exchange routine to accommodate delays due to invasive procedures and/or surgery.
7. Reminders about the need for thorough hand washing, wearing appropriate personal protective equipment (PPE) including a face mask, and observation of universal precautions.
8. Securing the PD catheter at all times during invasive procedures, surgery, and transfers to and from a bed to a stretcher or wheelchair.
9. Accurate and consistent documentation of the patient's PD therapy.
10. Preparation of a discharge plan.

D. Preparation for the discharge of a patient on PD.
1. The discharge planning process should be started early in the patient's hospitalization to facilitate a timely and smooth transition.
2. All the members of the patient's healthcare team may be involved, but the coordination is usually shared among renal/kidney case manager, the primary/bedside nurse, the home PD nurse, the nephrologist, the social worker, and the patient and family/significant other.
3. The discharge plan should include:
   a. Team discussion about safe discharge plan.
   b. Active patient and family involvement in the discharge plan.
   c. Identification of the PD unit that will resume patient follow-up.
4. Adequate supplies must be ordered and delivered to the patient's home prior to discharge.
5. A follow-up appointment should be scheduled with the nephrologist/APRN/PA and the PD unit.
6. If the patient is unable to resume self-care responsibility at discharge:
   a. Discuss options with the case manager, social worker, primary nurse, nephrologists, PD nurse, and the patient/family.
   b. Determine whether patient qualifies for either short- or long-term rehabilitation care.
   c. Evaluate the rehabilitation center for PD experience and patient safety.
   d. Provide in-service instruction and written references to rehabilitation staff if needed.
   e. Identify PD resource individuals among the rehabilitation staff.
   f. Use the above-mentioned criteria in evaluation for long-term care facility placement.
7. Document all plans in the patient's hospital record.
8. Send discharge summaries and follow-up with phone calls to all involved PD facility and healthcare team members.

II. Nursing management of the PD treatment in the acute care setting.

A. The PD experience of the acute care nursing staff will vary.
1. Identification of resources for the staff nurse is crucial in providing safe PD therapy.
2. Communication and collaboration of all involved healthcare providers is vital to achieve appropriate clinical outcomes for the patient on PD.
3. The acute care PD nephrology nurse may need to be the facilitator, educator, and coordinator of this process.
4. Clarify who will perform the PD procedures.
   a. A designated in-hospital team of nephrology PD nurses.
   b. An acute care hemodialysis nurse trained in PD.

c. An acute care dialysis technician with nurse supervision.

d. The critical care nurse trained in PD.

e. An expert medical/surgical floor nurse trained in PD (see Appendix 5.1).

f. A per diem or contracted nurse from a nursing agency or vendor trained in PD.

5. For general information regarding PD therapy, please refer to the following.

a. Module 3, Chapter 4, Section B, Peritoneal Dialysis Access.

b. Module 3, Chapter 4, Section C, Peritoneal Dialysis Therapy.

c. Module 3, Chapter 4, Section D, Peritoneal Dialysis Complications.

B. Initiating PD in the acute care setting.

1. Educate the patient and family about PD care in the acute care setting.

2. Evaluate the patient's need for a private room to limit exposure to possible infections and to provide privacy.

3. Identify the nursing staff's ability to safely perform PD services.

4. Identify the resources available to the nursing staff.

a. Expert PD nurses within the institution.

b. Outpatient home training PD nurses.

c. Acute care hemodialysis nurses who may cover inpatients on PD.

d. Nephrology clinical nurse specialists (CNS) or advanced practice registered nurses (APRN).

5. Inform the necessary healthcare team members of the patient's admission.

a. PD resource nurses, inpatient and outpatient.

b. Nurse manager or charge nurse on patient's unit to evaluate staff's ability to do the following.

(1) Safely perform PD.

(2) Provide appropriate staffing.

(3) Assess acuity of the patient on PD.

c. CNS or APRN to provide additional education and support.

d. Nephrologist/APRN/PA.

6. For the established patient on PD in the acute care setting, contact the home PD nurse and consult with the patient, family member(s), or significant other to obtain the following.

a. Current dialysis prescription.

b. Membrane transport characteristics.

c. Most recent Kt/Vurea results and blood urea nitrogen (BUN) results.

d. Medication list.

e. Infection history.

f. Allergies.

g. Other pertinent healthcare information.

C. Individualize prescription using the results of the peritoneal equilibration test (PET) to classify the patient's peritoneal membrane transport capability.

1. Rates of diffusion vary based on the following.

a. Vascularity.

b. Percent of perfused capillaries.

c. Distance of capillaries to dialysate.

2. Classic Test: 4 hour, 2.5% dextrose dwell.

a. 4-hour dwell.

b. Serum levels at 2 hours: BUN, creatinine, glucose, sodium.

c. Dialysate samples at 0, 2, and 4 hours.

d. Dialysate to plasma (D/P) ratio for urea, creatinine, and glucose calculated.

3. ISPD Guidelines: Modified PET recommends using a 4.25% dextrose solution to determine ultrafiltration (UF) failure.

4. Rule of 4's.

a. 4.25% dextrose.

b. 4 hours.

c. > 400 cc of UF.

5. Performing the PET should not begin until one month after starting PD due to minimal inflammatory changes.

6. The PET is not used to predict success, outcome, or survival but can help in individualizing prescriptions and in determining UF failure.

a. Low transporters – slow solute transport.

(1) Require longer dwells.

(2) Have sustained UF due to longer glucose osmotic gradient.

b. High transporters – rapid solute transport.

(1) Have better clearance with rapid exchanges.

(2) More rapid absorption of glucose/osmotic gradient compromising UF in longer exchanges (Guest, 2014; Ponferrada & Prowant, 2010).

7. Obtain, review, and follow pertinent hospital policies and procedures.

8. Obtain PD prescription orders.

9. Identify and obtain necessary PD equipment.

10. Order adequate supplies to prevent delays in providing dialysis.

11. Clarify how nursing management of PD will be communicated and documented, which is especially important when there are multiple nurses involved in providing PD therapy (see Appendices 5.1, 5.2, and 5.3 and Figure 5.1).

D. Ultrafiltration in PD.

1. Water and solute movement is driven by crystalloid or colloid osmotic gradients. If dialysate is hypertonic to blood, water will move from blood compartment to dialysate compartment.

Nursing Documentation for Hospitalized Patient on Peritoneal Dialysis

Education
Who was involved – Patient/family
Topic discussed
Assessment of understanding
Plan for further education

Procedure: Acute PD catheter placement at bedside
Pain assessment, intervention, and evaluation of
effectiveness
Catheter function (drain and fill), need for heparin
Exit-site dressing
Drainage:
Frequency of changes
Color of drainage
Check drainage for glucose
Secured:
Immobilization

Fluid balance
Schedule of exchanges: e.g., every 2 hours, every 4 hours
Fill volume of each exchange
Dextrose percentage used for each exchange
Medications added to dialysate solution bags
Number of exchanges completed
Amount of effluent drained (Ultrafiltration)
Intake and output of all fluids

Patient's disposition during exchanges
Positioning that facilitates infusion or drain
Comfort with exchange sensations
Presence of pain with infusion or draining of solutions
Presence of rectal pain, shoulder pain, and/or
abdominal pain
Unusual abdominal distention

PD effluent (drainage)
Color (clear, yellow)
Presence of fibrin
Clarity (clear, bloody, cloudy, tea colored)
Ease of infusion and drainage

Exit site
Color of site
Presence of exudate
Presence of pain
Leakage of dialysate at exit site
How catheter is secured

Infection

Peritonitis
Cloudy fluid
Abdominal pain
Nausea, vomiting, and/or diarrhea
Antibiotic therapy – medication, dose, route, and frequency
Color and clarity of solution
Collect PD fluid for cultures and sensitivity prior to 1st dose
of antibiotics
Organism causing the infection if known

Exit-site infection
Presence of:
Exudate
Erythema
Pain or tenderness
Any change or leaking at site
Pending cultures and antibiotics ordered

**Assessment of the serum laboratory levels of the 3 H's
associated with patients on PD**

1 Hyperglycemia
% dextrose of PD solution
Increase requirement of oral diabetes medication or insulin

2 Hypokalemia
Potassium loss into drained effluent can significantly
decrease serum potassium levels
Monitor serum potassium
Individualized nutrition consult

3 Hypoalbuminia
Protein loss with PD can be as high as 5–15 g/day and twice
as much with peritonitis
Does patient have nutritional support
Consult dietitian

Figure 5.1. Nursing documentation for hospitalized patient on peritoneal dialysis.
Courtesy of Maria Luongo. Used with permission.

2. How to increase diffusion in PD.
a. Maximize concentration gradient.
(1) Increase instilled volume.
(2) Increase frequency of exchanges.
(3) Alternative PD therapies (tidal regimen)
(Ponferrada & Prowant, 2008).
b. Increase contact area.
(1) Larger instilled volumes.
(2) Larger dwell volume.
3. As dextrose is absorbed and osmotic gradient
dissipates, net ultrafiltration ceases and dialysate is
reabsorbed.

E. Solute clearance involves two processes.
1. Diffusion is the movement of solute down
concentration gradients. It is influenced by:
a. The length of dialysate dwell.
b. Membrane surface area.
c. Vascularity of peritoneal membrane.
d. Inflammatory state.
e. Molecular size; i.e., the smaller molecular
weight substances diffuse more rapidly than
creatinine or middle molecules.
2. Convection.
a. The solute that is removed as a result of solvent
drag during ultrafiltration.

  b. Response to osmotic force.
  c. Provides clearance of middle molecules such as B2-microglobulin.
  3. The capillary vascular surface area is the most important determinant of solute transport.

F. A model of PD transport that is used to discuss methods of solute and water transport across the peritoneal capillary bed is called the three-pore model. The main barrier to solute transport is the peritoneal capillary endothelium.
  1. Transcellular aquaporins.
    a. Allow for only water transport.
    b. Complete barrier to any solutes.
  2. Small pores.
    a. Allow for transport of small solutes.
    b. Includes urea, sodium, potassium, and creatinine dissolved in water.
  3. Large pores.
    a. Allow for transport of larger macromolecules.
    b. Includes protein (Devuyst et al., 2010; Guest, 2014; Rippe, 2008).

G. Performing PD as kidney replacement therapy specific to the acute care setting.
  1. The nephrologist, renal fellow, APRN, PA, or attending physician should be notified of the following changes in condition.
    a. Severe abdominal pain or distention.
    b. Poor infusion or drainage.
    c. Leakage of dialysate from the exit site.
    d. Suspected exit-site or tunnel infection.
    e. Cloudy effluent.
    f. Grossly bloody effluent.
    g. Diminished ultrafiltration.
    h. Hyperglycemia.
    i. Rapid shifts in serum electrolytes.
    j. Increased respiratory distress.
    k. Unusual changes in abdominal girth.
    l. Suspected migration of catheter tip away from the left lower quadrant of the abdomen.
    m. Unintentional tubing disconnections.
  2. Inspection of effluent (drained dialysate).
    a. Color.
      (1) Colorless.
      (2) Light to dark yellow.
      (3) Pink, in female patient, may indicate menstruation.
      (4) Red indicates bleeding.
      (5) Tea colored may indicate old bleeding or certain medications.
    b. Clarity.
      (1) Clear.
      (2) Cloudy is a sign of peritonitis. Send effluent for cell count, Gram stain, and culture and sensitivity.
    c. Presence or absence of fibrin.

  d. Report unexpected changes to nephrologist.
  3. Monitoring the patient's weight. Daily weight is part of the global assessment of fluid balance.
    a. Obtain baseline weight prior to initiation of PD therapy.
    b. Weight should be obtained daily, consistently, either with or without fluid dwelling.
    c. Patient should use same scale and wear similar clothing.
    d. Daily weight and fill volume needs to be documented in progress notes, PD flow sheets, or other sites according to the institution's policy.
  4. Maintaining accurate documentation of intake and output. Document on unit specific PD treatment flow sheet (see Appendices 5.2 and 5.3).
    a. Frequency of exchanges, fill volume, and dextrose percent.
    b. The amount of dialysate fluid that was infused.
    c. The amount of dialysate fluid that was drained.
    d. Subtract amount of infused dialysate from the drained dialysate to determine if the patient has a net negative or positive ultrafiltration.
    e. Calculate intake.
      (1) Oral intake.
      (2) Intravenous infusions.
      (3) Tube feedings.
      (4) PD net negative ultrafiltration, i.e., retained dialysate.
    f. Calculate output.
      (1) Urine production.
      (2) Nasogastric tube drainage.
      (3) PD net positive ultrafiltration.
      (4) If catheter site is leaking, weigh saturated dressings for accurate accounting of dialysate.
  5. Facilitating infusion and draining of solution in the acute care setting.
    a. Secure catheter carefully to prevent kinking or occlusion.
    b. Use gravity.
      (1) Lower the patient or raise the dialysis solution to increase rate of infusion.
      (2) Raise the patient or lower the drain bag to increase rate of drainage.
    c. The patient may need to be turned from side to side to facilitate draining.
    d. If possible, elevate the patient's head and upper torso during infusion and draining of dialysis solution.
      (1) Assists in preventing respiratory compromise when infusing dialysate.
      (2) Maximizes the effect of gravity when draining dialysate.
    e. The patient may need to be carefully positioned with respect to other monitoring devices and/or ventilator connections.

6. If ultrafiltration is diminished, consider the following.
   a. Rule out problems related to issues with the catheter.
      (1) Obstruction from fibrin.
      (2) Kink in tubing or catheter.
      (3) Patient position.
      (4) Failure to open appropriate clamps on tubing set.
      (5) Failure to open frangible(s) in-line on tubing set.
   b. Assess abdominal wall for catheter exit-site leak or subcutaneous leaking.
   c. Assess for dehydration.
   d. Assess for constipation.
   e. Assess for unusual insensible loss of fluid.
   f. Consult with the nephrologist/APRN/PA.
7. Assessment of pain.
   a. A newly inserted temporary or chronic catheter may create pain perceived as cramping during infusion or draining.
   b. Slowing the rate of infusion or drainage may diminish the cramping sensation.
   c. Dialysis solution that is either too hot or too cold may cause cramping and pain.
   d. Warm dialysis solution bags according to established policy. Leaving solution bags at room temperature is acceptable for warming, while submerging solution bags in hot water or heating them in the microwave are not advised due to the possibility of creating hot spots in the fluid.

H. Dietary needs.
   1. The patient with diabetes.
      a. Consideration must be given to the glucose load that adds to daily caloric intake.
         (1) 1.5% dextrose – 15 to 22 grams of glucose absorbed.
         (2) 2.5% dextrose – 24 to 40 grams of glucose absorbed.
         (3) 4.25% dextrose – 45 to 60 grams of glucose absorbed.
      b. Diabetic gastroparesis and fullness can be exacerbated causing decreased appetite.
      c. Gastric emptying can be slowed down as the result of:
         (1) Autonomic neuropathy.
         (2) Uremia.
         (3) Reflux.
      d. Regularly monitor HbA1C.
      e. Visual impairments, manual dexterity problems, and/or amputations can impact not only access to food but also its preparation. These challenges are not restricted to those patients with diabetes.
   2. Dietary evaluation and intervention.

   a. Difficulties with dentition or swallowing must be considered. Monitor for periodontal disease.
   b. Protein supplements may be indicated.
   c. Lower volume exchanges at meal times with larger volumes at night while recumbent.
   d. Smaller feedings may be beneficial.
   e. Sodium restriction will reduce UF requirements.
   f. The use of hypertonic solutions should be avoided.
   g. Encourage exercise (Cotovio et al., 2011; Guest, 2014).
3. Protein losses.
   a. Protein losses can be as high as 5 to 15 g/day.
   b. To maintain neutral nitrogen balance, targets for patients on PD are 1.2 to 1.3 g/kg/day.
   c. nPNA.
      (1) Reflective of dietary protein intake in a stable patient.
      (2) Urea generation is proportional to protein breakdown, termed the normalized protein equivalent of nitrogen appearance (nPNA).
   d. Chronic inflammation may lower albumin concentration.
   e. High peritoneal membrane permeability can lead to hypoalbuminemia.
4. Managing potassium (K+).
   a. There are ongoing potassium losses into the dialysate.
   b. The intake of dietary K+ should be 70 mmol/day.
   c. The patient may require K+ supplementation.
   d. Chronic hypokalemia may precipitate peritonitis by impacting bowel motility, allowing for bacterial growth and transmural migration of enteric organisms into the peritoneum.
   e. Hypokalemia is marker of nutritional deficits.
   f. Foods rich in potassium, but low in phosphorous, should be encouraged.
      (1) Bananas.
      (2) Oranges.
      (3) Tomatoes.
      (4) Potatoes.
      (5) Spinach.
   g. Hyperkalemia is rare in patients who are on PD and adherent, but it can occur.
      (1) Missed exchanges.
      (2) Transcellular shifts due to metabolic acidosis.
      (3) Dietary nonadherence.
      (4) Tumor lysis syndrome.
      (5) Rhabdomyolysis.
      (6) Hemolysis.
      (7) Hepatitis.
      (8) Severe hyperglycemia (Guest, 2014).

I. Infectious complications of PD seen in the acute setting (Li et al., 2010; Piraino et al., 2011).
   1. For information regarding infections, refer to the following.
      a. Module 3, Chapter 4, Section C, Peritoneal Dialysis Complications, for infectious complications and treatment.
      b. Module 3, Chapter 4, Section C, for complications of peritoneal dialysis.
      c. Module 3, Chapter 4, Table 4.7, Evidence-Based Practice Guidelines for PD-Associated Peritonitis.
   2. Nursing assessment.
      a. Examine, clean, and dress exit site; observe for signs of infection.
      b. Recognize early signs of peritonitis.
         (1) Cloudy effluent.
         (2) Increased fibrin in effluent.
         (3) Abdominal pain.
      c. Assess for signs and symptoms of infection.
         (1) Assess patient for the following.
            (a) Abdominal pain or tenderness.
            (b) Constipation/diarrhea.
            (c) Nausea/vomiting.
            (d) Elevated temperature.
            (e) Blood leukocytosis, i.e., elevated white blood cell count.
         (2) Assess exit site and tunnel for the following.
            (a) Erythema.
            (b) Pain or tenderness.
            (c) Inflammation.
            (d) Exudate at exit site.
            (e) Purulent drainage (may be gently expressed from tunnel).
            (f) Elevated skin temperature over tunnel.
            (g) Fluid or fluctuance over the catheter tunnel.
            (h) Dialysate leak.
            (i) Edema over the catheter tunnel.
         (3) Assess PD effluent for the following.
            (a) Elevated white blood cell count, i.e., > 100/mL.
            (b) Cloudiness.
            (c) Blood.
            (d) Fibrin.
      d. Document and report any of the above changes to the nephrologist/APRN/PA (see Appendix 5.2 and Appendix 5.3).
         (1) Send effluent sample for cell count, gram stain, and culture and sensitivity, including fungal culture, as ordered.
         (2) Send swab of drainage from the catheter's exit site for culture and sensitivity as ordered.
         (3) Anticipate initiating antibiotics.
            (4) Communicate change in plan of care to hospital nurse assigned to patient.
   3. Patient and nursing safety issues.
      a. Careful, thorough hand washing is mandated to protect both patient and caregiver from transmission of infection.
      b. A mask should be worn by patients. All caregivers and/or family members present must wear a mask when patient is doing PD exchanges or procedures, or be given the option to step out of the room while the patient is connecting and disconnecting from the system (refer to Appendix 5.2).
      c. Nurses and caregivers must use universal precautions when performing PD therapy.
      d. Effluent must be disposed of as a hazardous waste. Receptacles and procedures will vary with each institution.

J. Noninfectious complications of PD seen in the acute setting.
   1. Leak – subcutaneous/retroperitoneal/pericatheter-disruption in integrity of deep cuff.
      a. Abdominal and flank swelling.
         (1) Boggy skin.
         (2) Pitting at beltline.
         (3) Weight gain without pedal edema.
      b. Scrotal or labial edema.
      c. Diminished effluent return.
      d. Pericatheter leak: wetness or swelling at exit site.
         (1) Hold PD for a couple of days, then restart night PD with day dry.
         (2) Reintroduce low-pressure, low-volume PD.
         (3) May need temporary HD to allow healing to occur.
   2. Hydrothorax – presence of peritoneal dialysis fluid in pleural cavity.
      a. May be asymptomatic.
      b. Shortness of breath (SOB) or dry cough.
      c. Worsening SOB with hypertonic dialysate.
      d. Diminished effluent return.
      e. Right-sided pleural effusion on chest x-ray.
      f. High glucose concentration.
         (1) Thoracentesis or pleurodesis may be helpful if SOB.
         (2) Lower volume PD recumbent or may need to stop PD.
         (3) Temporary hemodialysis.
         (4) Video assisted thoracoscopic surgery (VATS) – correct diaphragmatic leak.
   3. Hemoperitoneum – bloody-tinged PD fluid.
      a. Benign causes: menstruation, ovulation, ruptured renal or ovarian cysts, trauma, coagulopathy.
         (1) Assess hemodynamic stability.

(2) Unwarmed, several rapid exchanges to induce vasoconstriction.

(3) Consider intraperitoneal heparin 500 to 1000 units per 2L dwell to prevent clotting that can lead to catheter failure.

b. Serious causes: ischemic bowel, hepatic or colon cancer, pancreatitis, encapsulating peritoneal sclerosis, kidney cancer, vascular aneurysm, or splenic laceration. Laparoscopic intervention may be required.

4. Chyloperitoneum – milky white drained dialysate, negative bacterial culture.

a. Causes: trauma, surgery, inflammatory process, constrictive pericarditis, malignancy, lymphoma, amyloidosis, cirrhosis, pancreatitis, adenitis in systemic lupus erythematosus (SLE), calcium channel medications, or peritonitis.

(1) Spontaneous resolution.

(2) Low-fat, low-triglyceride diet to reduce lymph flow.

5. Back pain – related to mechanical stress on the lumbar spine.

a. Weight of dialysate and weakened abdominal muscles.

(1) Lower back strengthening exercises.

(2) Reduction in ambulatory dwell.

(3) Recumbent cycler regimen.

6. Hernia and increased intraabdominal pressure.

a. Lump or swelling in abdomen that may be tender.

(1) Umbilical and inguinal hernias are most common.

(2) Truss or lower dialysate volume if easily reducible.

(3) Reduce day dwell volume, especially in polycystic kidney disease.

b. Bowel incarceration or strangulation requiring surgical repair (Guest, 2014).

K. Components of the PD prescription and orders (see Appendices 5.4, 5.5, 5.6, and 5.7).

1. Fill volume: Average fill is 2 to 2.5 liters.

a. 500 mL to 1000 mL for initial exchanges on patients with new catheters.

b. 2000 mL to 2500 mL for maintenance therapy.

c. 3500 mL or greater only for unusual situations, since larger fill volumes may contribute to respiratory difficulty.

2. Frequency of exchanges will depend on the following.

a. Current patient fluid balance.

b. Need for emergent fluid removal.

c. Need for emergent correction of electrolyte imbalance.

d. Hemodynamic instability.

e. Membrane transport characteristics.

f. Metabolic stability or instability.

g. Manual PD: 4 to 12 exchanges per 24 hours.

h. Automated Peritoneal Dialysis (APD): 4 to 12 exchanges per 24 hours.

i. In unusual circumstances, exchanges may be done every 60 to 90 minutes, but this increases the risk of developing dialysis disequilibrium syndrome in patients with advanced uremia.

j. Tidal Peritoneal Dialysis.

(1) APD regimen.

(2) Dwell volume not completely drained before next fill cycle.

(3) Leaves reservoir 250 mL, 500 mL, or 1000 mL. Overfill needs to be avoided.

(4) Used if pain at beginning of fill or if draining very slowly (Guest, 2014).

3. PD solutions.

a. 1.5% dextrose.

b. 2.5% dextrose.

c. 4.25% dextrose.

d. Either low calcium (2.5 mEq/L) or regular calcium (3.0 mEq/L) formulation.

e. Extraneal® (Baxter, Deerfield, Illinois): icodextrin 7.5%.

(1) Nonglucose polymer.

(2) Used for selected patients for fluid removal.

(3) Used for only one exchange every 24 hours.

(4) Used as a long dwell exchange (10 to 12 hours).

(a) With manual PD, it is typically used for the overnight dwell.

(b) With APD, it is typically used for the long daytime dwell.

(5) Can interfere with select glucose monitoring devices. The Federal Drug Administration (FDA) warning indicates, "Blood glucose measurement in patients receiving Extraneal® must be done with a glucose-specific method (monitor and test strips) to avoid interference by maltose, released from Extraneal®. Glucose dehydrogenase pyrroloquin-olinequinone (GDH PQQ) or glucose-dye-oxidoreductase-based methods must not be used. If GDH-PQQ or glucose-dye-oxidoreductase-based methods are used, using Extraneal® may cause a falsely high glucose reading. Additionally, falsely elevated blood glucose measurements due to maltose interference may mask true hypoglycemia and allow it to go untreated. The maltose released from Extraneal® may be present in the patient's blood for up to 72 hours after exposure to Extraneal®." Check manufacturer's warnings and recommendations.

4. The addition of medication to the PD solution.

a. Refer to Module 3, Chapter 4, Section C, Peritoneal Dialysis Therapy.
b. Meticulous sterile technique must be used to prevent bacterial or fungal contamination of the solution bag.
  (1) Anyone instilling medications into a PD solution must be specifically trained to do so.
  (2) Alternatively, the pharmacy may instill medications into the PD solution using a laminar airflow hood.
c. Vials without preservative must not be reused.
d. After the medication is added, the solution bag must be labeled with name and dose of the medication, time and date of the addition, the initials of person who added the medication, and whether refrigeration is needed.
e. Any added medication must be documented on the PD flow sheet and on the medication record.
f. When medication(s) is added to the bag of PD solution, it is essential to mix the solution by inverting the bag several times.
g. Heparin.
  (1) Used to treat formation of fibrin in the effluent and to prevent fibrin accumulation in the catheter.
  (2) Typical dose is 500 to 1000 units per liter of solution.
  (3) For patients with heparin-induced thrombocytopenia (HIT), consult with the nephrologist/APRN/PA for anticoagulation alternatives.
h. Antibiotics.
  (1) Refer to Module 3, Chapter 4, Section D, Peritoneal Dialysis Complications.
  (2) Collect all specimens (culture and/or cell count of drainage or effluent) prior to the addition of antibiotics to the PD solution.
  (3) Clarify the route of administration.
    (a) Oral (PO).
    (b) Intraperitoneal (IP).
    (c) Intravenous (IV).
  (4) Clarify dosage and frequency of administration.
  (5) If antibiotic is administered IP, clarify length of dwell time of that solution bag to facilitate absorption of antibiotic.
i. Potassium.
  (1) If patient is unable to take oral potassium, or if vascular access prohibits IV administration, it can be added to the PD solution bags.
  (2) Clarify the dose and frequency of administration.
  (3) Obtain order for monitoring serum potassium levels.

(4) Infuse slowly as potassium can be irritating to the peritoneum.
j. Insulin.
  (1) Refer to Module 3, Chapter 4, Section C, Peritoneal Dialysis Therapy.
  (2) Insulin is absorbed from the peritoneal cavity and enters the systemic circulation via the hepatic portal system mimicking insulin delivery of the true pancreas.
  (3) Insulin should be added immediately before infusion.
  (4) Peak insulin levels are reached 20 minutes later than with endogenous insulin, and are sustained longer.
  (5) Frequent monitoring of blood glucose is imperative.
  (6) The needles on conventional insulin syringes may be too short to consistently and completely penetrate the medication port of the dialysis solution bags.
    (a) A 1 mL syringe with a larger needle may only be used if the insulin is manufactured as 100 units per mL.
    (b) When adding insulin to the PD solution, use extreme caution; double-check the dosage with a second RN.
  (7) Intraperitoneal insulin administration alone may be used to control serum glucose for patients on continuous forms of dialysis. It is more difficult to calculate insulin dosage and control glucose for patients on APD or continuous cycling peritoneal dialysis (CCPD) than on CAPD. Most of the caloric load takes place during the day when there is only one long dwell exchange; this is what makes insulin calculation difficult with APD or CCPD.
  (8) Only regular insulin is utilized.
  (9) Higher doses of insulin are required due to the dilution of the insulin and potentially a 10% absorption rate of insulin into the plastic of the bags.
  (10) Regular insulin can be added to icodextrin solutions. It is a nonglucose solution, so the insulin dose should be reduced by as much as 50% compared to standard glucose solutions.
  (11) Conversion from subcutaneous to intraperitoneal insulin should be individualized.
  (12) In patients with acceptable glucose control on subcutaneous regimen, it may be advisable to not convert to IP dosing due to the following.
    (a) Effort is required to adjust IP dosing.
    (b) There is a potential risk of peritonitis.

(c) The larger doses of insulin required come with cost implications.

(d) There is a conceivable chance of developing hepatic subcapsular steatosis (Ponferrada & Prowant, 2008).

5. Specimens.
   a. Send PD solution effluent sample when ordered.
      (1) For suspected peritonitis.
         (a) Cell count.
         (b) Gram stain.
         (c) Culture and sensitivity.
         (d) Fungal culture.
      (2) For suspected exit-site or tunnel infection.
         (a) Culture and sensitivity.
         (b) Gram stain of exudate or drainage.
   b. Follow the institution's clinical laboratory procedures for appropriate containers and documentation.

L. Documentation of PD therapy in the acute setting (see Appendices 5.2 and 5.3 and Figure 5.1).
   1. Documentation of PD therapy may be required with each exchange, on each nursing shift, or daily.
   2. The requirements should be part of the policy and procedures established by the hospital and/or the patient care unit in collaboration with the nephrology nursing team.
   3. Documentation may be accomplished by the use of a daily treatment flow sheet, a nursing kardex tool, progress notes, or a combination of methods.
   4. May be written, electronic, or a combination.
   5. Components that should be included.
      a. Patient assessment.
         (1) Vital signs.
         (2) Lung sounds and oxygenation status.
         (3) Presence of the following.
            (a) Nausea and vomiting.
            (b) Constipation and diarrhea.
            (c) Abdominal pain and tenderness.
            (d) Edema.
      b. PD effluent.
         (1) Color.
         (2) Clarity.
         (3) Presence or absence of fibrin.
         (4) Ease of infusion and drainage.
      c. Dialysate and fluid balance.
         (1) Schedule of exchanges.
         (2) Fill and drain volume of each exchange.
         (3) Dextrose percentage used for each exchange.
         (4) Medications added to dialysate solution bags.
         (5) Number of exchanges prescribed and completed.
         (6) Intake and output of all fluids.
         (7) Calculation of ultrafiltration and net fluid balances.

      (8) Exchange dwell time.
   d. Patient's disposition during exchanges.
      (1) Positioning that facilitates infusion and/or drainage.
      (2) Comfort with PD exchanges.
      (3) Pain with infusion and/or drainage.
      (4) Presence of rectal pain, shoulder pain, and/or abdominal pain.
      (5) Unusual abdominal distention.
   e. Exit-site and tunnel condition and care.
      (1) Appearance of exit site and tunnel.
      (2) Presence or absence of the following.
         (a) Exudate or drainage.
         (b) Pain or tenderness.
         (c) Leakage of dialysate.
      (3) Exit-site care with hypertonic saline or other agent.
      (4) How catheter is secured.
      (5) Dressing condition or dressing change performed.
   f. Infection.
      (1) If the patient has peritonitis demonstrated by cloudy effluent, document the following.
         (a) Color and clarity of effluent.
         (b) Presence or absence of fibrin.
         (c) Acquisition of laboratory specimens.
         (d) Administration of prescribed antibiotic therapy.
      (2) If patient has an exit-site or tunnel infection, document the following.
         (a) Antibiotic therapy.
         (b) Changes in local care.
         (c) Presence or absence of exudate.
         (d) Erythema.
         (e) Pain.
         (f) Tenderness.
         (g) Edema.

M. Supplies needed at the bedside in the acute care setting.
   1. PD solutions with prescribed additives.
   2. Dialysis tubings, transfer sets, drain bags, and cycler supplies if doing APD or CCPD.
   3. Masks.
   4. Clamps for tubing.
   5. Spring scale.
   6. IV pole.
   7. Dry heat source.
   8. Povidone iodine for medication port prep.
   9. Unsterile gloves for universal precautions.
   10. Specimen containers.
   11. Dressing supplies.
   12. PD treatment flow sheets or required forms for documentation in that institution.

III. Nursing management of the patient with emergent needs for PD.

A. Indications.
1. Urgent/emergent need for kidney replacement therapy with limited or absent vascular access or the need to avoid a vascular access complication (e.g., hemorrhage, thrombosis, or infection).
2. Treatment of hypothermia.
3. Treatment of hemorrhagic pancreatitis.
4. Treatment of toxic and/or metabolic abnormalities.

B. Urgent start PD.
1. Early initiation of PD in a patient with chronic kidney failure.
2. Patient population.
   a. Late referrals with CKD stage 5 without overt symptoms.
   b. Selected patients with AKI.
   c. Has functioning peritoneum but no long-term plan for dialysis.
   d. The patient with chronic kidney failure or a transplant recipient whose transplant has failed requires dialysis in less than 2 weeks, but has no plan for a long-term choice of modality.
   e. Urgent start PD is not appropriate for acute PD or as the initial modality for patients who need emergent dialysis, such as someone in congestive heart failure (CHF) with severe electrolyte imbalances or overt uremic symptoms that would require emergent dialysis.
   f. Patient made aware of all available options and informed consent obtained.
3. Access.
   a. Surgeon or interventional nephrologist initiates urgent placement of PD catheter.
   b. Patient is educated on preprocedure and postprocedure instructions.
   c. Initiate treatments in a hospital or out-patient facility. Minimize risk of early leak.
4. Peritoneal dialysis catheter laparoscopic placement orders.
   a. NPO night before procedure.
   b. All anticoagulants and antiplatelet agents should be held.
   c. Preoperative labs should include: PT-INR, PTT, CBC, CMP, and active type and screen.
   d. Preoperative antibiotics and bowel prep determined by surgical team.
   e. Once catheter placed, patient can resume normal diet.
   f. Do not remove or replace catheter dressing for 7 days (unless soiled or soaked with blood or stool).
   g. Pain control with acetaminophen, tramadol, or acetaminophen-hydrocodone as needed.
   h. Assess catheter function on day 1.
      (1) Infuse and drain 500 mL of 1.5% dextrose solution while patient is supine.
      (2) If effluent is blood-tinged, repeat exchanges with 500 unit/L of heparin until effluent clears.
      (3) If effluent is grossly bloody, do not use heparin but continue exchanges. If effluent remains bloody after 4 exchanges, report to nephrologist/APRN/PA.
   i. Physician/APRN/PA should be informed for the following.
      (1) Severe pain.
      (2) Bleeding.
      (3) Malfunction of the catheter.
      (4) Nausea, vomiting, constipation.
5. Prescription for urgent start peritoneal dialysis (see Figure 5.2). Precautions.
   a. All exchanges when the patient is supine.
   b. Patient should use the bathroom prior to being connected to cycler.

Prescription for Urgent Start Peritoneal Dialysis

1. An assessment of residual kidney function must be performed with a 24-hour urine with urea and creatinine clearance. If the residual kidney function ≥ 0.24 daily Kt/V patients can be initiated on CAPD with 1L exchanges every 4–6 hours with the patient remaining supine.

2. The % dextrose solution used will depend upon the volume status of the patient with 1.5% exchanges used for those with little edema and no shortness of breath. 2.5% exchanges for those with greater degrees of edema and shortness of breath. 4.25% exchanges will require physician approval.

3. For those patients with poor residual kidney function or uremic symptoms, the following prescriptions will be used (IPD with alternate in-center thrice weekly PD with cycler).

	BSA < 1.65	BSA 1.65 – 1.8	BSA > 1.8
MDRD GFR > 7 mL/min	500 mL 4 cycles	750 mL 5 cycles	1000 mL 6 cycles
MDRD GFR ≤ 7 mL/min	500 mL 6 cycles	750 mL 6 cycles	1250 mL 6 cycles

Dialysis times:

4 cycles: minimum 5:00 hours

5 cycles: minimum 6:40 hours

6 cycles: minimum 8:00 hours (staffing and time permitted)

Figure 5.2. Urgent start peritoneal dialysis prescription.
Courtesy of Mitchell Rosner, MD. Used with permission.

c. If the patient needs to sit-up or stand, he/she should be drained.

d. Cough may require a suppressant.

e. Patients should be on a stool softener to avoid straining.

f. Eating during the procedure should be confined to the drain periods.

g. Diuretics should be attempted in those with issues of volume overload.

6. Benefits.

a. Preserves vascular access.

b. Avoids temporary access and need for later permanent access. A dual cuff catheter can be used for both acute and urgent initiations.

c. Reduces the number of patients initiating dialysis with a central venous catheter (CVC).

d. Better preservation of residual kidney function.

e. Improved quality of life.

f. Early survival advantage.

g. Lower risk of sepsis and hepatitis B and C transmission.

7. Contraindications.

a. Inability for self-care and no capable caregiver to assist with PD on discharge.

b. Recent major intraabdominal surgery. Extra-peritoneal procedures, such as nephrectomy, are not necessarily a contraindication.

c. Severe morbid obesity (BMI > 40).

C. Urgent PD in AKI.

1. Contraindications.

a. Ileus.

b. Appendicitis.

c. Ischemic bowel.

d. Intestinal obstruction or perforation.

e. Bacterial or fungal peritonitis.

f. New aortic grafts.

g. Abdominal/diaphragmatic fistulae.

h. Abdominal burns.

i. Cellulitis.

j. Severe hypercatabolic states or profound metabolic acidosis.

k. Drug intoxications are better suited for hemodialysis.

2. Access.

a. Stiff acute catheter – intraumbilical midline.

b. Double-cuff Tenckhoff catheter – paramedian.

3. Complications.

a. Blind placement of catheter can result in puncture of abdominal vascular structures or abdominal organs encased in the visceral layer of the peritoneal membrane.

b. A bladder catheter may be used to reduce a distended abdomen.

c. Pericatheter dialysate leaks may occur, requiring bulky compression dressings to contain the peritoneal fluids.

4. Benefits.

a. Avoidance of temporary vascular access and heparinization.

b. Greater hemodynamic stability.

c. Cost-effective.

5. Prescription.

a. Small initial dialysate volumes of 500 mL to 1 L.

b. Supine position.

c. Dwell times ranging from 30 to 50 minutes.

(1) More rapid initial urea saturation.

(2) 50% urea saturation in 30 minutes.

d. APD.

6. Ultrafiltration and the amount of potassium and calcium in the PD solution need to be individualized.

a. 1.5% dextrose PD solution.

b. 2.5% dextrose PD solution.

c. 4.25% dextrose PD solution.

(1) Careful glucose monitoring required.

(2) If rapid fluid removal needed, perform several 4.25% exchanges with minimal dwell times of 10 to 15 minutes and warm solution.

7. Careful monitoring.

a. Standardized flow sheets.

b. Complete documentation.

(1) Orders.

(2) Actual dwell times.

(3) Concentration of PD solution.

(4) Net ultrafiltration.

(5) Medications administered.

c. Monitor signs and symptoms of peritonitis (Ghaffari, 2012; Mehrota, 2012).

(1) Cloudy effluent.

(2) Abdominal pain.

(3) Nausea, vomiting, or diarrhea.

(4) Elevated temperature.

D. Contraindications for use of PD.

1. Traumatic injury to the abdomen, either surgical or accidental.

2. Traumatic injury to the diaphragm and pulmonary cavity.

3. Acute diverticulitis with or without peritonitis.

4. Suspected bowel perforation or traumatic puncture.

5. Recent abdominal surgeries.

6. Severe gastrointestinal reflux disease.

7. Recent cardiothoracic surgery.

8. Life-threatening electrolyte and/or metabolic imbalance.

9. Recent fungal peritonitis.

10. Documented inadequate peritoneal clearances.

11. Lack of experienced nurses who can safely manage PD.

E. Initiating emergency PD with a temporary PD catheter.
 1. Rarely if ever performed, only consider in the absence of better alternative such as acute hemodialysis.
 2. Educate the patient and family about PD management.
  a. Catheter insertion procedure.
  b. PD as a kidney replacement therapy.
  c. PD exchange routine.
  d. Prevention of infection.
  e. Use of masks and hand washing.
  f. Provide time for questions.

F. Peritoneal dialysis catheter placement.
 1. Refer to Module 3, Chapter 4, Section C, Peritoneal Dialysis Therapy, for information on acute catheters and their insertion, surgical complications, and exit-site infection.
 2. Care of the patient with a temporary PD catheter.
  a. The temporary catheter is inserted, ideally, in the interventional radiology (IR) suite or the operating room (OR) where visualization will minimize the risk of complications (e.g., bowel or other organ perforation or trauma). Bedside or blind placement should only be performed in the absence of a better alternative.
  b. Staff nurse or nephrology nurse may need to assist with bedside PD catheter placement.
   (1) Obtain and organize catheter insertion equipment.
   (2) Set up sterile field for physician and assistants.
   (3) Position patient and complete skin preparation.
   (4) Assist with first exchange of dialysate while positioning catheter and/or after catheter placement.
   (5) Dress and secure catheter.
   (6) Initiate PD exchanges as ordered.
  c. Temporary catheters are often rigid and need to be carefully secured to the abdominal wall.
  d. The less rigid temporary catheter may or may not be sutured to the abdominal wall.
  e. The right angle component of the catheter requires a multilayered dressing to support and immobilize the catheter.
  f. Temporary catheters are intended for short-term use (48 to 72 hours).
  g. Lack of subcutaneous tunnel can result in leaking of dialysate, leading to the development of exit-site infection or peritonitis.
  h. Dressing changes must be done promptly when wet or bloody and performed per hospital policy and procedure.
  i. Observe and document characteristics of effluent.

   (1) May be bloody due to the trauma of catheter insertion or possible perforation of the abdominal viscera.
   (2) May be cloudy due to infection or bowel perforation.
  j. Assessment of pain.
   (1) A newly inserted temporary or chronic catheter may create pain perceived as cramping during infusion or draining.
   (2) Slowing the rate of infusion or drainage may diminish the cramping sensation.
   (3) Dialysis solution that is either too hot or too cold may cause cramping and pain.
   (4) Warm dialysis solution bags according to established policy. Leaving solutions bags at room temperature is acceptable for warming, while submerging solution bags in hot water or heating them in the microwave are not advised due to the possibility of creating hot spots in the fluid.
   (5) The patient may experience incisional or exit-site pain with a newly placed PD catheter.
    (a) Obtain appropriate pain medication orders.
    (b) The conscious patient should rate pain using the institution's pain scale assessment tool.
    (c) The unconscious patient should be assessed for pain according to his/her physical responses.
     i. Unusual movement or restlessness.
     ii. Facial grimacing.
     iii. Changes in vital signs.
      [a] Increased pulse rate.
      [b] Increased respiratory rate.
     iv. Agitation.
 3. Complication of PD associated with emergent temporary catheter placement.
  a. Refer to Module 3, Chapter 4, Section D, Complications of Peritoneal Dialysis.
  b. Additional issues that may specifically occur with temporary catheters include the following.
   (1) Referred pain to shoulders, primarily related to free air in the abdomen.
   (2) Accidental disconnection of temporary catheter and/or tubing.
   (3) Migration of catheter tip with difficulty filling or draining.
   (4) Bowel or other organ perforation or trauma.
 4. Chronic catheter placement and associated management of care.
  a. A chronic catheter can be inserted for emergent PD or for early initiation for late referrals.
  b. The procedure is usually done in the operating

room (OR) by surgical dissection or by laparoscopy.
  c. Refer to Module 3, Chapter 4, Section B, Peritoneal Dialysis Access.
  d. Refer to Module 3, Chapter 4, Section C, Peritoneal Dialysis Complications.
5. Development of disequilibrium syndrome.
  a. Usually associated with hemodialysis, but can also be seen in patients with a serum urea nitrogen ≥ 100 mg/dL receiving frequent PD exchanges with a 4.25% dextrose dialysis solution.
  b. Etiology. Different theories include the following.
    (1) Plasma solute level is rapidly lowered during dialysis.
    (2) Cerebral edema occurs due to a lag in osmolar shift between blood and brain.
    (3) An acute increase in cerebral water content.
  c. Manifestations.
    (1) Nausea.
    (2) Vomiting.
    (3) Headache.
    (4) Restlessness.
    (5) Seizures.
    (6) Obtundation.
    (7) Coma.
  d. Prevention of disequilibrium syndrome.
    (1) Reduce elevated serum urea slowly with less frequent PD exchanges.
    (2) More likely to occur in patients with advanced uremia.

References

Bernardini, J., Price, V., & Figueiredo, A. (2006). Peritoneal dialysis patient training. *Peritoneal Dialysis International, 26*, 625-632.

Blake, P. (2006). The importance of the dialysis nurse. *Peritoneal Dialysis International, 26*, 623-624.

Cotovio, P., Rocha, A., & Rodrigues, A. (2011). Peritoneal dialysis in diabetics: There is room for more. *International Journal of Nephrology, 2011.* doi: 10.4061/2011/914849

Czajkowski, T., Pienkos, S., Schiller, B., & Doss-McQuitty, S. (2013). First exposure to home therapy options – Where, when, and how. *Nephrology Nursing Journal, 40*(1), 29-34.

Devuyst, O., Margetts, P., & Topley, N. (2010). The pathophysiology of the peritoneal membrane. *Journal of the American Society of Nephrology, 27*, 1077-1085.

Farina, J. (2008). Peritoneal dialysis: Strategies to maintain competency for acute and extended care nurses. *Nephrology Nursing Journal, 35*, 271-275.

Ghaffari, A. (2012). Urgent-start peritoneal dialysis: A quality improvement report. *American Journal of Kidney Diseases, 59*(3), 400-408.

Guest, S. (2014). *Handbook of peritoneal dialysis* (2nd ed.). CreateSpace Publishing.

Li, P., Szeto, C., Lye, W., Piraino, B., Bernardini, J., Figueiredo, A.E. … Struijk, D.G. (2010). ISPD guidelines/recommendations. *Peritoneal Dialysis International, 30*, 393-423. doi:10.3747/pdi.2010.00049

Mehrotra, R. (2012). Expanding access to peritoneal dialysis for incident dialysis patients. *American Journal of Kidney Diseases, 59*(3), 330-332.

Piraino, B., Bernardini, J., Brown, E., Figueiredo, A., Johnson, D., Lye, W., … Szeto, C. (2011). ISPD position statement on reducing the risks of peritoneal dialysis-related infections. *Peritoneal Dialysis International, 31*, 614-630.

Piraino, B. (2006). Nurses and physicians working together. *Peritoneal Dialysis International, 26*, 641-642.

Ponferrada, L., & Prowant, B. (2008). Peritoneal dialysis therapy. In C.S. Counts (Ed.), *Core curriculum for nephrology nursing* (5th ed., pp. 795-823). Pitman, NJ: American Nephrology Nurses' Association.

Prowant, B., Moore, H., Twardowski, Z., & Khanna, R. (2010). Understanding discrepancies in peritoneal equilibration test results. *Peritoneal Dialysis International, 3*, 366-370.

Rippe, B. (2008). Free water transport, small pore transport and the osmotic pressure gradient three-pore model of peritoneal transport. *Nephrology Dialysis Transplant, 23*, 2147-2153.

Yip, T., Tse, K., Lam, M., Cheng, S.W., Lui, S.L., Tang, S., … Lo, W.K. (2007). Risks and outcomes of peritonitis after flexible colonoscopy in CAPD patients. *Peritoneal Dialysis International, 27*, 560-564.

Appendix 5.1. CAPD Daily Checklist.

Courtesy of Western Nephrology Acute Dialysis, Denver, Colorado. Used with permission.

Daily Bedside Inservice Checklist for CAPD Patient Care

1. Review the patient's prescription
   - _____ a. Number of exchanges per day
   - _____ b. Volume of exchanges
   - _____ c. Dextrose and Calcium concentrations
   - _____ d. Effect of dextrose on fluid removal
   - _____ e. Medications to be added
   - _____ f. Where to get supplies needed for treatment
   - _____ g. Mask everyone, close the door, and wash your hands

2. Review the steps in performing a CAPD exchange - Tri-fold reference sheet
   - _____ a. Connect and drain
     - - Assess effluent for color, clarity, fibrin
     - _____ - Length of drain time
     - _____ - Difficulty or pain with draining
   - b. Fill
     - _____ - Length of time to fill
     - _____ - Difficulty or pain with filling
   - c. Disconnect and cap off the catheter
     - _____ - Weighing the effluent
     - _____ - Disposing of the effluent

3. Exit site and tunnel assessment
   - _____ a. Exit site care
   - _____ b. Tunnel palpation
   - _____ c. Securing the catheter

4. Documentation on the CAPD Treatment Record
   - _____ a. Exchange Record - out and in
   - _____ b. Patient Volume Net
   - _____ c. Effluent Characteristics
   - _____ d. Exit Site and Tunnel
   - _____ e. Observation of patient exchanges
   - _____ f. Labs
   - _____ g. Vital signs
   - _____ h. Patient assessments

5. When to call the nephrologist:
   - _____ a. If the effluent becomes cloudy or has fibrin in it.
   - _____ b. If the lab values are out of the normal range for a dialysis patient.
   - _____ c. If the catheter exit site or tunnel appear inflamed, sore, or draining.
   - _____ d. If the patient's fluid status is changing and the prescription for ulltrafiltration needs to be adjusted.

_____
Hospital Staff

_____
Western Acute Dialysis Staff

_____
Date   Time

Appendix 5.2. Acute Care PD Flow Sheet.

Courtesy of Maria Luongo. Used with permission.

Acute Peritoneal Dialysis Flow Sheet											

Patient Name **John Doe** Medical Record # **000-00-00**
Nephrologist **Dr. G.F. Rate**

Date	Time	Ex.#	Previous Fill Vol. (PFV)	% Dex.	Medication Added	Drain Vol. (DV)	Description Of effluent	(PFV)-(DV)= Ex. Balance	24hr.bal.	Daily Wt.
12-5-14	2 AM	1	2000 ml	1.5 %	none	2100 ml	Clear, no fibrin	2000-2100=-100	-100	169 lbs.
12-5-14	6 AM	2	2000 ml	2.5 %	none	2500 ml	Clear (+) fibrin	2000-2500=-500	-600	
12-5-14	10AM	3	2000 ml	1.5%	Heparin 2000u	2700 ml	Clear, no fibrin	2000-2700=-700	-1300	
"	2 PM	4	2000 ml	2.5 %	Heparin 2000u	2200 ml	Clear, no fibrin	2000-2200=-200	-1500	
"	6 PM	5	2000 ml	2.5 %	Heparin 2000u	2700 ml	Clear, no fibrin	2000-2700=-700	-2200	
"	10PM	6	2500 ml	2.5 %	Heparin 2000u	2700 ml	Clear, no fibrin	2500-2700=-200	-2900	
12-6-14	2 AM	7	2500 ml	2.5 %	Heparin 2000u	2800 ml	Clear, no fibrin	2500-2800=-300	-300	166 lbs.
12-6-14	6 AM	8	2500 ml	2.5%	Heparin 2000u					

Appendix 5.3. CAPD Treatment Record.

Courtesy of Western Nephrology Acute Dialysis, Denver, Colorado. Used with permission.

Western Acute Dialysis Peritoneal Dialysis Record

Date: _____ Date PD Initiated: _____ Hosp Day# _____

Hospital: _____ Patient Name: _____

Primary Diagnosis: _____ Set up:_____ Nurse visit:_____ On call:_____
Pager:_____

Out Patient Unit/Contact: _____ Phone: _____ Supplies: Adequate _____
Order placed _____

Physician CAPD Orders:

Number of exchanges _____
Volume: 2500ml or _____ml x2
Dianeal: 2.5mEq Ca or _____mEq Ca
: Add K+ _____mEq/L
Dry Weight _____

1. 6am _____%
2. 10 am _____%
3. 2 pm _____%
4. 6 pm _____%
5. 10 pm _____%

1. 8am _____%
2. 1 pm _____%
3. 6 pm _____%
4. 10 pm _____%

CAPD EXCHANGE RECORDS:

				OUT			IN			
Date	BP	Exch No	Time	ml's drained	Drain Time	Dextrose Solution % Selected	Meds added	ml's infused	Patient Volume Net	Staff Signature

Daily Total Net

Labs:

	Prev	Today
Na		
K+		
Cl		
C02		
BUN		
Cr		
Gluc		
Ca		
Alb		
Phos		
WBC		
Hgb		
Hct		
Plt		

Cell Count:

Gram Stain:

Culture Results:

Assessment:

	Prev	Today
BP		
HR		
Temp		
Weight		
02		
Lungs		
Edema		
Muscle Cramping		

Effluent Characteristics:

Time	Color	Clarity	Fibrin

EXIT SITE:		TUNNEL:
Skin Color		Red
Clean		
Crusted		Warmth
Tender		
Drainage		Tender
Cleaned with		
Ointment applied		
Dressing		

Mental Status	
Mobility	
Dexterity	
Appetite	
N/V	
Pain	
Observed Technique	
Mask	
Washed Hands	

Comments:

Appendix 5.4. Peritoneal Dialysis Orders.

Courtesy of Maria Luongo. Used with permission.

Peritoneal Dialysis Orders for the Hospitalized Patient   Date_____

Patient Name:_____   Diagnosis:_____

Nephrologist: _____   PD RN Resource phone # _____

CAPD orders:

Dialysate Solution   Low Ca+ 2.5 mEq/1L solution _____
1.5%_____   Reg. Ca+ 3.5 mEq/L solution _____
2.5% _____
4.25% _____
or alternate_____% and _____ %

Fill volume (FV) per exchange _____mL

Frequency of exchange: Every _____hrs. or _____ times per day

Assess drained effluent past each exchange. Report cloudy or bloody drainage.

Dialysate specimens to lab:
(Baseline upon admission and prn cloudy fluid)

Hematology – Cell count _____and differential_____

Microbiology – Gm Stain_____and C & S_____

Medications Added to Dialysate Bag: **Allergies:**_____

Heparin _____units per solution bag prn fibrin

Antibiotic:_____Start Date_____ Frequency_____
Antibiotic:_____Start Date_____ Frequency_____

Potassium Chloride (KCl) _____ mEq per bag

Other medications: _____

Exit-Site Care:

Keep catheter secured to abdomen with tape.

Change tape and dressing daily and more frequently if needed.

Wash exit site daily with soap and water.

Apply: Bactroban ointment_____ Gentamycin ointment_____

Report signs and symptoms of infection of exit site to nephrologist.

Send swab for: Gm stain_____ C & S _____

Diet: High protein and low concentrated sweets

Appendix 5.5. CAPD Orders.

Courtesy of Western Nephrology Acute Dialysis, Denver, Colorado. Used with permission.

CONTINUOUS AMBULATORY PERITONEAL DIALYSIS (CAPD) STANDING ORDERS

1. CAPD #_____ Exchanges/day of 2500 ml or _____ ml x2 Dianeal with 2.5 mEq or _____ mEq C

    Exchanges:
    1. 6 am _____%
    2. 10 am _____%
    3. 2 pm _____%
    4. 6 pm _____%
    5. 10 pm _____%

    1. 8 am _____%
    2. 1 pm _____%
    3. 6 pm _____%
    4. 10 pm _____%

2. Reassess weight gain or loss with Nephrologist and adjust % of dextrose prn.

3. Measure drain volume and record on flow sheet for each exchange every day.

4. Check peritoneal dialysis drainage bag with each exchange for fibrin, blood, or cloudiness. If present, notify nephrologist.

5. If peritonitis is present, the initial antibiotic regimen is as follows:
    __a. Vancomycin _____ mg per bag one 6-hour dwell (15–30 mg/kg I.P. with maximum dose of 2000 mg). Note: This is a one-time dose order.
    __b. Ciprofloxacin 500 mg p.o. bid or equivalent available on Formulary.
    __c. Once the organism is identified, narrow the antibiotic spectrum to cover the specific organism.

6. If fibrin is present, add Heparin_____ units per bag (recommended range of 500-1000 units Heparin/Liter of dialysate solution) after checking with nephrologist.

7. Pharmacy only to add any medication to dialysis bag.

8. Daily weight and record on graphic and CAPD flow sheet. (Weight should be done at the same time each day with abdomen full.)

9. If patient has had no bowel movement for 2 days, contact Nephrologist for prn laxative/stool softener order.

10. Diet: 1.3-1.5 g protein/kg/day, no added salt, no potassium restriction.

11. Daily exit-site care should be done by cleansing with liquid soap via pump dispenser. Follow by applying Gentamicin 1% cream to site daily and covering with nonocclusive dressing. If new (fresh postop) exit site, use sterile technique to change dressing once a week or if dressing is soiled (bloody). Continue for first 3 weeks postop.

12. Call Western Acute Dialysis team for nursing issues:
    M-F from 0600-1600 at 303-595-2660 and after hours 303-231-6552

    MD Signature_____ Date_____

Appendix 5.6. CCPD Orders.

Courtesy of Maureen Craig, University of California, Davis Medical Center, Sacramento, California. Used with permission.

UNIVERSITY OF CALIFORNIA, DAVIS
MEDICAL CENTER
SACRAMENTO, CALIFORNIA

PHYSICIAN'S ORDERS

CONTINUOUS CYCLING PERITONEAL DIALYSIS

Directions: Check (√) and complete those orders to be carried out on this patient.

Date:	For Date:
Time:	For Time:
1.	√ Fax orders to Tower Four x43505 and call x43333
2.	□ Daily Weight in Kg
3.	□ Daily exit site care with 3% saline followed by mupirocin 2% ointment at time of disconnection
4.	□ Number of 5 liter dialysate bags____ 1.5% dextrose ____ 2.5% _____ 4.25% (Only one fill volume will be used from a loading dose bag) □ Delflex dialysate concentrations (mEq/L) **Ca^{++}** 2.5 **Na^{+}** 132 **Lactate** 40 **K^{+}** 0 **Mg^{++}** 0.5 **Chloride** 95
5.	□ Fills _____ (6-7) (includes last fill) Total daily Fill volume_____ liters
6.	□ CCPD volume _____ (2 - 3) liters (single fill volume)
7.	□ Last Fill volume _____(2 - 3) liters (zero if patient to be left dry)
8.	□ Fill Time 15 minutes
9.	□ Dwell Time _____(1-3) hours (shorter dwell times increases ultrafiltration)
10.	□ Drain Time 30 minutes
11.	□ Manual drain of last fill volume at _____(4-6) hours post CCPD last fill
Laboratory:	
12.	□ Dialysate effluent cell count (send 5 ml sample of first drain in lavender top tube)
13.	□ Dialysate effluent gram stain, culture and sensitivity (send 100 ml sample of first drain)
14.	□ Catheter exit site culture and sensitivity (swab exit site with culturette swabstick)
15.	□ __________________(antibiotic) serum level (draw if suspected bacteremia)
Medications:	Complete the antibiotic order from for any antibiotics ordered below.
16.	□ Heparin _____(1000) units / liter Intra peritoneal
17.	□ Deliver Antibiotics as follows: During first Fill cycle Loading bag is open and all Maintenance bags are clamped. After first Fill cycle, clamp Loading bag, and unclamp all Maintenance bags.
18.	□ Loading Bag (LB): Antibiotic:__________ _______ mg / liter Intraperitoneal ____% dextrose Antibiotic:__________ _______ mg / liter Intraperitoneal
19.	□ Maintenance Bags (MB): Antibiotic:__________ _______ mg / liter Intraperitoneal Antibiotic:__________ _______ mg / liter Intraperitoneal

Dosing guide in mg/L: Gentamicin LB 60 (max LB volume = 2L) MB 4, Cefazolin LB 500 MB 125, Vancomycin LB 1000 MB 25, Ceftazidime LB 500 MB 125

Nephrologist (signature/print name):	P.I.:	Pager:
Nephrology Nurse(signature/print name):	Date/Time:	

AR4098 (9/07) **CONTINUOUS CYCLING PERITONEAL DIALYSIS ORDERS** **MR#07/00566**

Appendix 5.7. CCPD Suspect Peritonitis Orders.

Courtesy of Maureen Craig, University of California, Davis Medical Center, Sacramento, California. Used with permission.

UNIVERSITY OF CALIFORNIA, DAVIS
MEDICAL CENTER
SACRAMENTO, CALIFORNIA

PHYSICIAN'S ORDERS

CONTINUOUS CYCLING PERITONEAL DIALYSIS "SUSPECT PERITONITIS"

Directions: Check (√) and complete those orders to be carried out on this patient.

Date:	For Date:
Time:	For Time:

1.	√ Fax orders to Tower Four x43505 and call x43333
2.	☐ Daily exit site care with 3% saline followed by mupirocin 2% ointment at time of disconnection

3.	☐ Number of 5 liter dialysate bags _____ 1.5% dextrose
	☐ Delflex dialysate concentrations (mEq/L)
	    Ca⁺⁺ 2.5 **Na⁺** 132 **Lactate** 40
	    K⁺ 0 **Mg⁺⁺** 0.5 **Chloride** 95

4.	☐ Fills _____ (3) (includes last fill) Total daily Fill volume_____ liters
5.	☐ CCPD volume _____ (1- 2) liters (single fill volume)
6.	☐ Last Fill volume _____(1 - 2) liters (membrane is typically more permeable during peritonitis)
7.	☐ Fill Time 15 minutes
8.	☐ Dwell Time 5 minutes
9.	☐ Drain Time 20 minutes
10.	☐ Routine CCPD orders should begin within 4 hours

Laboratory:

11.	☐ Dialysate effluent cell count (send 5 ml sample of first drain in lavender top tube)
12.	☐ Dialysate effluent gram stain, culture and sensitivity (send 100 ml sample of first drain)
13.	☐ Catheter exit site culture and sensitivity (swab exit site with culturette swabstick)

Catheter Inflow / Outflow Treatment:

14.	☐ _____ (50) units of Heparin in 50 ml normal saline in syringe for flushing.
15.	☐ Vigorously flush PD catheter with ordered flush solution. Flush in and out to reestablish flow.
16.	☐ If poor flow, abdominal X-ray 2 views to check Peritoneal Dialysis catheter placement.
17.	☐ If poor flow fill PD catheter with Alteplase 5mg/5ml (use volume to fill catheter) Dwell for 2 hours and aspirate Alteplase. Repeat heparinized saline flush above.
18.	☐ If flow is not reestablished call Nephrologist.
19.	☐ Lactulose 30ml by mouth, twice a day, until stooling occurs.

Nephrologist (signature/print name):	P.I.:	Pager:
Nephrology Nurse (signature/print name):	Date/Time:	

AR5937 (9/07)   **CCPD "SUSPECT PERITONITIS" DIALYSIS ORDERS**   MR 08/05993

The Patient with a Ventricular Assist Device

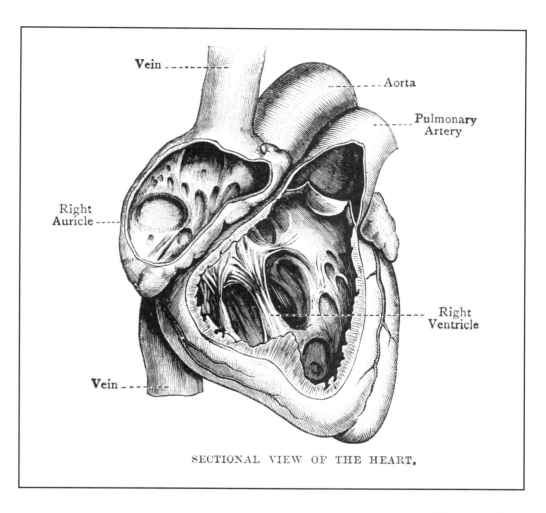

SECTIONAL VIEW OF THE HEART.

Chapter Editor
Helen F. Williams, MSN, BSN, RN, CNN

Author
Mary Alice Norton, BSN, FNP-C

CHAPTER **6**

The Patient with a Ventricular Assist Device

This offering for **1.5 contact hours** is provided by the American Nephrology Nurses' Association (ANNA).

American Nephrology Nurses' Association is accredited as a provider of continuing nursing education by the American Nurses Credentialing Center Commission on Accreditation.

ANNA is a provider approved by the California Board of Registered Nursing, provider number CEP 00910.

This CNE offering meets the continuing nursing education requirements for certification and recertification by the Nephrology Nursing Certification Commission (NNCC).

To be awarded contact hours for this activity, read this chapter in its entirety. Then complete the CNE evaluation found at **www.annanurse.org/corecne** and submit it; or print it, complete it, and mail it in. Contact hours are not awarded until the evaluation for the activity is complete.

Example of reference for Chapter 6 in APA format. One author for entire chapter.

Norton, M.A. (2015). The patient with a ventricular assist device. In C.S. Counts (Ed.), *Core curriculum for nephrology nursing: Module 4. Acute kidney injury* (6th ed., pp. 143-160). Pitman, NJ: American Nephrology Nurses' Association.

Interpreted: Chapter author. (Date). Title of chapter. In ...

Illustration from iStock, Getty Images.

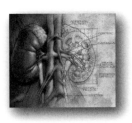

CHAPTER 6

The Patient with a Ventricular Assist Device

Purpose

The purpose of this chapter is twofold. First, it is to provide an overview of heart failure (HF) in the United States. It attempts to define HF, HF etiologies, patient symptoms, patient assessment, and medical therapies used in the treatment of HF. Second, it focuses on one therapy for those with advanced HF: mechanical circulatory support with the HeartMate II® Left Ventricular Assist Device (LVAD).

Indications for LVAD support, patient selection criteria, and an overview of pump components are discussed. Additionally, the chapter reviews outpatient management, medical therapy, device management, and pump troubleshooting, along with special considerations for LVAD patients during hemodialysis. Last, discussion includes monitoring during procedures, emergency care, and safety issues specific to patients with LVADs.

Objectives

Upon completion of this chapter, the learner will be able to:
1. Relate the most common symptoms that patients experience with acute heart failure to the causes of the heart failure.
2. Discuss the focus of treatment for patients with heart failure, including the LVAD.
3. Name the four pump parameters and discuss the nurse's responsibility for monitoring.
4. Describe assessment of the patient with an LVAD.

I. Overview of heart failure in the United States.

A. Definition of heart failure.
   1. Heart failure (HF) has been defined and redefined over the years with no consensus on one encompassing definition.
   2. It is difficult to define because it is a complex syndrome with many causes, different degrees of clinical manifestation, and pathophysiologic responses.
   3. The 2010 Heart Failure Society of America (HFSA) Guidelines define heart failure as a "syndrome caused by cardiac dysfunction, generally resulting from myocardial muscle dysfunction or loss and characterized by either left ventricular dilation or hypertrophy or both. Whether the dysfunction is primarily systolic or diastolic or mixed, it leads to neurohormonal and circulatory abnormalities, usually resulting in symptoms such as fluid retention, shortness of breath, and fatigue, especially with exertion" (Lindenfeld et al., 2010).

4. HFSA describes the syndrome of HF as progressive and usually fatal, but with appropriate therapies, patients can be stabilized and the effects of neurohormonal activity and cardiac dysfunction can be improved and sometimes reversed (Grady et al., 2000; Lindenfeld et al., 2010).
5. Multiple terms are used to describe the characteristics of HF. Those terms are often based on the presence or absence of fluid congestion, but may also be based on the following:
   a. Acute or chronic HF.
   b. Right-sided vs. left-sided.
   c. Systolic and/or diastolic.
   d. With or without other organ involvement as in cardiorenal syndrome (Grady et al., 2000).
6. It is important to understand the cause of a patient's HF in order to prevent disease progression and correctly diagnose, treat, and educate the patient.
7. The term systolic dysfunction means there is impairment in the contractile function of the heart

muscle when blood is ejected, whereas diastolic dysfunction is impairment in the relaxation ability of the heart muscle during filling.

8. Further classification of systolic heart failure is described as either preserved left ventricular ejection fraction (pLVEF) or reduced left ventricular ejection fraction (rLVEF).
   a. The LVEF is a measurement of how much blood is pumped out of the ventricles with each heartbeat.
   b. Normal LVEF is > 55% and normal right ventricular ejection fraction (RVEF) is approximately the same as LVEF with only small differences (Marving et al., 1985).
   c. When LVEF is reduced (rLVEF) or less than normal, it may be reported as mildly reduced (40% to 50%), moderate (26% to 39%), and severely reduced (< 25%).
   d. LVEF can be measured by echocardiography, cardiac catheterization, and radionuclide imaging. Results can vary based on the test used, method of analysis, and the operator (Yancy et al., 2013).
9. Data is limited on patients with HF and pLVEF as it has not been studied as extensively as those with systolic dysfunction with reduced EF.
   a. According to a report from the Acute Decompensated HF National registry (ADHERE), patients with pLVEF are more often older, women, and most often obese.
   b. HF with pLVEF accounts for one half of all hospitalizations for heart failure (Yancy et al., 2013).
10. Patients with impairment in the relaxation of the heart often experience the same symptoms as those with systolic dysfunction and a low ejection fraction.

B. Incidence, prevalence, and survival with HF.
   1. Heart failure affects approximately 5.1 million people in the United States and accounts for about 650,000 new cases annually.
   2. It is the number one cause of hospitalization for people 65 years and older (Lindenfeld et al., 2010).
   3. Over the past 30 years, the incidence and prevalence of HF has increased. Contributing factors to this increase include:
      a. The aging population.
      b. Improved survival for patients with cardiovascular disease.
      c. Advances in diagnostic abilities.
      d. Improved medical and surgical treatments.
   4. As a result of living longer, there is increased incidence of comorbidities such as kidney failure, coronary artery disease, and diabetes complications.
      a. Data analysis involving 10,311 subjects from 50 years of follow-up of the Framingham Study found HF occurred in 1,075 participants during the study period. Of these participants with HF, 51% were women.
      b. The mean age of HF onset during the period between 1950 and 1999 was 62.7 ±8.8 years with men's rates slightly higher than women's (Ho et al., 1993).
      c. Survival after the onset of HF was noted to improve over the decades studied.
         (1) During the four consecutive periods of participant follow-up (1950 to 1969, 1970 to 1979, 1980 to 1989, and 1990 to 1999), the 1-year mortality rates were 30%, 41%, 33%, and 28% respectively among men and 28%, 28%, 27%, and 24% among women.
         (2) Five-year mortality for men decreased from 70% to 59% and declined from 57% to 45% in women from the first to the last time period. In addition, the Framingham study found a prevalence of HF in men of 8 per 1000 at age 50 to 59 years; the prevalence increased to 66 per 1000 by age 80 to 89 years. Similar findings of 8 per 1000 and 79 per 1000 were found in women (Ho et al. 1993).
   5. Despite the improved survival and technologic advances, the incidence and prevalence of HF increases with age and the mortality rates remain about 50% within 5 years of being diagnosed (Yancy et al., 2013).

C. Etiologies.
   1. People at risk for cardiovascular (CV) diseases are at risk for heart failure (HF) (Lindenfeld et al., 2010).
   2. In the United States, the lifetime risk for developing HF is 20% in those ≥ 40 years of age (Yancy et al., 2013).
   3. Identifying and treating the risk factors associated with developing HF are crucial to prevention. Many of those predisposing conditions are modifiable if diagnosed and treated appropriately.
      a. Hypertension, both systolic and diastolic, is probably the single most important modifiable risk factor. The lifetime risk of developing hypertension in the United States is > 75%, so early diagnosis and long-term treatment are essential to decrease the risk of HF (Yancy et al., 2013).
      b. Dilated cardiomyopathies (DCM) are a large group of disorders also known as nonischemic cardiomyopathy, usually classified as:
         (1) Idiopathic.
         (2) Valvular.
         (3) Familial.
         (4) Restrictive.
         (5) Hypertrophic.

c. Patients with atherosclerotic disease, whether it is coronary artery, cerebral, or peripheral arterial disease, are at increased risk for HF.

d. Other metabolic and endocrine conditions that can cause cardiomyopathies are obesity, thyroid disease, diabetes mellitus, and insulin resistance. These comorbidities increase the risk for HF in patients with or without structural heart disease and negatively affect those who already have HF (Yancy et al., 2013).

e. Toxic cardiomyopathy can be caused by external factors.

(1) Chronic alcoholism, cocaine abuse, and several cytotoxic antineoplastic medications used to treat certain cancers are cardio toxic.

(2) The anthracyclines tend to be quite cardio toxic and can lead to long-term cardiac problems (Yancy et al., 2013).

(3) Other cardiac toxic agents include ephedra, amphetamines, cobalt, catecholemines, and anabolic steroids.

(4) Nutritional deficiencies related to eating disorders, AIDS, and pregnancy, although rare, can lead to cardiomyopathies.

(5) Tachycardia-induced cardiomyopathy from increased ventricular heart rate is most often reversible depending on the duration and rate of the tachyarrhythmia (Yancy et al., 2013).

(6) Myocarditis is an inflammation of the heart often seen after a viral infection and seen in systemic lupus, HIV, and peripartum cardiomyopathies.

4. Whatever the cause for the onset of HF, the pathophysiology begins with an initial cardiac injury that results in a decrease in heart function.

a. This initial injury stimulates activation of neurohormonal cascade from the renin-angiotensin/aldosterone system (RAAS), the sympathetic nervous system (SNS), and antidiuretic hormone release.

b. Over time these initial compensatory mechanisms cause remodeling of the ventricles, dilation of heart chambers, worsening of systolic or diastolic dysfunction, peripheral vasoconstriction, and eventually symptoms of HF that increase morbidity and mortality the longer left untreated.

D. Assessment of patients.

1. Obtaining a thorough history and physical examination on someone with established HF is the first step in assessing a patient.

2. One must be alert to the original cause and any additional contributing factors that could exacerbate cardiac dysfunction.

3. Factors such as angina, myocardial ischemia/infarction, viral infection, pneumonia, uncontrolled hypertension, or drug abuse could contribute to an acute decompensation or exacerbation of symptoms.

4. The focus for routine assessment of outpatients with HF should be their circulatory status and functional capacity at rest and with activity.

5. Symptom assessment includes questioning patients about episodes of:

a. Shortness of breath.

b. Orthopnea.

c. Paroxysmal nocturnal dyspnea.

d. Activity tolerance.

e. Chest pain.

f. Weight gain.

g. Fatigue.

h. Dizziness.

i. Weakness.

j. Symptoms related to arrhythmias such as palpitations.

k. Syncope.

l. Visual or speech disturbances.

m. Delivery of cardiodefibrillator shock.

6. Hemodynamic status is evaluated by looking for evidence of elevated filling pressures and adequate tissue perfusion.

a. Is there evidence of hypoperfusion (cold) or congestion (wet), or are they warm (perfused) and dry (euvolemic)?

b. Orthopnea is the most sensitive and specific symptom of elevated filling pressures, and jugular venous distention is a sensitive sign for resting elevated filling pressures (Grady et al., 2000).

c. A cough at night or with exertion could indicate volume overload.

d. Some patients have peripheral edema while only a few with chronically elevated filling pressure have rales (Grady et al., 2000).

7. Two classification systems used to evaluate development and progression of HF and evaluate symptom burden and exercise capacity are the American College of Cardiology Foundation/American Heart Association (ACCF/AHA) stages of HF and the New York Heart Association (NYHA) functional classes.

a. NYHA Functional Classification.

(1) Class I: No limitation of physical activity. Ordinary physical activity does not cause symptoms.

(2) Class II: Slight limitation of physical activity. Comfortable at rest, but ordinary physical activity results in symptoms.

(3) Class III – IIIA: Marked limitation of physical activity causes symptoms.

(4) Class IIIB: Marked limitation of physical activity. Comfortable at rest but minimal exertion causes symptoms.

(5) Class IV: Unable to carry on any physical activity without discomfort. Symptoms present at rest.

b. ACCF/AHA stages.

(1) Stage A: At high risk for HF but without structural heart diseases or symptoms of HF.

(2) Stage B: Structural heart disease but without signs or symptoms of HF.

(3) Stage C: Structural heart disease with prior or current symptoms of HF.

(4) Stage D: Refractory HF requiring specialized interventions.

E. Current focus of medical therapy for HF.

1. Pharmacology, implantable cardio defibrillators (ICDs)/cardiac resynchronization therapy (CRT), patient education, mechanical circulatory support, and heart transplantation are the main therapies available in the care of HF patients today.

2. The latter two are reserved for those with end-stage HF who have no other options but advanced therapies or hospice. Several different classes of medications are used in the treatment of HF.

a. The ACCF/AHA guidelines recommend goal directed therapies with medications that target the neurohormonal responses noted above.

b. Treatment will depend on the stage and functional class of HF, etiology of HF, and whether EF is preserved or reduced.

c. Recommendations for treatment of those with HF with preserved EF.

(1) Control systolic and diastolic blood pressure (BP) with beta-blockers (BB), angiotensin converting enzyme inhibitors (ACE-I), or angiotensin receptor blockers (ARBs).

(2) Use diuretics for symptom relief due to volume overload.

(3) In those with coronary artery disease who have angina or are experiencing ischemia, revascularization should be considered.

(4) Management of arrhythmias with rate control and maintenance of sinus rhythm would be a goal of therapy (Yancy et al., 2013).

3. For those with reduced EF, first line treatment recommendations as noted above with addition of aldosterone antagonists, potassium sparing or thiazide diuretics, nitrates, hydralazine, and/or digoxin are recommended.

4. To prevent sudden cardiac death (SCD), placement of implantable cardio defibrillators is appropriate for selected patients if they meet established criteria.

5. Guidelines from the ACCF/AHA recommend that patients with advanced heart failure should be considered for an ICD as primary prevention.

6. All patients with HF should be educated on their individual disease process and taught self-management skills to prevent further progression, decompensation, and hospitalizations, such as:

a. Maintaining a low-salt diet.

b. Daily self-weights.

c. Monitoring symptoms.

d. Adhering to medications and prescribed therapies.

e. Follow-up appointments.

f. Exercising routinely.

7. When HF progresses and functional capacity declines to NYHA class IIIB & IV, more advanced therapies, such as mechanical circulatory support (MCS) or cardiac transplantation, may be recommended.

II. Mechanical circulatory support: left ventricular assist device (LVAD).

A. Indications for LVAD support.

1. The HeartMate II® LVAD is FDA approved for bridge to transplant (BTT), destination therapy (DT), and postcardiotomy recovery.

2. It is indicated for patients with NYHA class IIIb-IV, stage D AHA/ACCF HF, and those meeting the criteria outlined in the INTERMACS profiles (Stevenson et al., 2009).

a. Profile 1: Critically ill with hemodynamic compromise and cardiogenic shock that is life threatening. Sometimes referred to as "crash and burn scenario."

b. Profile 2: Decreasing functional capacity with worsening end organ function despite inotropic support and maximal medical therapies. Sometimes referred to as "sliding on inotropes."

c. Profile 3: Stable hemodynamics, organ function, symptoms and nutritional status, and inotrope dependent. Several failed attempts to wean from support due to compromised organ function or symptom worsening. Sometimes referred to as "dependent stability."

d. Profile 4: Patient has symptoms at rest or with minimal activities. Diuretic doses usually high and change frequently due to volume status and compliance to medications and dietary restriction. Some patients may move between Profile 4 and 5.

e. Profile 5: Patient is comfortable at rest but not able to participate in usual daily activities without symptoms. May have kidney dysfunction and/or increased volume status and nutritional deficits which increases risk for further intervention.

   f. Profile 6: Patient is comfortable at rest and with usual activities, but experiences fatigue with more strenuous activities. EVO2 exercise test and hemodynamic monitoring my be necessary to confirm degree of cardiac dysfunction. Sometimes referred to as "walking wounded."

   g. Profile 7: Patients without current or any recent episodes of decompensated heart failure. Fluid status is stable and patient is living comfortably with mild physical activity. This profile is for those who may need future advanced therapies. Considered Advanced NYHA class III.

3. The goals of LVAD therapy are to improve symptoms, quality of life, and prognosis in patients with advanced HF.

4. Two of the most important factors for improving outcomes after LVAD implant are patient selection and timing of the implant.

5. Patients are selected for LVAD therapy based on the following inclusion and exclusion criteria.

B. Inclusion criteria.

1. NYHA class IV HF/Stage D AHA/ACCF HF (DT) or NYHA class IIIb-IV HF (BTT) despite optimal medical therapy for at least 45 of the last 60 days, or intraaortic balloon pump (IABP) dependent for 7 days, or inotrope-dependent for > 14 days.

2. ICD/CRT device, if indicated.

3. LVEF <25%.

4. SBP 80 to 90 mmHg, or cardiac index (CI) < 2 L/min/m^2 or declining kidney or RV function.

5. Exercise VO$_2$ < 14 mL/kg/min unless IABP or inotrope dependent or physically unable.

6. High 1-year mortality due to HF.

7. Listed for heart transplant at a Medicare approved transplant center (BTT).

8. Ineligible for transplant candidacy secondary to: advanced age, end organ damage due to diabetes, chronic kidney disease with creatinine > 2.5 mg/dL, moderate but not prohibitive peripheral vascular disease (DT).

9. BSA > 1.2 m^2.

10. There is a committed social support system at home. The patient and/or family member is/are willing and able to learn and manage the device.

11. Relatively preserved RV function as assessed by recent echocardiogram and RV hemodynamics including CVP, PCWP, PAP, etc.

C. Exclusion criteria: Medical and surgical contraindications to LVAD therapy.

1. Predicted very high risk on INTERMACS Profiles.

2. Noncardiac terminal illness that would limit survival to less than 1 year.

3. Liver failure or hepatic cirrhosis (biopsy proven).

4. Kidney failure requiring hemodialysis.

5. Irreversible pulmonary disease or severe COPD (FEV1 < 1.0 L).

6. Severe hemodynamic compromise and unable to be corrected or stabilized with inotropes or IABP.

7. Multiorgan system failure.

8. Active infection.

9. Recent cerebrovascular accident.

10. Severe RV dysfunction.

11. Severe deconditioning or malnutrition.

12. Pregnancy.

13. Metastatic or advanced cancer.

14. Impaired cognitive function, confirmed by Neurology.

15. Unable to tolerate anticoagulation.

16. Inability to undergo complete preimplant evaluation process for LVAD.

D. Interagency Registry for Mechanically Assisted Circulatory Support (INTERMACS).

1. This database is sponsored by the National Heart, Lung and Blood Institute (NHLBI), the U.S. Food and Drug Administration (FDA), and the Centers for Medicare and Medicaid Services (CMS).

2. Patient enrollment and data collection began June 2006 for patients who had an FDA-approved mechanical circulatory support device implanted.

   a. The Thoratec HeartMate II® and the Heartware HVAD® are the only approved adult devices (Kirklin et al., 2013).

   b. As of December 16, 2013, there are 152 active participating sites and 11, 255 subjects enrolled in the INTERMACS registry (INTERMACS, http://www.uab.edu/medicine/intermacs).

   c. Clinical data is collected at 1 week, 1 month, 3 months, 6 months, and every 6 months thereafter.

   d. Outcomes postimplant such as explant, death, hospital readmits, and adverse events are recorded at these intervals and are the major endpoints collected. The data is reviewed, analyzed, and reported annually.

   e. The fifth INTERMACS annual survival report for continuous flow pumps is 80% at 1 year and 70% at 2 years (Kirklin et al., 2013; INTERMACS website).

   f. Long-term data from INTERMACS has resulted in patient profiles that help identify risks associated with timing of the implantation (Slaughter et al., 2010). The profiles allow for improvement in risk stratification and patient selection.

E. Pulsatile vs. continuous flow pumps.

1. Pulsatile, volume displacement pumps have been replaced by continuous flow rotary pumps (see Figure 6.1).

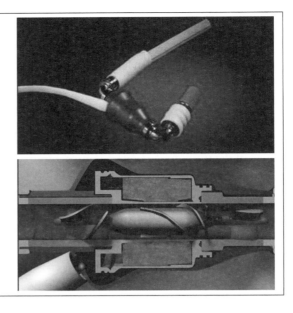

HeartMate II pump

- Smaller size
  - 60% smaller than XVE
  - 35 mm diameter
  - 70 mm long
  - 400 grams

- No requirement for venting
  - 40% reduction in the size of percutaneous driveline

- Enhanced patient comfort

- Near noiseless operation

- Ease of surgical implantation
  - Standard sternotomy vs. extended midline excision
  - Smaller preperitoneal pocket

Figure 6.1. Continuous flow, rotary pumps.
Used with permission from Thoratec Corporation.

2. Continuous flow pumps offer smaller size, quieter operation, and less surgical intervention; only one moving part makes them more durable than the pulsatile design.
3. Percutaneous lead dimensions are 40% smaller, thereby reducing infection rates and improving patient comfort.

F. Overview of HM II® LVAD.
   1. The HM II® LVAD is an electric, continuous flow pump that uses a rotary blood pump to generate flow and assist the left ventricle.
   2. The pump is implanted in front of the peritoneum, below the left rectus muscle and above the rectus sheath.
   3. The rotor, the only moving part, spins on two synthetic ruby bearings at either end of the assembly and sits in ceramic cups immersed in blood. It has blood flow capacity up to 10 L/min, is preload dependent, and afterload sensitive.
   4. The electric motor operates by creating a magnetic field that produces torque, spinning the rotor and moving blood forward.
   5. Components of the pump.
      a. The inflow conduit is attached to the apex of the left ventricle (LV) and is pointed up toward the mitral valve (see Figure 6.2).
      b. Blood enters the inflow conduit and exits via an outflow conduit that is sewn into the ascending aorta. Both conduits have internal textured surfaces designed to stimulate tissue growth and create a pseudo intima, which helps decrease thrombus formation.
      c. The percutaneous lead (driveline), attached to the implanted pump, exits the skin on either

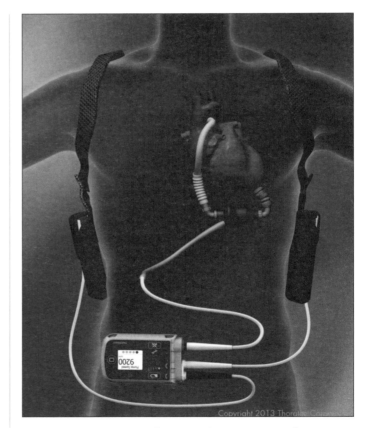

Figure 6.2. HeartMate II inflow cannula in LV apex, outflow to ascending aorta, tunneled percutaneous lead, external percutaneous lead, SC, power leads, batteries in holster.
Used with permission from Thoratec Corporation.

the right or left upper abdominal quadrant. The lead contains six wires, three for the primary and three for the backup system, which carry power to the pump.

d. The tunneled internal part of the percutaneous lead is covered with woven polyester that encourages tissue ingrowth to help stabilize the driveline and prevent infections and damage to the line.

e. The external driveline then plugs into the system controller (SC), which controls LVAD operation and functions.

f. The system controller.
   (1) Controls motor power and speed.
   (2) Diagnoses problems.
   (3) Provides alarms.
   (4) Monitors, interprets, and responds to the system.
   (5) Records and stores events and transfers system performance data to the system monitor (SM) and display module (DM) (Thoratec, 2010).

g. One black and one white power lead connect the SC to a power source. The white power lead also contains a data link cable that transmits information from the SC to the SM or DM.

h. The SC has a user interface keypad with two buttons: a test select button to perform daily system checks and a silence alarm button. Either of these buttons can be pressed and held for 2 seconds to restart the pump if it doesn't start automatically.

i. Other keypad symbols are four battery fuel gauge lights, battery symbol (yellow or red warning), red heart symbol, controller battery cell, and a green power symbol.

j. Thoratec has come out with a smaller HM II® pocket controller with a different interface keypad and improved safety features, which consist of a backup battery that will power the pump for 15 minutes if all power is disconnected or lost (see Figure 6.3).

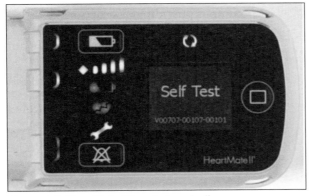

Figure 6.3. HeartMate II® pocket controller.
Photo courtesy of Mary Alice Norton.

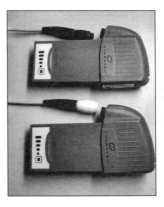

Figure 6.4.
Two 14-volt lithium-ion batteries.
Photo courtesy of Mary Alice Norton.

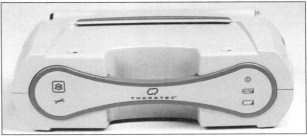

Figure 6.5.
Power module (PM) which supplies AC power during tethered operation.
Photo courtesy of Mary Alice Norton.

k. Two sources of power for the pump are either two 14-volt lithium-ion batteries (see Figure 6.4) worn in holsters or the power module (PM), which supplies AC power during tethered operation (Figure 6.5).

l. AC power provides display of pump parameters and monitoring information via the SM or DM when connected to the PM.

m. Two fully charged batteries provide 6 to 12 hours of power and allow patients to be independent with many activities outside of the home.

n. The HM II® universal battery charger tests, calibrates, and charges four batteries at a time.

6. Principles of operation.
   a. Blood flow through the HM II pump follows the native cardiac cycle and differs during systole and diastole. The LVAD is synchronous with the contraction of the patient's heart and follows the Frank Starling curve.
   b. The amount of flow across the pump is determined by the set speed and by the pressure gradient across the pump. At a given speed, flow varies inversely with pressure.
   c. The pressure gradient is the aortic pressure (outflow conduit) minus the LV pressure (inflow conduit). "Typically, a patient's aortic pressure is within a normal range, and the net cannula pressure drop, although related to flow

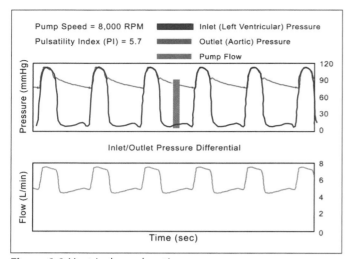

Figure 6.6. Ventricular and aortic pressures.
Reprinted with permission from Thoratec Corporation

(for example, 10 mmHg at 6 L per minute), is low and does not greatly affect the overall differential pressure. Therefore, the dynamic parameter that determines pump differential pressure is left ventricular pressure, which in turn is dependent upon the contractile state of the ventricle. Even a severely depressed heart will have some residual rhythmic contraction that will create a pressure pulse" (Thoratec, 2013).

  d. Even hearts that are severely depressed will have some contractile activity that provides a pressure pulse that can vary depending on the patient's heart rate and rhythm, activity level, and physiologic responses to life.
    (1) The tracings in Figure 6.6 show ventricular and aortic pressures.
    (2) The dark blue waveform represents the pressure at the pump inlet, which is the left ventricular or LV pressure.
    (3) The gray waveform represents the pressure at the pump outlet, which is the aortic pressure.
    (4) The difference between these two pressures, indicated by the thick, vertical, shaded blue bar, is the pressure difference across the pump. This difference varies over the cardiac cycle, with the largest pressure difference occurring in ventricular diastole and the smallest pressure difference occurring during ventricular systole (Thoratec, 2010).
  7. Pump parameters. The system's parameters are the primary source of proper LVAD function. There are four parameters displayed on the SM during tethered operation to the PM and also viewed on the pocket system controller screen. Those parameters are pump speed, flow, power, and pulsatility index.

  a. Pump speed is initially set in the operating room by the surgeon with a transesophogeal echo.
    (1) Visualization of LV cavity size, opening/closing of the aortic valve, position of intraventricular septum, blood pressure, and RV geometry and function are all assessed while increasing pump speed to determine the best level of support.
    (2) The usual fixed speed range for patients is 8,600 to 9,800 revolutions per minute (rpm's) and is optimally determined postop once the patient is hemodynamically stable, has returned to euvolemia, and vasoactive and inotropic drugs have been discontinued.
    (3) The low speed limit (LSL) is the lowest speed the LVAD can operate while maintaining patient stability and is usually set at 400 to 800 rpm below the fixed speed.
  b. Pump flow is not directly measured but is an estimate determined from the pump power and pump speed.
    (1) If fixed speed is increased, flow increases.
    (2) Certain conditions that can cause an increase in power, but are not related to increased flow, will display an erroneously high flow; for example, a thrombus on the rotor or bearings can cause this situation.
  c. Pump power is a direct measurement of the motor voltage or current. Gradual increases in power from usual baseline numbers could indicate thrombus formation inside the pump. Any abrupt changes should be investigated.
  d. Pulsatility index. During systole when the LV contracts, there is an increase in LV pressure which increases pump flow. These flow pulses (native heart contractions) are measured and averaged over 15-second intervals and a pulsatility index or number is produced.
    (1) The numbers usually range from 1 to 10.
    (2) Generally, higher numbers mean more ventricular filling and higher PI means the pump is providing less support.
    (3) Lower numbers mean less ventricular filling and lower PI which means the pump is providing more support.
    (4) Baseline PI numbers should not change significantly during normal activities, so any significant decreases could indicate a decreased blood volume. Likewise, any significant increases in PI should be concerning.

III. Outpatient management of LVAD patients.

A. Long-term management of LVAD patients takes a multidisciplinary team approach.
1. Discussion and education about LVADs should begin early in the progression of HF.
2. To help patients and significant others make an informed decision, it is essential to provide them the opportunity to visualize the pump, learn how it functions, and see how it is going to change their lives.
3. Meeting an LVAD recipient is helpful with that decision making. Early education provides the practitioner an opportunity to assess for any learning barriers and make appropriate modifications to the teaching process.
4. Most implanting centers have a multidisciplinary team approach with monthly meetings where patient cases are presented and all members participate in the decision of whether or not they are appropriate candidates.
5. VAD coordinators are the professionals assigned the bulk of education and training of the patient and family, coordination of the patient's equipment, follow-up appointments, and discharge. They are also responsible for educating EMS/paramedics regarding outpatient anticoagulation and blood pressure management.

B. Blood pressure monitoring.
1. Immediate postoperative blood pressure measurement is done using an arterial catheter. Once the catheter is removed, the most accurate way to obtain mean arterial pressure (MAP) is by using a Doppler probe.
2. Because the LVAD is a continuous flow pump and the patient's pulse is often not palpable, blood pressure is most accurately obtained by using a manual cuff, sphygmomanometer, and a Doppler probe, using the brachial or radial artery. See Table 6.1 for instructions on how to obtain a mean arterial pressure (MAP) using the Doppler method. A normal MAP is 70 to 90 mmHg.
3. Hypertension needs careful monitoring after LVAD implant and should be controlled with beta blockers, ACE inhibitors, and/or ARBs as previously discussed.
4. Mean arterial pressures (MAPs) higher than 90 mmHg (increased afterload) affect pump function by decreasing support and cardiac output.
5. Hypertension can increase stroke risk and bleeding, so maintenance of a "normal" MAP is paramount to preventing these complications.
6. Diuretics are often needed to maintain euvolemia.
7. Volume status needs continual monitoring with patient's recording of daily weight and maintenance of a low sodium diet.

Table 6.1

How to Measure Blood Pressure in Patients with an LVAD

1.	Apply a correct size B/P cuff in correct position over brachial artery.
2.	Apply conducting gel to brachial artery (antecubital) area.
3.	Turn on Doppler, grasp Doppler probe, and place probe tip on gel.
4.	Listen for the continual "swishing or whooshing" sound.
5.	Once found, inflate cuff until sound stops and pump about 40 mmHg above that.
6.	Slowly release air from B/P cuff while closely watching the pressure gauge.
7.	Record the pressure when the first "swish or whoosh" is heard.
8.	This is the **mean arterial pressure** and ideally should be 70–90 mmHg

C. Anticoagulation.
1. Candidates for LVAD therapy must be able to tolerate anticoagulation therapy. Whether they are BTT or DT, they will need anticoagulation for the duration of LVAD support.
2. Post implant prior to leaving the operating room (OR), anticoagulation is completely reversed to prevent postop bleeding. It is resumed usually 24 to 48 hours later or when chest tubes are discontinued.
3. Maintenance of an INR range of 2 to 3 is standard with the higher end range for those with comorbidities (e.g., atrial fibrillation, previous stroke, etc.). For those at risk of bleeding, consideration is given to increasing antiplatelet medications and decreasing anticoagulation for an INR range of 1.7 to 2.3.
4. In addition to warfarin, daily aspirin is used for antiplatelet therapy at doses of 81 mg to 325 mg daily and/or dipyridamole 75 mg three times a day.
5. INR and hematology testing are done routinely; and, because of an increased risk of hemolysis, lactate dehydrogenase (LDH) and plasma-free hemoglobin are monitored.
6. The most frequent site for bleeding is the gastrointestinal (GI) track; it becomes important to assess and educate patients on signs of GI bleeding.

7. Anticoagulation during hemodialysis may need adjustment based on the patient's risk for bleeding.

D. Device management.
 1. Patient education.
  a. All members of the HF team contribute to preparing the patient and the family for discharge. The bedside nurses, coordinators, social workers, physicians/consults, dietitians, pharmacists, physical therapists, and occupational therapists all work together to provide comprehensive care and help transition the patient to home.
  b. Assessment of the patient's living situation is completed to assure a safe, clean environment with adequate electric and telephone services.
  c. Communication with the primary care physician and the patient's local EMS is mandatory, and educational materials and/or in-services on the LVAD are provided by the coordinators as needed.
  d. Coordinators provide intense education to the patient and main care provider on all LVAD equipment, alarms, emergencies, driveline/equipment care and maintenance, activity restrictions, medications, daily documentation of vital signs and parameters; they also provide resources for emergencies.
  e. Patients do not leave the hospital until they demonstrate competency with power lead connections/disconnections and are independent with all aspects of LVAD maintenance.
 2. Driveline care and management.
  a. Proper percutaneous lead exit-site care and maintenance is paramount to preventing damage and infection.
  b. Postoperatively, patients cannot shower until the tunneled part of the driveline and the exit site has healed.
  c. Once the exit site has healed, a special shower bag is used for keeping the system controller and batteries dry and preventing electric shock.
  d. Most centers anchor the external portion of the percutaneous lead and advise patients to wear an abdominal binder to protect it from getting kinked, twisted, pulled, or damaged, thereby disrupting the healing that has taken place.
  e. Patients also need to secure the SC and batteries so they don't drop and pull on the driveline, which in turn tears the subcutaneous tissue.
  f. Patients and significant others learn proper dressing change technique and report any signs or symptoms of infection immediately.
  g. Prompt treatment of superficial exit-site infections is essential to preventing pump pocket involvement that could require pump exchange.
 3. Follow-up care.
  a. The frequency of follow-up depends on several factors including medical issues, any concerns, and how far they are from the implant center.
  b. Those who have just been discharged will be seen in outpatient LVAD clinic weekly, then every 2 weeks, then monthly. Then, as the patient recovers, the visits will be extended.
  c. Keeping in touch by phone is helpful. Patients are given emergency numbers as well as office numbers for general concerns and questions.
  d. Communication is generally frequent. INR monitoring is done routinely, and problems can be discussed at the same time.
  e. Whenever there are changes in baseline parameters or the driveline site, patient is symptomatic, or pump is alarming, they are seen in clinic. It is important that patients have access to the LVAD team at the implanting center for any issues and equipment needs.
  f. Close monitoring of blood pressure, anticoagulation, driveline exit site, parameters and alarms, vital signs, weight, equipment tracking, and emotional well-being are all part of the comprehensive follow-up care plan that clinicians and patients must adhere to for improved quality of life and long-term survival.

E. Troubleshooting pump problems.
 1. Pump parameters are used to evaluate patient and pump conditions.
 2. Baseline parameter ranges are determined, and trends in those parameters are monitored.
 3. Abrupt changes in parameters that are not associated with normal physiologic changes require further investigation, especially if there is a change in the patient's clinical status (Slaughter et al., 2010).
 4. The SC continually monitors the LVAD for any changes and alarm conditions.
 5. Alarms and emergency responses.
  a. Emergency situations include when the pump stops or is unable to move an adequate amount of blood. When this happens, the red heart or red battery symbol illuminates and a continuous audio tone is heard on the system controller.
  b. A red heart symbol with a continuous audio tone is an emergency situation that needs to be addressed immediately. The possible causes of red heart alarms and the messages displayed on the SM include: LOW FLOW, PUMP OFF, and/or PUMP DISCONNECTED.

(1) When the estimated flow is < 2.5 L/min, the SC activates the red heart symbol and alarm. Resolving the alarm will depend on identifying the cause of the low flow hazard.

(2) If after checking connections, the percutaneous lead is connected and auscultation over the pump reveals the pump is running, the next step is to assess for other potential causes, including:
  (a) Hypovolemia.
  (b) Bleeding.
  (c) Right heart failure.
  (d) Arrhythmia.
  (e) Hypertension.
  (f) Obstruction of the inflow or outflow cannula with thrombus.

(3) The pump off and/or disconnected message means the pump has stopped.
  (a) If the pump stops for more than a few minutes, depending on the anticoagulation status of the patient, there is a risk of stroke or thrombus if it is restarted.
  (b) For correction:
    i. Reconnect the perc lead to the SC or check connections between SC and pump, then between SC and power source (e.g., batteries or PM).
    ii. If the alarm continues, change the power source.
    iii. If still not corrected, change system controller and call for help.

(4) A low-flow alarm could also be related to an interruption in power or a perc lead disconnection. Therefore, checking connections is usually the first action taken.

c. A continuous audio tone and red BATTERY symbol means low voltage and indicates there is only 5 minutes of battery power remaining. Batteries need to be replaced immediately or connected to another power source, the power module (PM).

d. A yellow battery symbol with one beep every 4 seconds means there is < 15 minutes of battery power left.

e. A rapidly flashing green power symbol and four flashing green battery fuel gauge lights with a beep every second indicates a power lead is damaged or disconnected. Inspect for damage or reconnect the lead to resolve the advisory alarm.

f. A continuous audio tone and no warning lights with no message on the SM means the SC is not receiving power. To correct, check connections, change power source, change SC, and call for assistance.

F. Safety issues specific to LVAD patients.
  1. Safety is paramount when instructing patients, healthcare providers, EMS/paramedics, and others involved in caring for LVAD recipients.
  2. Patients must always have backup equipment with them.
    a. System controller (SC).
    b. Battery clips.
    c. Two charged batteries.
    d. Alarm card.
    e. Emergency numbers.
  3. Activity restrictions and specific procedures and tests to be avoided.
    a. No chest compressions. They could dislodge the inflow/outflow conduits. If cardiopulmonary resuscitation (CPR) is required, defibrillation, airway management/resuscitation, and pharmacologic treatment should be instituted per protocol.
    b. No tub baths or swimming. Showering using shower bag is allowed when exit site is healed. All parts of the pump must be kept dry; using the shower bag protects external parts from water and moisture. If they were to get wet, the pump would stop.
    c. No magnetic resonance imaging (MRIs). The LVAD contains ferromagnetic parts, so an MRI could cause patient injury and pump failure.
    d. Never have therapeutic radiation that uses radio frequency (RF) energy sources. Therapeutic ionizing radiation can cause damage that might not be immediately detected. Chest x-rays and computed tomography (CT) scans are diagnostic tools that can safely be used.
    e. No contact sports or jumping activities, as both can lead to dislodgement of the inflow or outflow cannulas, resulting in bleeding.
    f. Never disconnect both power leads at the same time because the pump will stop.
    g. Pregnancy must be avoided since a developing fetus could dislodge the pump.
    h. Avoid static electric potentials such as vacuuming, touching TV or computer screen, and microwave, as these could damage the major parts of the system.
    i. The implanted pump's components should not be exposed to therapeutic levels of ultrasound energy used to alter or ablate tissue, as the device may inadvertently concentrate the ultrasound field and cause harm. This does not apply to diagnostic tests such as echocardiography.
    j. Never connect the power module (PM) or universal battery charger (UBC) to an outlet controlled by a wall switch, as power could be interrupted.

Table 6.2

Abbreviations Associated with LVAD Therapy

Administrative	
ACCF	American College of Cardiology Foundation
ADHERE	Acute Decompensated Heart Failure National Registry
HFSA	Heart Failure Society of America
AHA	American Heart Association
NHLBI	National Heart, Lung and Blood Institute
NYHA	New York Heart Association

Clinical	
BTT	Bridge to transplant
CRT	Cardiac resynchronization therapy
DT	Destination therapy
DCM	Dilated cardiomyopathies
DM	Display module
HF	Heart failure
ICDs	Implantable cardiodefibrillators
LSL	Low speed limit
LV	Left ventricle
pLVEF	Preserved left ventricular ejection fraction
rLVEF	Reduced left ventricular ejection fraction
MAP	Mean arterial pressure
MC	Mechanical ciculatory support
PI	Pulsatility index
PM	Power module
RF	Radio frequency
RV	Right ventricle
SC	System controller
SCD	Sudden cardiac death
SM	System monitor
UBC	Universal battery charger
UFR	Ultrafiltration rate

k. Never use extension cords or adapters. PM and UBC must be plugged directly into a 3-prong, grounded outlet.

l. Never transport a patient with an LVAD on PM. Transport only on batteries and always with backup equipment.

IV. Special considerations for patients with an LVAD during hemodialysis/plasmapheresis.

A. Differing degrees of kidney dysfunction are common in patients with advanced heart failure. For most of them, the kidney dysfunction is reversible.

B. Many studies have shown long-term improvement in kidney function after LVAD implantation. However, there remains a high incidence of acute kidney failure (ARF) postoperatively that contributes to increased morbidity and mortality.
   1. Reported incidence ranges from 10% to as high as 56% (Topkara et al., 2006).
   2. Several study outcomes concur that an unstable early postoperative period with hemodynamic instability can result in ARF.
      a. A single center retrospective analysis of two groups of patients who underwent LVAD implant from June 1996 to April 2004 were studied to determine predictors and outcomes of those who had ARF requiring continuous venovenous hemodialysis (CVVHD) and those who did not (Topkara et al., 2006).
      b. Patients who had kidney failure requiring CVVHD postoperatively had a high incidence of intraaortic balloon pump (IABP) use, were older, and had a higher preoperative LVAD score.
      c. The LVAD score was determined by using five clinical variables: postcardiotomy shock, previous LVAD use, ventilatory status, central venous pressure >16 mmHg and prothrombin time > 16 seconds.
      d. The investigators in this study concluded that multiple comorbid conditions and older age were risk factors for developing postoperative kidney failure.

C. The HM II® is preload dependent and afterload sensitive, so obtaining the MAP and documenting estimated pump flow, pulsatility index, power, and speed at baseline and during the procedure will bring attention to any potential problems.
   1. Pump flow can become retrograde if the pump is turned off or there is high afterload pressure and low pump speed.
   2. High negative pressures at the inflow conduit can cause changes in septal and right ventricular geometry.

3. Left ventricular collapse or "suction events" can occur when the pump speed is set higher than the available volume in the LV. This usually happens when the patient is hypovolemic (Slaughter et al., 2010).

4. Treatment for hypotension generally consists of decreasing ultrafiltration rate (UFR), gently placing patient in modified Trendelenburg, giving a normal saline bolus, and notifying the physician.

5. Other precipitating factors that can initiate a suction event are RV failure, pulmonary hypertension, or cardiac tamponade.

6. When a suction event is detected by the system, the pump speed automatically decreases to the low speed limit until resolution of the event. It will gradually increase back to the original fixed speed.

V. Monitoring during procedures.

A. LVAD therapy is standard of care for patients with end stage heart failure. For those who develop kidney failure, outpatient hemodialysis will be needed.

B. Establishing an ongoing relationship between the dialysis and implanting center is essential to ensure patient safety.

C. Developing protocols and processes for safe dialysis management and care of patients with LVAD should be completed prior to outpatient treatment and should consist of the following.
   1. Education of HD staff on care of patients with an LVAD, pump function/parameters, Doppler BP monitoring, addressing potential problems, safety concerns, and proper care and maintenance of equipment and driveline.
   2. Establishment of the frequency of competency requirements for staff and development of an orientation plan for new staff.
   3. Development of processes with the implanting center to receive ongoing information and education on LVADs, and establishment of a contact list for problems and emergencies that is easily accessible by all staff.
   4. Establishment of standing orders and documentation requirements.
   5. Determination of frequency of reassessment of patient's progress and goals.
   6. Development of standing orders specific to LVAD patients in addition to the usual dialysis prescription to help standardize care. Orders should state when to call a physician and specify:
      a. Target amount of volume removal: do not set target over 6 liters.
      b. Verification and documentation of predialysis and postdialysis weight.
      c. Vital sign criteria and when to call physician.

   d. Normal ranges for MAP, weight gain or loss, and when to notify physician or implant team.
   e. LVAD parameters, and when flow is < 2.5 LPM and/or pulse index is < 2.0, notify the physician or implant team.
   f. Procedures to avoid in case of cardiac or respiratory arrest, i.e., chest compressions.
   g. Notifying physician for any of the following:
      (1) Chest or back pain.
      (2) Neurologic deficits or signs of a stroke: slurred speech, facial droop, one-sided weakness, etc.
      (3) Cyanosis or signs of low perfusion.
      (4) Fever.
      (5) Shortness of breath.
      (6) Visual disturbances.
      (7) Nausea or vomiting.
      (8) Change in mental status or level of consciousness.
      (9) Lightheadedness, dizziness, or syncope.
      (10) Alarms or problems with the pump.

D. Hemodialysis nursing assessment takes into consideration the medical history and comorbidities of the individual patient.
   1. Once the protocols and orders for safe hemodialysis have been established and the HD staff members are educated on the special needs of a patient with an LVAD, initiation of HD can begin.
   2. Predialysis, intradialytic, and postdialysis nursing assessment and management of the patient with an LVAD maintain the established principles and techniques for safe and effective treatment.
   3. Additional assessment and management requirements specific to LVAD patients.
      a. Initial predialysis nursing assessment.
         (1) If needed or required by policy, a trained caregiver or significant other is present.
         (2) Confirmation that backup equipment is present and includes a second system controller, two charged batteries, battery clips, and alarm card.
         (3) The power module is plugged in and patient is tethered to AC power. Some HD centers allow patients to use battery power if they have the pocket system controller with visual display screen and extra charged batteries.
         (4) The display monitor or pocket system controller display screen is visible for parameter monitoring and documentation. The patient should be asked if the LVAD is functioning properly, if the parameters are at baseline, and if any alarms have occurred. Compare to previous baseline parameters.

(5) Obtain the predialysis weight; compare it to the previous postdialysis weight and the estimated dry body weight.

(6) Check the patient's temperature and the rhythm and rate of respirations per minute. Most patients with LVADs will not have palpable peripheral pulses.

(7) Auscultate the area over the left upper quadrant for continuous humming sound from the pump and over the left upper chest/subclavicular area for native heart sounds.

(8) Assess mental status: alert and oriented x 3, responding appropriately, gait stable.

(9) Observe the skin's color and assess its temperature and turgor.

(10) Perform a system's review and explore current complaints, including:
  (a) Fever.
  (b) Chills.
  (c) Pain including chest pain.
  (d) Dizziness.
  (e) Nausea or vomiting.
  (f) Diarrhea.
  (g) Bleeding.
  (h) Shortness of breath.
  (i) Palpitations.
  (j) Anorexia.
  (k) Fatigue.
  (l) Edema.

b. Review recent lab work.
  (1) CBC.
  (2) CMP.
  (3) INR.
    (a) Patients with an LAVD are anticoagulated with an ideal therapeutic INR range of 1.5 to 2.5.
    (b) Patients at higher risk, such as those with atrial fibrillation/arrhythmia, previous stroke, pulmonary embolism, deep vein thrombosis (DVT), etc., should ideally be in the 2.0 to 2.5 range.
    (c) The standard anticoagulation approach for HD cannot be used since the patient is on warfarin. Careful consideration must be given to each individual patient to determine the course of action for further anticoagulation.

c. Evaluate the vascular access site for signs of infection.

d. Change dressing on the dialysis access catheter using sterile technique with staff and patient donning masks.

e. Evaluate the patient's fluid status.

(1) Assess for ascites.
(2) Edema of lower extremities
(3) Skin turgor.
(4) Jugular venous distention (JVD).
(5) Breath sounds for rales, rhonchi, or wheezes.

f. Assess the prescribed HD treatment plan and orders based on predialysis assessment findings and report any abnormal findings.

g. Assess the blood flow rate and saline flush order based on heparin-free dialysis.

h. Do not initiate dialysis if the patient is unstable, the device or equipment is malfunctioning or not present, or the patient arrives without the required or needed trained caregiver or significant other.

4. The intradialytic assessment and management also require specific care.

a. The patient is assessed at regular intervals based on the facility's policies for review of systems (symptoms).

b. Record the MAP, temperature, respirations, and pump parameters every 30 minutes and compare to baseline numbers.

c. Notify the physician if the MAP is < 60 mmHg and the patient is symptomatic. Remember that the pump is preload dependent.
  (1) Assess for signs and symptoms of hypovolemia.
    (a) Hypotension.
    (b) Lightheaded.
    (c) Dizzyness.
    (d) Palpitations.
  (2) Low volume can cause left ventricular irritation leading to premature ventricular contractions and a suction event (left ventricular collapse) which can occlude the inflow cannula.
    (a) If this occurs, the pump will alarm and automatically decrease speed if flow is < 2.5 L/min.
    (b) When resolved, the pump will ramp back up to the fixed speed setting.
  (3) Hypovolemia treatment consists of:
    (a) Giving 200 mL saline boluses every 10 minutes up to 1000 mL.
    (b) Gently placing the patient in a MODIFIED Trendelenburg position and setting the UFR at a minimum until receiving further instruction from the physician.

d. Notify the physician if the MAP is consistently > 90 mmHg. Remember: continuous flow pumps are afterload sensitive, which can decrease pump output and/or cause backward flow through the LVAD.
  (1) The nephrologist should contact the LVAD

team for treatment of hypertension to improve pump function.

(2) Angiotensin converting enzyme inhibitors and angiotensin receptor blocker are the drugs of choice for patients with LVADs.

e. Notify the physician of any significant changes in parameters, especially a decrease in pulsatility index (PI) along with a decrease in pump flows. The PI reflects residual pulsatility of the native ventricle which during systole increases flow through the pump. A decrease in PI can indicate low preload from excessive ultrafiltration, arrhythmia, right heart failure, and/or sepsis.

f. Notify the physician if respirations are < 12 or > 30 per minute.

g. Notify the physician if temperature is > 100.5°F.

h. Continue the routine assessment of the vascular access site and HD equipment connections per the facility's policy.

i. Assess and document amount of fluid removed.

j. Assess the patient's complaints and report as needed.

5. The postdialysis assessment and management also require specific care.

a. The routine management and termination of treatment is carried out as per the facility's protocol and established criteria.

b. Assess the patient's fluid status including the weight as compared to the predialysis weight and estimated dry weight.

c. When the treatment is complete, perform the vascular access catheter care, including the instillation of the heparin lock per protocol/orders.

d. Compare the MAP, temperature, and respirations to baseline readings.

e. Parameters should be at baseline numbers; any abnormalities should be reported to the physician.

f. The patient or caregiver removes the patient from tethered PM operation and places the patient on the battery power for travel.

E. Understanding the effects of continuous blood flow perfusion on kidney function.

1. Results of recent studies reveal mortality from acute kidney injury (AKI) after LVAD implantation has declined but still remains high.

2. It remains unclear if AKI is a direct cause for the high mortality, or if sicker patients with heart failure and baseline kidney dysfunction (GFR < 60 mL/min) and multiple comorbidities are associated with the high mortality.

3 Some studies suggest the decrease in mortality is due to a more recent trend to implant patients before severe hemodynamic compromise occurs.

F. Special precautions are taken when a patient with an LAVD is undergoing any noncardiac procedure.

1. Transporting a patient with an LVAD is done only on batteries and then changed over to tethered operation prior to the procedure.

2. The patient must be tethered to the power module for monitoring of parameters, and all backup equipment should be available.

3. The established ranges of the baseline parameters should be recorded for evaluating significant changes. If the procedure requires sedation and/or intubation, an arterial line should be placed for monitoring MAP.

4. An outpatient dialysis treatment should not be initiated, and 911 and/or the LVAD center called when:

a. The patient is unstable, unresponsive, or unable to obtain MAP with Doppler.

b. The LVAD is malfunctioning or there are unresolved hazard alarms after attempts to resolve have failed.

c. Patient arrives without backup equipment (extra charged batteries and backup system controller).

d. Patient arrives without PM and does not have the pocket controller with ability to monitor parameters.

e. Since these criteria must be met before dialysis treatment can begin, it may be necessary to send the patient home to get the proper equipment or to contact the LVAD center to see if they have equipment that can be borrowed for the treatment time.

G. Other information.

1. Recent research studies of patients supported by continuous flow LVADs reveal fewer device-related problems due to the smaller size, increased patient comfort, and device durability.

2. Survival and quality of life indicators are also improving.

3. There are, however, persistent complications after LVAD implant due to preexisting conditions from chronic heart failure, the surgical implant of the pump, and the effects of the device itself.

4. Acute kidney failure in the early postoperative period remains a significant problem and appears to be related to RV failure, older age, being ventilated preimplant, and in some studies preoperative kidney dysfunction. Whatever the cause, kidney failure is a predictor of poor outcome and death in patients receiving LVADs.

5. Since the approval of continuous flow pumps for DT in 2010, there has been a significant increase in the number of DT designated implants.

a. According to the Fifth INTERMACS Annual

Report, more than 40% of implants were for DT in 2012 (Kirklin et al., 2013).

b. This fact highlights the importance of patient selection and the timing of the implant.

c. Further research is needed to better define predictors of those patients who are at the highest risk for complications postimplant.

6. Opportunity exists in the nursing field, especially with regard to evidence-based clinical management of continuous flow devices in patients requiring hemodialysis.

References

Grady, K., Dracup, K., Kennedy, G., Moser, D.K., Piano, M., Stevenson, L.W., & Young, J.B. (2000). Team management of patients with heart failure: A statement for healthcare professionals from the Cardiovascular Nursing Council of the American Heart Association. *Circulation, 102,* 2443-2456. doi:10.1161/ 01.CIR.102.19.2443

Ho, K.K., Pinsky, J.L., Kannel, W.B., & Levy, D. (1993). The epidemiology of heart failure: The Framingham Study. *Journal of the American College of Cardiology, 22*(4)(Suppl. A), 6A-13A.

INTERMACS. (2009). Retrieved from http://www.uab.edu/medicine/intermacs

Kirklin, J.K., Naftel, D.C., Kormos, R.L., Stevenson, L.W., Pagani, F.D., Miller, M.A., Baldwin, T., & Young, J.B. (2013). Fifth INTERMACS annual report: Risk factor analysis from more than 6,000 mechanical circulatory support patients. *The Journal of Heart and Lung Transplantation, 32*(2), 141-156. doi:10.1016/j.healun.2012.12.004

Lindenfeld. J., Albert, N.M., Boehmer, J.P., Collins S.P., Ezekowitzm, J.A., Givertz, M.M., ... Walsh, M.N. (2010). Executive summary: HFSA 2010 comprehensive heart failure practice guideline. *Journal of Cardiac Failure, 16*(6), 475-539. Retrieved from http://www.heartfailureguideline.org/_assets/document/ 2010_heart_failure_guideline_exec_summary.pdf

Marving, J., Hoilund-Carlsen, P.F., Chraemmer-Jorgensen, B., & Gadsboll, N. (1985). Are right and left ventricular ejection fractions equal? Ejection fractions in normal subjects and in patients with first acute myocardial infarction. *Circulation, 72*(3), 502-514. doi:10.1161/ 01.CIR.72.3.502

Slaughter, M.S., Pagani, F.D., Rogers, J.G., Miller, L.W., Sun, B., Russell, S.D., ... HeartMate II Clinical Investigators. (2010). Clinical management of continuous-flow left ventricular assist devices in advanced heart failure. *The Journal of Heart and Lung Transplantation, 29*(Suppl. 4), S1-S39. doi:10.1016/j.healun.2010.01.011

Stevenson, L.W. Pagani, F.D., Young, J.B., Jessup, M., Miller, L., Kormos, R.L., ... Kirklin, J.K. (2009). INTERMACS profiles of advanced heart failure: The current picture. *The Journal of Heart and Lung Transplantation, 28*(6), 535-541.

Thoratec Corporation. (2010). *HeartMate II LVAS operating manual.* Thoratec Corporate Headquarters, 6035 Stoneridge Drive, Pleasanton, CA 94588. Retrieved from http://www.thoratec.com/_assets/download-tracker/103884F-HMII-LVS-Operating-Manual.pdf

Thoratec Corporation. (2013). *HeartMate II LVAS operating manual.* ThoratecCorporate Headquarters, 6035 Stoneridge Drive, Pleasanton, CA 94588. Retrieved from http://www.thoratec.com/_assets/download-tracker/103884F-HMII-LVS-Operating-Manual.pdf

Topkara, V.K., Dang, N.C., Barili, F., Cheema, F.H. Martens, T.P., George, I., ... Naka, Y. (2006). Predictors and outcomes of continuous veno-venous hemodialysis use after implantation of a left ventricular assist device. *The Journal of Heart and Lung Transplantion, 25*(4), 404-408. PMID: 16563969

Yancy, C.W., Jessup, M., Bozkurt, B., Butler, J., Casey, D.E., Jr., Drazner, M.H., ... Wilkoff, B.L. (2013). ACCF/AHA guideline for the management of heart failure. A report of the American College of Cardiology Foundation /American Heart Association Task Force on Practice Guidelines. *Circulation, 128,* e240-e327.

CHAPTER **7**

Continuous Renal Replacement Therapies

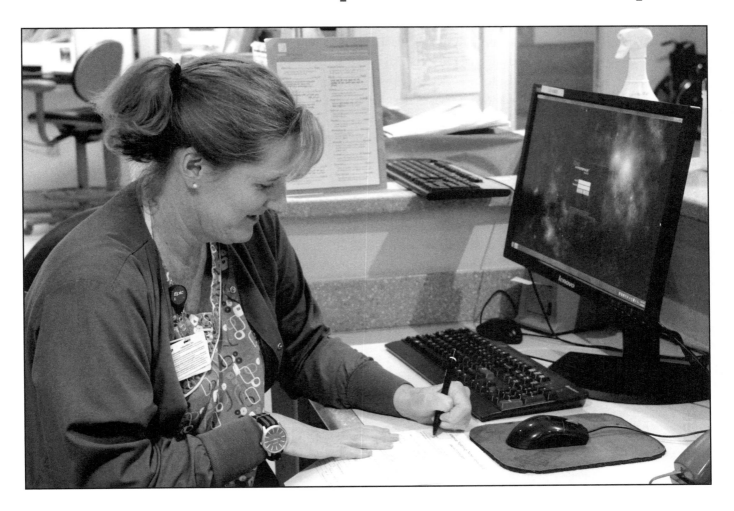

Chapter Editor and Author

Helen F. Williams, MSN, BSN, RN, CNN

CHAPTER **7**

Continous Renal Replacement Therapies

This offering for **1.7 contact hours** is provided by the American Nephrology Nurses' Association (ANNA).

American Nephrology Nurses' Association is accredited as a provider of continuing nursing education by the American Nurses Credentialing Center Commission on Accreditation.

ANNA is a provider approved by the California Board of Registered Nursing, provider number CEP 00910.

This CNE offering meets the continuing nursing education requirements for certification and recertification by the Nephrology Nursing Certification Commission (NNCC).

To be awarded contact hours for this activity, read this chapter in its entirety. Then complete the CNE evaluation found at **www.annanurse.org/corecne** and submit it; or print it, complete it, and mail it in. Contact hours are not awarded until the evaluation for the activity is complete.

Example of reference for Chapter 7 in APA format. One author for entire chapter.

Williams, H.F. (2015). Continuous renal replacement therapies. In C.S. Counts (Ed.), *Core curriculum for nephrology nursing: Module 4. Acute kidney injury* (6th ed., pp. 161-210). Pitman, NJ: American Nephrology Nurses' Association.

Interpreted: Chapter author. (Date). Title of chapter. In …

Cover photo by Counts/Morganello.

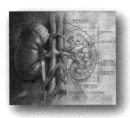

CHAPTER 7

Continuous Renal Replacement Therapies

Purpose

The purposes of this chapter are to define various forms of intermittent and continuous therapies available for patients with acute kidney injury or disease in the intensive care unit (ICU) setting, to provide examples of continuous renal replacement therapy (CRRT) equipment and coordinating documentation, to provide an outline for developing a new CRRT program in various ICU environments, and to define the nursing care necessary to ensure safe, effective therapy for patients receiving CRRT.

Objectives

Upon completion of this chapter, the learner will be able to:
1. Define the various forms of intermittent and continuous renal replacement therapies.
2. Describe the various anticoagulation options and parameters to monitor for a CRRT or intermittent treatment.
3. Define nephrology and ICU nursing responsibilities for collaborative patient management to provide safe, effective CRRT treatments.
4. Identify the role of administrators, nephrologists, intensivists, nephrology nurses, ICU nurses, pharmacists, nurse managers, and pediatric healthcare providers in the development of a program using intermittent or CRRT.

Significant Dates in the History of CRRT and SLEDD

1967   Pioneer work of Henderson and colleagues with hemodiafiltration using hemodialyzers.

1974   Silverstein used a technique to perform ultrafiltration isolated from hemodialysis by modification of a standard hemodialysis circuit and the addition of a hemofilter.

1975   Henderson proposed a hemofiltration technique by collecting an ultrafiltrate of plasma and then reconstituting the blood volume with a fluid composition similar to normal plasma.

1977   Kramer and colleagues in West Germany first used continuous arteriovenous hemofiltration (CAVH) to treat fluid overload.

1979   Continuous veno-venous hemofiltration (CVVH) was first used in acute kidney failure following a cardiac surgery in Cologne, Germany (Kellum et al., 2010).

1979–1982
        Paganini (MD) and Whitman (RN) used slow continuous ultrafiltration (SCUF) and CAVH at Cleveland Clinic.

1982   Food and Drug Administration (FDA) approved use of hemofilters for the management of acute kidney failure.

1983   Geronimus and colleagues started investigating clinical applications of continuous arterio-venous hemodialysis (CAVHD) and continuous arteriovenous hemodiafiltration (CAVHDF).

1982–1984
        Kaplan and colleagues extended work with CAVH using suction assistance to enhance ultrafiltration.

1987   Pump-assisted CRRT introduced.

1988	Regional citrate anticoagulation used as an alternative to heparin in CRRT.
1989-1991	Dirkes, Price, and Whitman made contributions to the CRRT literature helping improve and standardize nursing practice.
1990	CRRT considered state-of-the-art therapy for treatment of acute kidney failure.
1992	Continuous venovenous hemofiltration (CVVH), continuous venovenous hemodialysis (CVVHD), and continuous venovenous hemodiafiltration (CVVHDF) were widely accepted in clinical practice.
1993	Standards of Clinical Practice for CRRT published by ANNA and endorsed by American Association of Critical Care Nurses (AACN).
1995	Mehta (MD), assisted by Martin (RN), chaired the First International Conference on CRRT.
1998	Depner (MD) and Craig (RN) introduced Slow Low-Efficiency Daily Dialysis (SLEDD) at UC Davis Medical Center, Golper (MD) at University of Arkansas, and Amerling (MD) at Beth Israel in New York City as an alternative to CRRT in the ICU environment.
1999	Venovenous continuous therapies nearly replaced arteriovenous continuous therapies.
1900–2000	Machines developed specifically for CRRT; there was progression in the discussion of dose delivery and prescription
2000–present	CRRT used as support therapy in multisystem organ failure; Acute Dialysis Quality Initiative (ADQI) is an ongoing process to produce evidence-based recommendations for the prevention and management of acute kidney injury (AKI), including definition and classification of ARF and development of practice guidelines.

I. Definitions of intermittent kidney replacement therapy (KRT) for acutely ill patients in the ICU.

A. Intermittent hemodialysis (IHD).
  1. Intermittent hemodialysis can be used for chronic or acute care patients.
  2. Clearance can be by diffusion and/or convection depending on the fluid management and electrolyte parameters prescribed.
  3. Many patients in the ICU requiring KRT for acute kidney injury (AKI) are too hemodynamically unstable to tolerate the necessary ultrafiltration to achieve a euvolemic state during a 3- to 4-hour treatment. One of the slow or continuous therapy options may be more appropriate.

B. Slow low-efficiency daily dialysis (SLEDD) is a modification of traditional intermittent hemodialysis (IHD).
  1. Treatments can be performed using a variety of combinations of frequency, treatment time, blood flow rate, dialysis solutions, and ultrafiltration rates.
  2. These treatment modifications can result in larger net solute clearances and fluid removal than would be tolerated by the patient during shorter, more intense treatments.
  3. Commonalities among SLEDD programs.
    a. SLEDD can be customized to allow the time to achieve a euvolemic state by slowly removing the fluid intake the patient received during the previous 24-hour period.
    b. SLEDD extends the treatment time to 6 to 10 hours, which decreases the rate of both solute clearance and ultrafiltration (UF).
    c. The composition of the dialyzing solution is similar to that used in chronic hemodialysis.
    d. Adult SLEDD treatments are performed using high-flux dialyzers to maximize clearances.
    e. Clearance is largely by diffusion.
    f. Daily dialysis offers solute and volume control with fewer episodes of hypotension in comparison to IHD.

II. Definitions of continuous KRT.

A. Slow continuous ultrafiltration (SCUF) is the continuous removal of fluid from the blood achieved by a hydrostatic pressure gradient as it passes across a semipermeable membrane.
  1. SCUF is used for fluid management.
  2. The ultrafiltrate has solute concentrations matching plasma water for those solutes that are cleared by the semipermeable membrane.
  3. Solute clearance is minimal and convective in nature.
  4. SCUF can be performed with either an arteriovenous or venovenous circuit.

5. SCUF can be done independently or in combination with another extracorporeal circuit such as extracorporeal membrane oxygenation (ECMO).
   a. The hemofilter or hemodialyzer can be added to the ECMO circuit.
   b. The removed fluid is measured to maintain accurate intake and output (I/O).

B. Continuous arteriovenous hemofiltration (CAVH), continuous arteriovenous hemodialysis (CAVHD), and continuous arteriovenous hemodiafiltration (CAVHDF) all use the arteriovenous extracorporeal circuit.
   1. Blood is propelled from an artery through a filter and back to a vein, usually by the patient's own pump, i.e., the heart. Therefore, these therapies depend upon the patient's mean arterial pressure (MAP) to establish and maintain blood flow in the extracorporeal circuit.
   2. In addition, blood flow through the extracorporeal circuit varies with the patient's hematocrit (HCT). The higher the HCT, the slower the blood flow rate (BFR), secondary to the increased viscosity of the blood (see Figure 7.1).
   3. For many ICU patients with kidney injury/disease, the MAP is inadequate (≤ 60 mm Hg) or so variable that it is difficult to maintain the blood flow in an arteriovenous extracorporeal circuit. A blood pump can be added to the arteriovenous circuit to maintain the desired blood flow.
   4. While the simplicity of the arteriovenous circuit is an advantage for some ICUs, issues with the thermoregulation, hemoconcentration in the filter, and high doses of anticoagulants that will be required are disadvantages (see Figure 7.2).
   5. The potential complications from arterial access leave these therapies largely of historical interest.
   6. CAVH, CAVHD, and CAVHDF may be performed on the arteriovenous circuit used in ECMO. A hemofilter or hemodialyzer may be added to the ECMO circuit. Intravenous (IV) fluid may be given through another access to provide volume replacement, and/or dialysis solution may be pumped through the ultrafiltrate-dialysate compartment of the hemofilter or hemodialyzer depending on the solute clearance and/or fluid removal desired.

C. Continuous venovenous hemofiltration (CVVH) is the process where blood from a vein is propelled from a vein through a filter and back to the patient's vein using an extracorporeal blood pump.
   1. The hydrostatic pressure created as the blood moves through the filter forces plasma water across the membrane by the process of ultrafiltration.
   2. The ultrafiltrate produced is mostly replaced with IV fluids, also referred to as replacement or reinfusion fluids.

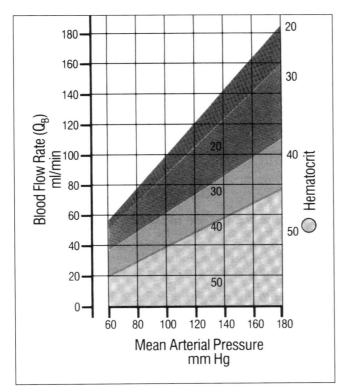

Figure 7.1. Blood flow rate related to mean arterial pressure and hematocrit.

Courtesy of Amicon, Inc.

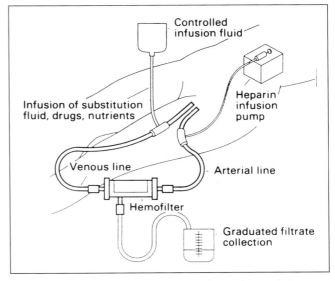

Figure 7.2. CAVH circuit: CAVH using a femoral cannulation.

Reprinted with permission from Millipore Corporation.

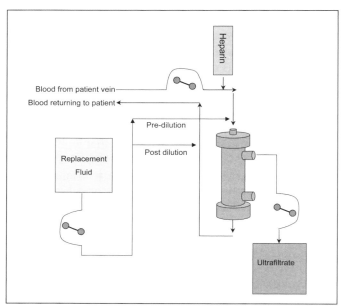

Figure 7.3. CVVH circuit: CVVH circuit with heparin anticoagulation.

Courtesy of Maureen Craig, UC Davis Medical Center, Sacramento, California.

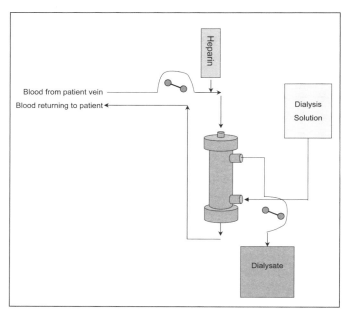

Figure 7.4. CVVHD circuit: CVVHD circuit with heparin anticoagulation.

Courtesy of Maureen Craig, UC Davis Medical Center, Sacramento, California.

3. Clearance is largely due to convection, as the ultrafiltrate carries the solvent across the membrane, in a process known as solute drag (see Figure 7.3).

D. Continuous venovenous hemodialysis (CVVHD) is also sometimes called continuous hemodialysis (CHD).
1. In this process, blood is driven by a pump through a hemodialyzer with blood access originating and terminating in a vein.
2. Dialysis solution is pumped through the ultrafiltrate-dialysate compartment of the hemodialyzer countercurrent to the blood flow.
3. Clearance is largely by diffusion with molecules moving across the membrane dependent on the concentration gradient, from an area of higher concentration to an area of lower concentration (see Figure 7.4).
4. Diffusion is an effective transport mechanism for the removal of relatively small solutes, such as urea.

E. Continuous venovenous hemodiafiltration (CVVHDF) is a modification of the CVVHD circuit achieved by the addition of sterile replacement solution to the blood.
1. Replacement solution can be administered either before (prefilter) or after (postfilter) the hemodialyzer.
   a. Prefilter administration will aid in prolonging filter life by diluting the concentration of hematocrit and total blood proteins going

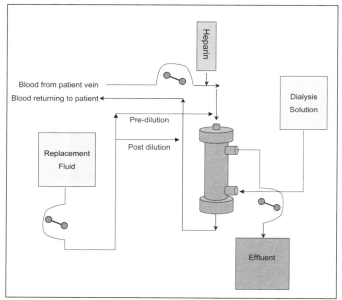

Figure 7.5. CVVHDF Circuit: CVVHDF circuit with heparin anticoagulation.

Courtesy of Maureen Craig, UC Davis Medical Center, Sacramento, California.

through the filter, but can also decrease the efficiency of clearance for the same reason.
   b. Postfilter administration may comparatively increase clearance, depending on the ultrafiltration rate, the blood solute concentration, and membrane sieving coefficients (Kellum et al., 2010).
2. Clearance is by both convection and diffusion (see Figure 7.5).

F. High volume hemofiltration (HVHF) is a relatively new modification of CVVHF (Cruz et al., 2009).
   1. The amount of fluid removed and replaced is much higher than the typical balance.
   2. This method uses from 6 to10 L/hr of replacement solution.
   3. The goal of this therapy is to increase the blood purification and to remove cytokines, components of sepsis. It can also remove water-soluble free toxic drugs like lithium or sodium valproate more efficiently than standard CRRT (Kellum et. al., 2010).
   4. Using this therapy requires close attention to the patient's fluid balance.

III. Indications for SLEDD or CRRT in the ICU.

A. Considering the improved patient management, SLEDD or CRRT should be considered for every ICU patient with kidney injury (whether AKI or CKD stage 5) and/or disease that requires KRT depending on the goals of that therapy (see Table 7.1 for advantages and disadvantages of intermittent vs. continuous renal replacement therapy).

B. Fluid removal: SLEDD or CRRT can provide effective fluid removal for a patient with compromised kidney function. It can also aid the patient in achieving a euvoluemic state, despite the relatively hemodynamic instability in an ICU patient who is receiving more IV intake than has urine output.

C. Solute removal: CRRT or SLEDD can provide excellent solute clearance in the catabolic ICU patient who has little or no residual kidney function.

D. Examples of patients that may benefit from intermittent or continuous KRT to assist in achieving volume and/or solute balance include:
   1. Patients with chronic kidney disease (CKD) stage 5 when they have other acute medical complications requiring an ICU stay.
   2. Patients with acute kidney

injury (AKI) who are catabolic and/or volume overloaded and would benefit from daily clearance of uremic toxins, management of fluid and electrolytes, and interventions to maintain acid-base balance (see chapter 2 regarding causes of ATN).
   a. Acute tubular necrosis (ATN) secondary to ischemic injury to the kidney.
      (1) Congestive heart failure.
      (2) Gastrointestinal bleed.
      (3) A recent myocardial infarction with or without cardiogenic shock.
      (4) Status postsurgery with intraoperative or postoperative hypotension.
      (5) Hepatic dysfunction.
      (6) Burn wounds.
      (7) Rhabdomyolysis due to release of myoglobin.

Table 7.1

Advantages and Disadvantages of Intermittent vs. Continuous Renal Replacement Therapy

	Intermittent hemodialysis	Continuous renal replacement therapy
Advantages	Lower risk of systemic bleeding	Better hemodynamic stability
	More time available for diagnostic and therapeutic interventions	Fewer cardiac arrhythmias
	More suitable for severe hyperkalemia	Improved nutritional support
	Lower cost	Better pulmonary gas exchange
		Better fluid control
		Better biochemical control
		Shorter stay in intensive care unit
Disadvantages	Availability of dialysis staff	Greater vascular access problems
	More difficult hemodynamic control	Higher risk of systemic bleeding
	Inadequate dialysis dose	Long-term immobilization of patient
	Inadequate fluid control	More filter problems (ruptures, clotting)
	Not suitable for patient with intracranial hypertension	Greater cost
	No removal of cytokines	
	Potential complement activation by nonbiocompatible membranes	

Source: Lameire, N., VanBiesen, W., & Vanholder, R. (2005). Acute renal failure. *The Lancet, 365*(9457), 417-430. Used with permission.

(8) Sepsis.

(9) Systemic inflammatory response syndrome (SIRS).

(10) Multisystem organ failure (MSOF).

b. Nephrotoxin exposure.

(1) Antineoplastic agents.

(2) Antimicrobial agents.

(3) Radiocontrast agents.

(4) Poisons, such as ethylene glycol.

3. Patients with acute kidney injury as well as acute brain injury or other causes of increased intracranial pressure or generalized brain edema (KDIGO, 2012).

4. Patients with acute rejection following kidney or other solid organ transplant.

5. Patients with cardiac dysfunction who are resistant to diuretics or oliguric despite inotropic support and have low plasma refill rates.

6. Patients with anuria or oliguria who require large volumes of intravascular fluids (IVF) including medications, hyperalimentation, and/or blood products.

7. Neonates with inborn errors of metabolism such as hyperammonemia.

8. Patients with hemolytic uremic syndrome (HUS).

9. Patients with tumor lysis syndrome (TLS) after receiving antineoplastic agents.

IV. Therapeutic mechanisms of KRT.

A. Initiate treatment early, before complications occur (Lameire et al., 2005).

1. KRT should be initiated when the patient's heart and kidneys are unable to adequately remove fluids or keep the patient in fluid balance or when the kidneys are unable to keep up with the solute load (e.g., the patient's blood urea nitrogen [BUN] and creatinine are rising each day).

2. Postponing KRT treatment initiation in these circumstances increases the likelihood that the patient will experience hypotension and/or multisystem organ failure (MSOF) and will struggle to survive the fluid and/or solute imbalances that ensue.

B. Fluid removal/balance: SLEDD or CRRT can achieve a net ultrafiltration rate (UFR) of 0 to 1000 mL/hr. The total volume of fluid removal in 24 hours using CRRT may be greater than during SLEDD due to the continuous nature of the therapy. Alternatively, a patient can be kept in a positive fluid balance if insensible fluid losses are large, as in a burn patient.

1. Ultrafiltration (UF) is the process whereby plasma water is forced across a semipermeable membrane by hydrostatic pressure (Tolwani, 2012). This occurs when a solution moving in a closed space puts pressure on the surrounding surfaces as it

comes in contact with them, such as blood moving through dialyzer fibers.

2. Rapid UF that occurs with IHD may be poorly tolerated in an ICU patient, resulting in hypotension and/or the inability to remove fluid. Hypotensive episodes have been linked to delays in recovering kidney function.

3. SLEDD or CRRT can achieve the desired volume of fluid removal. Since the necessary UF rate is lower when removing the fluid over a longer period of time, continuous therapy is generally preferred for extremely unstable patients.

4. CRRT is better able to provide larger total fluid removal and/or better fluid control over the entire 24-hour period, with overall improved hemodynamic stability, when compared to IHD (Bouchard et al., 2009).

5. When removing fluid, the filtration fraction can estimate the amount of hemoconcentration within the circuit.

6. The filtration fraction (FF) is the fraction of plasma water removed by ultrafiltration. This value can be calculated.

$$FF\ (\%) = \frac{UFR\ (mL/hr)}{BFR\ (mL/min)} \times \frac{100}{60\ (min/hr)} \times \frac{100}{(100-Hct)}$$

7. The FF should be no higher than 20% and ideally < 10% to minimize filter clotting.

C. Solute clearance: CRRT can gently and effectively clear solutes and/or toxins from the plasma and balance electrolytes, minimizing the risk of changes to intracranial pressure. Decreased rebound of solutes occurs after treatment termination following CRRT when compared to IHD.

1. Convection.

a. Convection is the process of transporting solutes dissolved in fluid across a membrane in response to the transmembrane pressure (TMP) gradient.

b. Small solutes freely pass across the semipermeable membrane into the ultrafiltrate in a concentration matching the concentration of that solute in the plasma (see Figure 7.6).

c. Increased solute size (5,000 to 50,000 daltons) may decrease convective solute removal depending on the permeability (porosity) of the membrane. In general, however, larger molecules move across the same membrane better by convection than by diffusion.

d. Convective clearance (CC) can be calculated.

$$CC\ (mL/min) = \frac{UFR\ (mL/hr)}{60\ min/hr} \times \frac{ultrafiltrate\ concentration}{plasma\ concentration}$$

2. Diffusion.

a. Diffusion is the process of transporting solutes

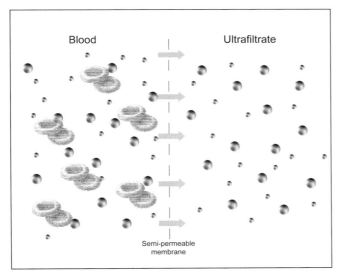

Figure 7.6. Convection: Solutes are transported across the semipermeable membrane together with fluid, which occurs in response to a transmembrane pressure gradient.

Courtesy of Maureen Craig, UC Davis Medical Center, Sacramento, California.

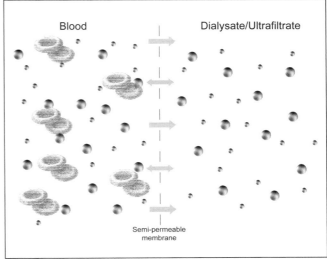

Figure 7.7. Diffusion: Solutes are transported across a semipermeable membrane from an area of higher solute concentration to an area of lower solute concentration.

Courtesy of Maureen Craig, UC Davis Medical Center, Sacramento, California.

across a semipermeable membrane from an area of higher solute concentration to an area of lower solute concentration (see Figure 7.7).

b. Diffusion occurs in response to the concentration gradient. The greater the difference between the two sides of the membrane, the faster solute moves across the membrane.

c. Dialysis solution flow is countercurrent to blood flow to maximize the diffusive gradient across the entire hemodialyzer.

d. Diffusive clearance (DC) is more dependent on molecular size than convective clearance and works well for smaller size molecules (less than 200 daltons).

e. DC can be calculated using the dialysis flow rate (DFR).

$$DC \text{ (mL/min)} = DFR \text{ (mL/min)} \times \frac{\text{dialysate concentration}}{\text{plasma concentration}}$$

3. Adsorption.

a. Adsorption is the removal of molecules from the blood by binding them to the filtering membrane.

b. Large pore synthetic membranes have been developed with a propensity for adsorbing plasma proteins (Kellum et al., 2013).

   (1) They are being studied for the treatment of sepsis by removing inflammatory mediators such as cytokines (Santoro & Guadagni, 2010).

   (2) They can remove some protein-bound uremic toxins (Karkar, 2013).

   (3) They can also bind relatively high

molecular weight proteins leading to loss of albumin.

   (4) Overall clearance may decrease as the pores on the filter membrane become "plugged" by proteins.

D. Medication clearance in CRRT: There may be notable variations in drug removal and dosing that should be considered on an individual basis.

1. Patients may have residual kidney function resulting in some medication clearance into the urine.

2. A pathway other than the kidney, such as the liver or lung, may clear medications.

3. Medications may be cleared through a hemodialyzer or hemofilter.

a. Clearance of any medication is impacted by the sieving coefficient (SC) of that substance as it passes across the membrane. As a result, it is different for different hemofilters or hemodialyzers with different membrane characteristics.

   (1) The sieving coefficient is the fraction of a substance that will pass through a semipermeable membrane in relation to the concentration of the substance in the patient's plasma (see Table 7.2).

   (2) SC can be calculated.

$$SC = \frac{\text{ultrafiltrate concentration}}{\text{plasma concentration}}$$

b. Several references predict medication clearance during dialytic therapies. Textbooks,

Table 7.2

Comparison of Serum and Ultrafiltrate Chemistries with Sieving Coefficients

Substance	Serum	Ultrafiltrate	Seiving Coefficient
Sodium	140 mEq/L	140 mEq/L	1.00
Potassium	3.9 mEq/L	3.9 mEq/L	1.00
Chloride	105 mEq/L	111 mEq/L	.94
Bicarbonate	26 mEq/L	28 mEq/L	1.07
Urea	81 mg/dL	80 mg/dL	.99
Creatinine	4.0 mg/dL	3.8 mg/dL	.95
Calcium	8.3 mEq/L	5.2 mEq/L	.62
Phosphate	4.0 mEq/L	3.9 mEq/L	.98
Albumin	3.6 g/dL	0 g/dL	0
Total protein	4.6 g/dL	.1 g/dL	.02
Uric acid	8.4 mg/dL	7.7 mg/dL	.92
Total bilirubin	1.9 mg/dL	.1 mg/dL	.05
Direct bilirubin	.6 mg/dL	0 mg/dL	0
Alkaline phosphatase	65 IU/L	10 IU/L	.15
SGPT	31 IU/L	3 IU/L	.10
SGOT	29 IU/L	3 IU/L	.10
LDH	311 IU/L	7 IU/L	.02
CPK	55 IU/LI	29 IU/L	.53
Cholesterol	89 mg/dL	8 mg/dL	.09
Glucose	89 mg/dL	108 mg/dL	1.21

pamphlets, drug information handouts, and charts are available to provide the clearance information for a particular medicine during a particular dialytic therapy.

c. The practitioner implementing SLEDD or CRRT should exercise caution when referencing these medication clearance resources due to the many variations among forms of dialysis or filtration and within a specific form of dialysis or filtration.

d. The more protein bound a medication is, the lower the clearance of that substance during CRRT. Albumin's molecular weight is 66,000 daltons, so solutes bound to albumin will be minimally cleared.

e. Due to the longer duration of CRRT, even those medications that are highly protein bound may be more readily removed than with intermittent therapies.

f. Medication clearance can occur via convection, diffusion, and/or adsorption.

g. Clearance can be increased or decreased by changes in the blood flow rate (BFR), dialysate flow rate (DFR), replacement fluid rate (RFR), ultrafiltration rate (UFR), size or type of membrane in the dialyzer/hemofilter, or available surface area of the membrane.

h. Clotting in the filter decreases the available membrane surface area so clearance may decrease with longer treatment times if clotting occurs.

4. Dose adjustment of medications.
   a. Medications such as vasopressors or sedatives may be titrated based on the effect on the patient.
   b. Medications such as heparin or citrate may be titrated based on patient laboratory parameters.
   c. Medications such as immunosuppressant medications or antibiotics may require monitoring of therapeutic serum levels.
   d. Achieving the desired level of a medication in the blood in a consistent fashion is challenging, and the assistance of the clinical pharmacist is essential.

V. Equipment and system components for intermittent and continuous KRT.

A. Machines capable of performing the various modalities within the definition of intermittent and continuous KRT are available internationally.
   1. Some machines are designed to provide intermittent hemodialysis and are capable of also doing SLEDD.
   2. Some machines are designed to only provide continuous therapies (CRRT).
   3. Some machines are capable of performing both intermittent or continuous therapies.
   4. This discussion will not include machines that can only perform intermittent hemodialysis.

B. There are two types of equipment available for these therapies in the United States: the scale-based fluid management of the Prismaflex® System (Gambro) and the Diapact® CRRT System (B. Braun Medical Inc.), or volumetric fluid management of the

NxStage® System machine (NxStage) (see Figures 7.8 and 7.9).

C. Because the functionality of the two types of systems are very different, they each have features that make them unique and offer the practitioner distinct choices in managing their CRRT program.
1. The volumetric system provides:
   a. Volumetric measurement of fluids administered as dialysate so volume in equals volume out.
   b. A wide range of choices in dialysis solutions to meet the specific needs of the individual patient.
   c. Several ports for connecting fluids to manage and achieve prescribed ultrafiltration.
   d. The options of continuous (CVVH or CVVHD), extended daily (SLEDD), or intermittent (HD or hemofiltration) therapies as well as therapeutic plasma exchange (TPE).
2. The scale-based systems.
   a. Provide a series of scales to manage fluid removal and administration.
   b. Provide a wide range of choices in dialysis solutions to meet the needs of the individual patient.
   c. See Table 7.3 for description of the characteristics of the scale-based systems.

D. All CRRT machines have three essential classes of components, which will vary in their particular adaptation and presentation depending on the manufacturer. They will each also include visual and audible alarm systems when preset limits are violated.
1. The communication system and monitoring screen.
   a. The communication unit is where the operator receives information and communicates with the system.
   b. The computer screen provides the operator with the treatment information updated every few minutes or in real time.
   c. Patient vital signs are usually visible on the main screen to allow constant adjustment of therapy based on changes in the patient's condition.
   d. The screen provides an interface so the user can adjust flow rates and monitor pressures.
      (1) Machine inlet (negative) pressure also called arterial pressure (AP) or access pressure.

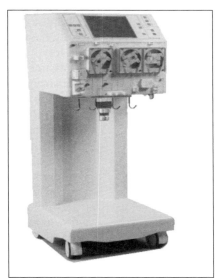

Figure 7.8. B Braun Diapact Machine.
Courtesy of B. Braun Medical Inc.

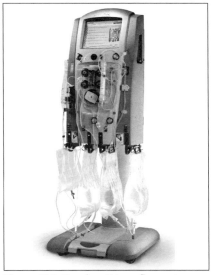

Figure 7.9. Gambro Prismaflex system.
Courtesy of Gambro.

      (2) Machine return (positive) pressure also called venous pressure (VP) or return pressure.
      (3) Transmembrane pressure (TMP).
      (4) Ultrafiltration (UF) port pressure.
      (5) Inlet and/or filter pressure.
   e. The screen will display fluid volumes administered, ultrafiltrate removed, and pump flow rate settings.
      (1) The blood pump moves blood through the system at the programmed BFR reflecting the prescription.
      (2) The dialysate pump moves dialysate through the hemofilter using a countercurrent flow path when performing CVVHD or CVVHDF. Co-current flow may be used to decrease the efficiency of the dialysis treatment in an attempt to avoid dialysis disequilibrium syndrome in patients with severely untreated high urea levels or in very small pediatric patients (Abra, 2010).
      (3) The replacement or reinfusion pump is used when performing CVVH or CVVHDF to pump sterile replacement solution to mix with the blood as it enters (prefilter) or as it leaves (postfilter) the filter.
      (4) A syringe pump may be available for administering anticoagulant with bolus and/or continuous infusion options.
   f. Time is reported in terms of treatment duration and, in some cases, the manufacturer's recommended machine disinfection schedule.
   g. Dialysate conductivity and temperature (if available) are monitored and displayed on the screen.

CRRT Machine Characteristics

Table 7.3

Company	Machine	Blood Flow mL/min	Dialysis Solution mL/hr	Replacement Solution mL/hr	Patient Fluid Removal Rate	Effluent Removal mL/hr	Heparin Pump	Reinfusion Pump	Built-in Dialysis Solution Heater	Recirc Time	Filter Membrane	Printer/ Sensors to Remote Monitor	Scales	CRRT Treatment Options
B. Braun	Diapact	10–500	0–12000	0–6000	0–300 mL/min	0–1400	n/a	n/a	0–40 C	per need	Universal	n/a	1	CVVH CVVHD CVVHDF SCUF
Gambro	Prismaflex	10–450	0–8000	0–8000	0–2000 mL/hr	0–10,000	Yes	Pre, Post, Pre-Post simultaneous & Pre-BP*	PrismaFloII/ Prisma-Therm	2 hours	AN69 or PAES	No/Yes	4 scales Gravi-metric	SCUF CVVH CVVHD CVVHDF TPE

* Additional pump, Pre-Blood Pump (PBP) flow = 4000 mL/hr

h. Graphic displays may also reflect the administration of anticoagulant and/or the blood volume processed in liters.

i. Pressure pods or transducers connect to a pressure sensor housing on the extracorporeal system. They provide noninvasive pressure measurements, preferably without an air-blood interface, to continuously monitor the system's pressures.

j. Safety monitoring includes a blood leak detector, an air bubble detector, and a return line clamp as well as alarm systems to notify the operator of pressures that have exceeded the pre-set pressure parameters.

k. Technology under development will use ultrasonic blood flow measurements that can be computer-linked to the blood pump to ensure correct blood flow. Development of online urea clearance measurement is also being considered (Mehta, 2005).

l. The service screens provide guidance for calibration and testing procedures for machine/biomed technicians and users.

2. The extracorporeal blood circuit.
   a. The blood is continuously circulated from the patient through the filter or dialyzer where fluid and toxins are removed before the blood is returned to the patient.
   b. The circuit is monitored for arterial pressure (also labeled as "access"), venous pressure (also labeled as "return"), transmembrane pressure (TMP), the presence of air in the blood, and the presence of blood leaking out of the filter into the circuit.
   c. Heparin or other anticoagulation may be administered into the blood circuit, using a syringe pump attached to the machine (if available) or by attaching an external medication pump tubing to one of the circuit's access ports.
   d. Blood volume monitoring, either as an internal function of the machine or by using an external monitor, may be a part of the blood circuit. This enables detection of changes in blood volume relative to the initial blood volume at the start of the treatment.

3. Dialysis solutions and their delivery system (Culley et al., 2006).
   a. Both dialysis and replacement solutions will contain glucose and electrolytes including at least sodium, potassium, magnesium, and possibly calcium in physiologic ranges. Adjustments of electrolytes may be needed to respond to clinical conditions (Tolwani, 2012).
   b. The use of preprinted CRRT order sets are important in maintaining the safety of the solutions and avoiding errors from illegible handwriting.
   c. Some facilities implement a two-nurse check of all the solutions that are recorded on the medication administration record (MAR) prior to administration to ensure consistency with the physician's orders.
   d. Solutions may be custom made by a hospital pharmacy or other custom solution vendor. The solutions are attached to the extracorporeal system using a delivery system of scales, pumps, and/or balance chambers that

deliver a range of possible volumes that varies with the functionality of the equipment being used.
(1) The advantage of these solutions is that they can be formulated with sodium, potassium, bicarbonate, calcium, and glucose concentrations that are prescribed to meet the patient's specific metabolic needs.
(2) The disadvantages.
  (a) Additional cost, considering the time and labor required of the local or the hospital's pharmacy.
  (b) The inherent risk of the solution being prepared with an unintended electrolyte composition leading to a risk to the patient's homeostasis and potential death.
  (c) Risk of infection if the solution gets contaminated.
(3) Custom solution vendors have safeguards and quality programs in place to ensure preparations are consistent with labeled content. Vendors undergo regular inspections by regulatory agencies to ensure safety.
e. The CRRT machine may produce solutions by proportionately mixing reverse osmosis water with acid and bicarbonate concentrates.
(1) A buffer is included in dialysis solutions or replacement solutions to normalize acidosis of patients without causing alkalosis (Kellum et al., 2010).
(2) Acetate has been shown to negatively affect myocardial contractility and is not currently in common use as a buffer.
(3) Lactate has been used as the buffer in dialysis solutions as well as in replacement solutions to correct acidosis. Hyperlactatemia can occur, especially when there is impaired liver function or tissue hypoperfusion (Kellum et al., 2010).
(4) Bicarbonate is the most commonly used buffer. In studies of replacement solution used in CVVH, it has been shown to be superior to lactate in treating patients with acute kidney failure, particularly if there is a previous history of cardiovascular disease or heart failure (Barenbrock et al., 2000).
f. Dialysis solution containing citric acid may be used for intermittent therapies (IHD or SLEDD).
(1) It is more effective than normal saline flushes as an anticoagulant (Ahmad, 2007).
(2) It does not adversely affect patient serum calcium levels.
g. Some machines can heat the dialysis solution to

decrease the risk of hypothermia.
(1) For patients less than 10 kg, the dialysis solution may need to be warmed to 38°C to maintain the patient's temperature in the normal range.
(2) Alternatively, for dialysis solution flow rate of 100 mL/min, insulating the dialysis tubing lines with foam insulation or attaching a blood warmer device to the return line can reduce the heat loss to the environment.
h. The temperature of the dialysis solution may be adjustable. A temperature of 35° C may decrease the incidence of hypotension.

E. Replacement solutions. Some machines have the capability to perform CVVH or CVVHDF using replacement solutions, also called reinfusion solutions.
1. Normal saline, by itself or mixed with selected electrolytes, can be used as a replacement fluid.
2. Pharmacy prepared replacement solutions.
  a. Selecting a pharmacy or solutions vendor for replacement solutions needs to be done with consideration of the same alternatives as a dialysis solution vendor.
  b. At lower flow rates (1800 mL/hr or less), replacement solutions may be composed to correct electrolyte imbalances (e.g., potassium).
3. The more rapid the replacement solution flow, the more critical the electrolyte composition becomes, as the patient's serum chemistry will more quickly begin to match the electrolyte composition of the replacement solution. Sodium, potassium, bicarbonate, chloride, calcium, magnesium, and phosphorus electrolyte content all need to be considered.
  a. Some electrolytes, such as calcium and bicarbonate, will precipitate above certain concentrations, so care needs to be taken when customizing a solution with a hospital pharmacy.
  b. The pharmacy can custom mix solution to include 0.45% NaCl with 35 mEq NaCl, 35 mEq $NaHCO_3$, 3 mEq KCl, and 1.5 mEq $MgSO_4$. In a separate line infuse $CaCl_2$ 40 mEq in 125 mL D5W at 1% of the replacement fluid rate. This results in a replacement fluid that mimics the normal plasma water with the exception of phosphorus. A solution of this ratio can be prepared in 3 to 5 liter bags to avoid frequent bag changes on the system.
  c. Alternatively, the pharmacy can provide a combination of replacement solutions to be administered simultaneously when rates are greater than 1200 mL/hr or alternating between the two solutions using a Y-connector

Table 7.4

Electrolyte Composition of Commercially Available Replacement Fluids

Replacement Solution	Normocarb 25 HF	Normocarb 35 HF	PrismaSol BK 0/3.5	PrimsaSol BGK 2/0	PrismaSol BGK 2/3.5	PrismaSol BGK 4/2.5	PrismaSol BGK 0/2.5
Sodium (mEq/L)	140	140	140	140	140	140	140
Potassium (mEq/L)	0	0	0	2	2	4	0
Chloride (mEq/L)	116.5	106.5	109.5	108	111.5	113	109
Bicarbonate (mEq/L)	25	35	32	32	32	32	32
Lactate (mEq/L)	0	0	3	3	3	3	3
Calcium (mEq/L)	0	0	3.5	0	3.5	2.5	2.5
Magnesium (mEq/L)	1.5	1.5	1	1	1	1.5	1.5
Phosphorus (mg/dL)	0	0	0	0	0	0	0
Dextrose (mg/dL)	0	0	0	100	100	100	100

Courtesy of Maureen Craig, UC Davis Medical Center, Sacramento, California. Used with permission.

on the replacement infusion line for lower rates. Two solutions commonly used are:
(1) 1L 0.9% NaCl + 5 mL 10% $CaCl_2$.
(2) 1L 0.45% NaCl + 75 mL 8.4% $NaHCO_3$.

4. Another custom formulation includes citrate in the replacement solution.
   a. This solution provides adequate regional anticoagulation with a dilute concentration of citrate administered through a prefilter tubing set.
   b. Calcium is then infused postfilter through a separate central line.
   c. When administering citrate in this fashion, a customized dialysis solution is also required. Since the citrate provides a bicarbonate source, the bicarbonate level in the dialysate must be decreased.
5. Commercially available solutions (Culley et al., 2006).
   a. PrismaSol® (Gambro, Stockholm, Sweden) is a commercially available sterile electrolyte replacement solution available in several different formulations to meet the needs of patients with a variety of electrolyte replacement needs on either heparin or citrate anticoagulation (see Table 7.4).
   b. Normocarb (NC) HF™ (Dialysis Solutions INC., Richmond Hill, Ontario, Canada) is a commercially available sterile electrolyte concentrate. This 240 mL concentrate is available as NC 25 HF or NC 35 HF and must be diluted into 3 L of sterile water for injection to make 3.24 L of infusate solution. Normocarb

HF™ is dextrose, calcium, and potassium-free (see Table 7.4 for the final electrolyte composition).
   c. Other dialysis vendors produce their own dialysis and/or replacement solutions that have not yet been approved by the FDA for these uses.
   d. Replacement fluid can be put into the CRRT circuit either prefilter/predilution or postfilter/ postdilution. Many arguments have been made supporting one over the other, but advocates of both still stand by the option they prefer.
      (1) Many of today's CRRT systems accommodate either option.
      (2) Adding replacement fluid into a CRRT circuit increases the volume of ultrafiltrate and thereby increases convective clearance.

F. Hemofilters, hemodialyzers, and blood tubing.
   1. Membranes. Hollow fiber hemofilters and hemodialyzers are available with membranes composed of polysulfone, polyamide, polycarbonate, polyacrylonitrile (PAN), polymethylmethacrylate (PMMA), polyaryl ether sulfone (PAES), polyvinylpyrrolidonee (PVP), or a blending of these membranes.
      a. Depending on the equipment being used, nearly any hemofilter or hemodialyzer with a biocompatible membrane can be used for CRRT.
      b. Synthetic membranes have increased biocompatibility and minimized patient complement activation. These membranes may

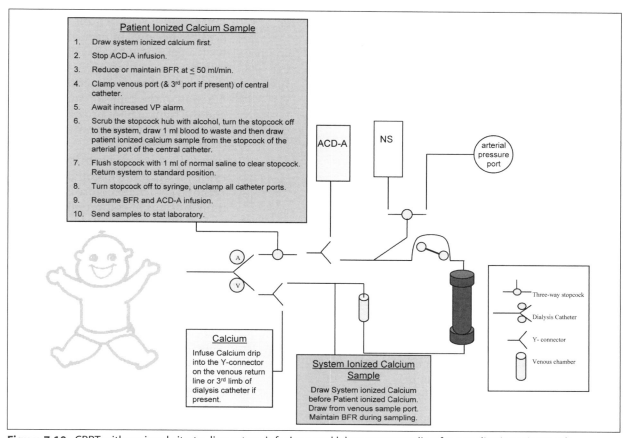

Patient Ionized Calcium Sample

1. Draw system ionized calcium first.
2. Stop ACD-A infusion.
3. Reduce or maintain BFR at ≤ 50 ml/min.
4. Clamp venous port (& 3rd port if present) of central catheter.
5. Await increased VP alarm.
6. Scrub the stopcock hub with alcohol, turn the stopcock off to the system, draw 1 ml blood to waste and then draw patient ionized calcium sample from the stopcock of the arterial port of the central catheter.
7. Flush stopcock with 1 ml of normal saline to clear stopcock. Return system to standard position.
8. Turn stopcock off to syringe, unclamp all catheter ports.
9. Resume BFR and ACD-A infusion.
10. Send samples to stat laboratory.

Calcium
Infuse Calcium drip into the Y-connector on the venous return line or 3rd limb of dialysis catheter if present.

System Ionized Calcium Sample
Draw System ionized Calcium before Patient ionized Calcium. Draw from venous sample port. Maintain BFR during sampling.

- Three-way stopcock
- Dialysis Catheter
- Y- connector
- Venous chamber

Figure 7.10. CRRT with regional citrate: line set up, infusions, and laboratory sampling for a pediatric patient with only a dialysis catheter.

Courtesy of Maureen Craig, UC Davis Medical Center, Sacramento, California.

decrease infection, morbidity, and mortality rates associated with AKI.

c. Low-flux dialyzers and filters clear solutes ≤ 5000 daltons, while high-flux dialyzers and filters clear solutes ≤ 50,000 daltons. The size of the solute that needs to be cleared may impact the dialyzer or filter choice.

d. Choosing a high-flux dialyzer assists in maximizing clearance. Hemofilters have essentially the same coefficient membrane properties as high-flux dialyzers, thus are able to achieve significant ultrafiltration and clearance.

2. Volumes. Hemofilters and hemodialyzers range in volume from about 20 mL to 120 mL. Blood tubing ranges in volume from 20 mL to 140 mL.

a. When providing SLEDD/CRRT to smaller patients, volume may be a concern.

b. The smaller tubing sets minimize volume by reducing the lumen of the tubing and/or eliminating the arterial chamber. When no arterial chamber is present, AP monitoring should be accomplished by using two 24" pressure-tubing lines. The first one is filled with normal saline and attached to a three-way stopcock on the saline line of the extracorporeal blood circuit. The second pressure tubing line is filled with air and connects the first pressure tubing line to a transducer protector and then to the AP port on the CRRT machine (see Figure 7.10).

c. Dialyzer and tubing combinations can be selected based on patient weight (see Appendix 7.1).

G. Vascular access.

1. A well functioning vascular access is essential for effective CRRT.

2. In general, AVF or AVG are not appropriate for use with CRRT due to the risk of needle dislodgement, needle migration with hematoma formation, or other needle trauma and permanent damage to the access (Vijayan, 2009).

3. Patients who have an AVF or AVG and require SLEDD must be constantly observed during treatment.

a. The access should be kept visible at all times and protected during the ICU stay.

b. If circumstances absolutely require its use, the AVF or AVG should not be used any longer than 12 to 24 hours. and protected during the ICU stay.

4. If CRRT is needed, a temporary nontunneled hemodialysis catheter (HDC) may be used for up to 3 weeks. If the need for KRT extends past 3 weeks, a tunneled cuffed central venous catheter (CVC) should be placed (NKF-K/DOQI, 2000).

   a. Other studies have found that there is an increased risk of infection if the temporary catheter is in place longer than 14 days (Weijmer, Vervloet, & Piet, 2004).

   b. The KDIGO Guidelines (2012) do not recommend a specific time to remove the temporary catheter, but suggest changing to a more permanent access when it becomes unlikely that kidney function will return, while weighing the concerns regarding infection risk with non-tunneled catheters and the technical and practical considerations of tunneled line insertion.

5. Catheters should be placed using strict sterile technique to prevent catheter-related bloodstream infections (CRBSI). Ultrasound-guided procedure for central vein catheter placement is recommended (Kellum et al., 2010; Tolwani, 2012).

   a. CAVH, CAVHD, and CAVHDF require cannulation of both an artery and a vein for extracorporeal blood flow.

     (1) Single-lumen dialysis catheters (8 FR x 15 cm) may be placed in a femoral artery and femoral vein (preferred) or subclavian vein for the arteriovenous circuit.

     (2) Femoral artery to an introducer for a pulmonary artery catheter will support the extracorporeal flow if the MAP is continuously maintained at greater than 70 mm Hg.

   b. For venovenous therapies, a standard dual or triple-lumen hemodialysis catheter is placed. The vessel used for catheter placement will depend on the adult patient's body characteristics, local infection, and coagulopathy.

     (1) Placement in the right internal jugular (IJ) vein is preferred over the left IJ (Tolwani, 2012) due to ease of placement, better blood flow, and lower complication rate.

     (2) A right IJ usually requires a 15 or 16 cm length catheter.

     (3) A left IJ usually requires a 19 to 20 cm length catheter.

     (4) Femoral vein usually requires a 24 cm length catheter.

     (5) Use of the subclavian vein may result in a lower infection rate but is more likely to

cause central vein stenosis, resulting in a possible negative impact should the patient need a permanent access placed in the future.

     (6) Placement of the catheter tip at the junction of the superior vena cava (SVC) and the right atrium provides the best blood flow and avoids cardiac trauma (Vijayan, 2009).

     (7) Internal jugular and subclavian catheters must have placement confirmed by x-ray.

     (8) Femoral catheters require assessing the limb for signs of compromised blood flow each shift. The leg with the catheter in the femoral vein should remain relatively still, which can be challenging for pediatric patients.

   c. For neonates, the umbilical artery or umbilical vein is an alternative choice for vascular access.

   d. For pediatric patients, smaller indwelling catheters are available, such as 4 or 5 Fr single lumen or 7, 8, 9, or 11.5 Fr double lumen, but the same arterial and/or venous sites should be used.

     (1) Cuffed catheters are made with softer material and have better memory, so will resume manufactured shape and preserve intralumenal space even after kinking.

     (2) They can be inserted and left untunneled for use during SLEDD or CRRT, resulting in more dependable blood flow rates over time compared to tunneled catheters.

     (3) It can be challenging to achieve adequate blood flow rates in the pediatric catheters. These catheters must be carefully placed to achieve desired blood flow so as not to limit the effectiveness of the treatment. Access difficulties should be corrected immediately.

     (4) Blood flow rates should be ≥ 50 mL/min for systemic heparinization and ≥ 20 mL/min when using regional citrate anticoagulation to minimize patient and system complications such as clotting from an elevated filtration fraction.

6. Good blood flow in a hemodialysis catheter is critical to a successful KRT treatment.

   a. Blood flow in the catheter can be compromised because of poor location in the blood vessel or because of a kink in the catheter or bloodline.

   b. Frequent (more than three per hour) equipment alarms related to poor blood flow in the catheter results in blood stasis in the hemofilter or hemodialyzer, increasing the risk for a clotted system.

   c. If good blood flow cannot be maintained

consistently, the catheter must be replaced to accomplish an effective SLEDD or CRRT treatment.

7. Recirculation occurs when blood that has just left the venous or return line is drawn back in through the arterial port for another pass through the filter instead of returning to the patient's systemic circulation.
   a. Some recirculation occurs with any hemodialysis catheter.
   b. When recirculation is ≥ 15%, the SLEDD/CRRT treatment effectiveness begins to be compromised.
   c. Recirculation should be checked when:
      (1) The patient does not achieve the expected change in solutes related to the treatment.
      (2) The hemofilter or hemodialyzer clots easily with hemoconcentration of recirculated blood.
      (3) Recirculation can be calculated using any freely diffusible small molecule such as BUN.

$$\text{Recirculation (\%)} = 100 \times \frac{(BUN_{peripheral} - BUN_{arterial})}{(BUN_{peripheral} - BUN_{venous})}$$

      (4) If excessive recirculation is occurring (>15%), the catheter should be changed over a guide wire or placed in a new location depending on the reason for the increased recirculation.
8. Catheter exit-site and site care.
   a. For a standard, nonocclusive gauze dressing, a sterile dressing change should be performed every other day or as needed to keep the site clean and dry. When using a chlorhexidine gluconate (CHG) sponge disc with a transparent semipermeable occlusive dressing, the dressing should be changed every 7 days or as needed to keep the site clean and dry.
      (1) The old dressing should be removed, taking care not to tug at the exit site.
      (2) The exit site should be cleansed with an approved antibacterial solution.
      (3) The catheter can be anchored with Steri-Strips™ and then covered with a nonocclusive dressing.
   b. The hemodialysis catheter should be accessed for treatment using aseptic technique to minimize the chance of microorganisms entering the patient via the lumen of the catheter. (For more details, refer to Module 3, Chapter 3: Vascular Access.)
   c. Patients with a hemodialysis catheter should be monitored for signs and symptoms of local and/or systemic infection.
   d. Alternatives for catheter "locks" include:

      (1) Heparin.
      (2) Sodium citrate 4% and trisodium citrate 30%. These have been proven to reduce catheter-related bacteremia. They are available in Canada and Europe but are not FDA approved in the United States for this function.
      (3) Devices that provide needle-free access to catheters as well as those that have a disinfecting cap have been developed.
      (4) Antibiotic or antiseptic lock solutions might reduce catheter related infections but carry a risk of toxicity and bacterial resistance.

VI. Anticoagulation.

A. Anticoagulation may be avoided with the use of saline flushes.
   1. When treating patients for whom anticoagulation is not feasible, 25 to 200 mL normal saline flushes every 30 to 60 minutes should be performed.
      a. The frequency can be adjusted based on the condition of the hemofilter.
      b. It is especially important in patients who may be auto-anticoagulated with low platelet counts.
   2. The flush volume needs to be calculated into the volume to be removed from the patient.
   3. Adding a predilution solution and/or increasing the BFR may decrease the need for anticoagulation as well, but flushing may accomplish a better result than predilution using the same volume of saline.

B. Heparin is the most commonly used anticoagulant for CRRT or SLEDD systems.
   1. There is increasing evidence calling into question the safety of heparin in critically ill patients, such as:
      a. Heparin resistance, requiring higher doses of heparin to achieve the desired prolongation of the activated partial thromboplastin time (APTT) into the therapeutic range (Anderson & Saenko, 2002).
      b. Bleeding due to systemic as well as circuit anticoagulation.
      c. Proinflammatory effects resulting in adverse effects on the microcirculation in sepsis (Oudemans-van Straaten et al., 2011).
      d. Heparin-induced thrombocytopenia (HIT).
   2. When using heparin as an anticoagulant, it is important to heparinize the systemic circulation with a bolus dose (10 to 30 units/kg) 5 minutes prior to connection to the SLEDD or CRRT system.
   3. The patient's PTT will rise during those 5 minutes, minimizing the clotting on the first few passes of blood through the circuit.

4. PTT should be drawn immediately upon starting treatment to determine if the patient is in the desired range (45 to 65 seconds or based on unit protocol).
   a. PTT is the preferred form of monitoring heparin anticoagulation as activated clotting time (ACT) monitoring is not reliable in this lower target range of heparin therapy.
   b. Smaller repeat boluses may be necessary to bring the PTT values into range.
   c. A heparin infusion (10 to 25 units/kg/hr) should be given to maintain the patient in the desired PTT range. This may be titrated using the cardiac or the neuro protocol depending on the patient's condition and the hospital's policies.
   d. The PTT should be rechecked after each heparin bolus, 4 hours after any heparin dosing changes, and immediately after blood product administration.
5. Heparin is highly protein bound; therefore, it is not readily removed during CRRT or SLEDD treatments.
6. Heparin may be administered in the syringe pump on the machine if available or, alternatively, may be diluted (5000, 10,000 or 20,000 units/L normal saline) and infused into the heparin line on the extracorporeal blood circuit using a standard IV pump.
7. Patients with HIT cannot be exposed to heparin because of the danger of white clot syndrome, which results in a drop in the patient's platelet count and potentially lethal clot formation. Alternative forms of anticoagulation must be used for these patients.
8. When using heparin, some users deliver an hourly flush of the system with 25 to 200 ml of normal saline to observe patency. The saline can be connected to a Y port, med port or stopcock on the access line.

C. Citrate is an anticoagulant and a buffer, leading to increased complexity of management compared to heparin.
   1. Citrate provides regional anticoagulation of the CRRT system.
   a. Citrate is administered either through a Y-port or stopcock attached to the access line. Calcium is administered through a central line, the third port on the dialysis catheter if available, or a Y port on the venous bloodline as the blood is returned to the patient.
      (1) Calcium binds to the citrate, interrupting the clotting cascade and forming a calcium/citrate molecule. This molecule can be removed from the blood either by diffusion when it goes back through the dialyzer or by liver metabolism into bicarbonate.
      (2) The calcium infusion also replaces the calcium lost from the patient in this process to prevent systemic hypocalcemia.
      (3) A poorly placed catheter with low blood flow will increase calcium recirculation resulting in the need to increase the citrate infusion, leading to the need for increasing the calcium infusion to reverse the citrate effect. This vicious cycle makes it difficult to deliver a safe and effective KRT treatment.
      (4) Ideally, the patient should have a well functioning dialysis catheter, a separate central line for calcium, and an additional line, such as an arterial line, for blood draws (see Figure 7.11).
   2. The patient with limited vascular access, e.g., neonate, pediatric, or vascular-compromised patient, may present with only a dialysis catheter. Although more challenging, this patient can still receive regional citrate.
   3. When using citrate anticoagulation, it is essential that IV infusions of calcium and citrate stop whenever the blood pump stops. This prevents backflow, which would result in direct administration of citrate and/or calcium to the patient.
   4. When using citrate anticoagulation, the dialysis solution should not contain calcium. This allows for effectiveness of the citrate and the diffusion of the calcium/citrate bound molecules.
   5. The BFR, DFR, IV citrate, and IV calcium must be initiated and terminated together to avoid undesired changes in the patient's serum chemistry.

D. Other anticoagulants.
   1. Alternative anticoagulation agents are available, including warfarin, argatroban, bivalirudin, r-hirudin, and fondaparinux.
   2. These forms of anticoagulation are not likely to be used to manage SLEDD or CRRT. However, a patient receiving one of these less common anticoagulants could require SLEDD or CRRT. When this occurs, the anticoagulation for the intermittent SLEDD or continuous CRRT treatments needs to be adjusted to accommodate any additive influences there may be from the other anticoagulants.

VII. Standards of nursing care for KRT.

A. CRRT guidelines.
   1. CRRT has existed in various forms for nearly 40 years. In 1993, the American Nephrology Nurses'

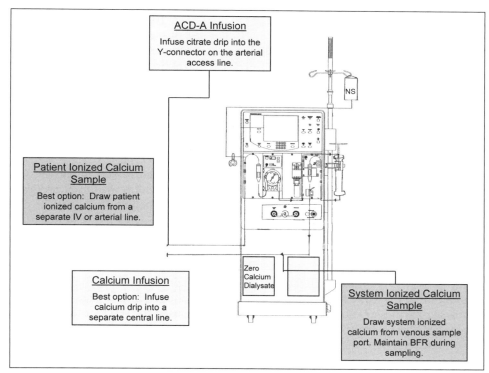

Figure 7.11. CRRT with regional citrate: infusions and laboratory sampling.
Courtesy of Fresenius and Maureen Craig, UC Davis Medical Center, Sacramento, California.

Association (ANNA) established and published *Nephrology Nursing Guidelines for Care: CRRT*.

2. These guidelines are endorsed by the American Association of Critical Care Nurses (AACN) and were updated in 2011.

3. These guidelines are a reference for all nephrology and ICU nurses looking for guidance in providing care for patients on CRRT.

4. *Nephrology Nursing Process of Care: Apheresis and Therapeutic Plasma Exchange and Continuous Renal Replacement Therapy* © 2011.

   a. This publication contains two sections reprinted from the *Nephrology Nursing Scope and Standards of Practice*, 7th edition. The contents deal with the nephrology nursing process for continuous renal replacement therapy, apheresis, and therapeutic plasma exchange. The book is published by the American Nephrology Nurses' Association and is endorsed by the American Association of Critical-Care Nurses.

   b. A copy can be ordered from the ANNA website, https://www.annanurse.org/resources/products/publications

B. SLEDD standards.

   1. This intermittent therapy has essentially the same standards for nursing care as apply to IHD.

      a. Differences include the variations in the involvement of the ICU nurse at the bedside

and the additional equipment being utilized.

      b. Similarities include the regular and intensive patient assessment shared by the nephrology nurse and the ICU nurse incorporated in following and adjusting the plan of care, frequently in response to changes in the patient's condition.

   2. As SLEDD therapy evolves further, additional acceptable variations will undoubtedly be expressed in the literature.

VIII. Collaboration between the nephrology nurses and the ICU nurses.

A. Nursing care for the patient, whether on intermittent or continuous therapy, is delivered differently in different settings.

   1. Nursing care provided to the patient on CRRT may be predominately nephrology or ICU driven.

      a. Collaboration between the nephrology and ICU disciplines leads to opportunities for excellent care and outcomes for the patient.

      b. For those facilities that do not have nephrology nursing backup, the ICU nurses deliver the CRRT treatment. Ideally, these nurses are trained and supported by a clinical nurse specialist (CNS) or advanced practice registered nurse (APRN) with a strong nephrology background.

      c. The nephrologists, intensivists, nephrology

nurses, and ICU nurses must all work together to meet the needs of the patient on CRRT.

   d. The input from a pharmacist and nutritionist is extremely valuable in optimizing the delivery of care to the patient on CRRT.

   e. The social worker/case manager provides support to patients and families as well as guidance on how to access needed community resources.

2. Nursing care for patients on SLEDD treatments also requires collaboration between the nephrology and ICU nurses.

   a. The nephrology nurse provides more of the direct patient care and documentation, in some cases staying at the bedside for the duration of the treatment just as they do for an IHD treatment.

   b. In larger institutions with multiple SLEDD treatments going on at the same time, the nephrology nurse provides a bedside in-service and then is physically away from the bedside of the ICU patient between the 30-minute to 60-minute checks.

   c. The ICU nurse responds to the patient's needs as indicated in the bedside in-service and has the nephrology nurse available by pager or phone for bedside response within 5 minutes.

   d. By design, SLEDD is intended to provide a planned period of time in which the patient is off treatment so that other interventions can occur. Therefore, some facilities run SLEDD during the day so the patient is off during the night; others run the treatment during the night so the patient is available during the day.

   e. Since SLEDD is a modification of IHD with extended time and slower rate of solute clearance and UF, management of the treatment is familiar to most nephrology nurses.

3. Ongoing communication between the nephrology and ICU nurses is a critical element to effective and safe KRT treatments.

B. Education and training in the collaborative setting between ICU and nephrology.

1. A successful KRT program must have an ongoing educational component to establish and maintain competency of all the nurses providing the treatment.

2. CRRT is frequently a collaboration between the ICU nurse and the nephrology nurse; in other facilities the ICU nurse assumes complete responsibility for doing the CRRT treatments. CRRT should only be performed by an ICU and nephrology nurse who have both successfully completed a class on CRRT.

   a. Some facilities require attendance at an 8-hour or 10-hour CRRT class taught by a nephrology nurse skilled in CRRT.

   b. Some facilities only offer time for a more abbreviated class of 1 to 2 hours with written materials providing a self-learning module for ongoing education and reference. This elevates the importance of the bedside in-service provided by the nephrology nurse for every shift of ICU nurses, whether on site or by phone.

   c. Regular review of patient outcomes should be audited in the QAPI program to analyze the cost-benefit that could be obtained with more extensive ICU staff education.

3. KRT education sessions for nephrology nurses.

   a. The acute care nephrology nurse will be able to learn the SLEDD treatment options and provide this therapy with either a 1-hour to 2-hour SLEDD class if the same equipment is used for IHD; or they may choose to attend a full CRRT class.

   b. To learn CRRT, they will need to attend a full CRRT class with additional time at the bedside with an experienced nephrology nurse preceptor.

   c. For either procedure, the nephrology nurse should be mentored by an experienced nurse providing backup for at least their first patient care assignment.

4. KRT theory for ICU nurses.

   a. The SLEDD class/in-service should include theoretical content that includes the definition of SLEDD and how it accomplishes solute clearance and ultrafiltration for the ICU patient. For the nephrology nurse, emphasis should be placed on the similarities and differences between SLEDD and IHD.

   b. The CRRT theory class should have theoretical content that covers the definitions of CRRT and related concepts, indications for CRRT, and benefits, challenges, and monitoring of the patient on CRRT as well as troubleshooting the equipment.

5. KRT equipment training.

   a. Typically the equipment used to perform SLEDD is the same equipment the nephrology nurse uses to perform IHD.

     (1) The SLEDD class/in-service should emphasize the importance of not exceeding the prescribed maximum BFR, DFR, and UFR.

     (2) Slowing the dialysis therapy, as is done during SLEDD, minimizes hemodynamic instability and reduces alarm conditions, allowing the nephrology nurse to walk away from the bedside after in-servicing the ICU nurse.

(3) The ICU nurse must have enough of an understanding of the SLEDD treatment and equipment used to independently:
   (a) Respond to the patient's hypotension.
   (b) Respond to arterial and venous pressure alarms.
   (c) Titrate anticoagulation.
   (d) Assess system clotting.
   (e) Respond immediately and appropriately to air in the system.
   (f) Return the patient's blood using normal saline for the total rinse-back procedure.
(4) The ICU nurse's response to other less common alarms or concerns should be to call or page the nephrology nurse and troubleshoot the situation together.

b. The CRRT equipment to be used should be reviewed and demonstrated in the CRRT class along with related system components such as vascular access, hemofilters or hemodialyzers, replacement solutions, dialysis solutions, and anticoagulation.
(1) The equipment review should emphasize the most frequently asked questions and most common alarm conditions.
(2) References and personnel resources should be identified for more uncommon alarm conditions or concerns and a standard approach sought.
(3) Each class participant should have hands-on time with a system setup as close to a patient scenario as possible (use a catheter in a fluid bag to simulate a "patient" and +/– pressures). This helps develop some familiarity with interacting with the CRRT equipment and serves to decrease anxiety and build confidence as understanding expands.
(4) The equipment time should include a review of the bedside in-service checklist with an opportunity for the learner to initiate and resolve alarm conditions.

6. CRRT bedside in-service: The importance of the bedside in-service for CRRT cannot be overemphasized (Baldwin & Fealy, 2009).
a. Several months may have passed since the ICU nurse has taken the CRRT class or managed a CRRT treatment.
b. The bedside in-service is provided just in time and includes:
(1) A refresher of all the major points of the CRRT class.
(2) Reason for treatment.
(3) How treatment is to be accomplished.
(4) How to respond to and care for the patient and CRRT system in a particular time frame.

(5) How to document the care provided.
(6) When and how to contact the nephrology nurse.
c. A bedside in-service checklist is a critical tool for both the nephrology and ICU nurse to make certain the in-service is as comprehensive as the ICU nurse desires.
d. The bedside in-service is best provided by the nephrology nurse who will be covering the CRRT call over the next shift.
e. The in-service can last up to 1 hour depending on the educational needs.
f. The bedside in-service should be repeated by the nephrology nurse daily or near the beginning of each shift. This can be coordinated with the time the nephrology nurse comes to do a patient/system assessment and to restock solutions and supplies needed for the CRRT treatment.

7. SLEDD bedside in-service. SLEDD treatments must also include a bedside in-service if the ICU nurse is going to directly help manage the treatment without the nephrology nurse constantly at the bedside.
a. The SLEDD bedside in-service should include the reason for treatment, how to respond to changes in the patient, and the management of the SLEDD system.
b. Emphasis should be placed on how to respond to the essential elements of a SLEDD treatment.
(1) Hypotension.
(2) Arterial or venous pressure alarms.
(3) Titration of anticoagulation.
(4) Assess system clotting.
(5) Respond immediately and appropriately to air in the system.
(6) Return the patient's blood using normal saline for the total rinse-back procedure.
(7) When and how to contact the nephrology nurse.

8. Samples of the bedside in-service documentation can be found in the appendix as follows.
a. CRRT Bedside in-service checklist (see Appendix 7.2).
b. CRRT with regional citrate bedside in-service checklist (see Appendix 7.3).
c. SLEDD bedside in-service checklist (see Appendix 7.4).

9. Documentation training.
a. Documentation for the patient on CRRT must be taught to both the nephrology and the ICU nurse.
b. Some facilities use the ICU nurse's regular documentation form and incorporate the patient's I&O, system pressures, and anticoagulation into that form. This might initially require revising the ICU flowsheet or

the electronic medical record (EMR).

c. Other facilities develop specific tracking logs for recording all the elements related to CRRT.

d. Documentation examples and scenarios improve effective and accurate documentation. Ideally, two shifts of a patient scenario should be documented during the 8-hour CRRT class to show how I/O are totaled and documented at change of shift.

   (1) Elements of adjusting the UFR or BFR in response to changes in patient I/O or condition should be emphasized.

   (2) Examples of resolving patient/system condition changes, such as hypotension and equipment alarms, should be included.

e. SLEDD documentation. The nephrology nurse provides most of the documentation for the patient on SLEDD.

   (1) The documentation is very similar to that associated with an IHD treatment and should occur every 30 to 60 minutes with both patient and system assessments.

   (2) The nephrology nurse is familiar with the documentation required during the mentored SLEDD treatment since it is so similar to IHD.

   (3) The ICU staff will document that the SLEDD treatment was initiated and terminated and the volume changes that occurred during the treatment, similar to the way they might document following an IHD treatment.

   (4) Additionally, during treatment the ICU nurse may document alarm conditions and the action taken.

f. Documentation should be developed emphasizing the principle of simplicity.

   (1) When introducing new documentation, there is a tendency to "double document" to "just make sure."

   (2) Each entry and calculation creates another chance for an error simply because humans are performing this task.

   (3) Increasing the number of entries or calculations increases the likelihood of errors.

   (4) A simple method of documentation that minimizes calculations is best and more likely to be implemented by staff.

   (5) The area of documentation of fluid balance and I/O during CRRT is especially challenging for the beginner.

      (a) The best way to keep the patient safe is to keep the nurse's eyes on the patient and the patient's parameters as the patient responds to treatment.

      (b) Correlating the documentation to the

order in which tasks are performed and to the principles taught in the training program will facilitate learning, accuracy, and efficiency.

C. Samples of standing orders for different combinations of elements and equipment as well as Intake and Output flow sheets for calculating fluid management are included in the appendices as follows.

   1. SLEDD/CRRT orders with regional citrate anticoagulation (see Appendix 7.5).

   2. CRRT orders with heparin or no anticoagulation (see Appendix 7.6).

   3. Pediatric CRRT orders with regional citrate anticoagulation (see Appendix 7.7).

   4. Pediatric CRRT orders with heparin or no anticoagulation (see Appendix 7.8).

   5. CRRT orders with regional citrate anticoagulation (see Appendix 7.9).

   6. CRRT orders with heparin or citrate anticoagulation (see Appendix 7.10).

   7. Pediatric CRRT orders with regional citrate anticoagulation (see Appendix 7.11).

   8. Nephrology nursing flowsheet (see Appendix 7.12).

   9. Nephrology nursing flowsheet (see Appendix 7.13).

   10. ICU nursing kardex for CRRT with regional citrate (see Appendix 7.14).

   11. ICU nursing I&O flowsheet for CRRT (see Appendix 7.15).

D. Competency.

   1. If a nurse's exposure to the SLEDD/CRRT equipment and therapy is less than once every 6 months, a competency program should be added that includes an equipment demonstration lab. The review/demonstration should occur preferably every 6 months but at least every 12 months.

   2. A competency assessment should include a written examination and a demonstration checklist on equipment and documentation similar to the modality's bedside in-service.

   3. Maintaining the nephrology and ICU nurse competency without performing treatments is challenging, time consuming, and costly.

   4. Every effort should be made when planning a KRT program, that once the initial training has occurred, treatments should be routinely ordered and supported by all the nephrology and ICU providers, nurses, and administration.

   5. Initially, challenging experiences should be buffered by the fact that repetition smooths and improves the road of experience. Do not stall a new program with the "paralysis of analysis."

IX. CRRT treatment overview and schedule coordination for a collaborative program (Craig, 1998a).

A. When a CRRT treatment is ordered by a nephrology physician/APRN/PA, a nephrology nurse will set up the CRRT system and initiate therapy in collaboration with the ICU nurse.

B. The nephrology and ICU charge nurses should both be made aware of the pending treatment as soon as possible to take into consideration the staffing that the CRRT treatment will require.
1. Most facilities practice a 1:1 nurse-to-patient ratio for the patient who is on CRRT. In pediatric programs, the staffing ratio for patients < 10 kg may be increased to 2 RNs:1 patient (one RN to monitor the patient and one to monitor the machine).
   a. This planned 1:1 ratio is preferred, especially in new and growing programs where the group's expertise is still emerging and several nurses may be involved to assist with the treatment or to learn from the more experienced nurses caring for the patient.
   b. As the group's expertise grows and the CRRT program becomes simpler and more systematic, the ICU charge nurse will make staffing assignments based on the overall level of care the patient will require, and the application of CRRT to the patient's treatment plan will be one of many factors taken into consideration.
2. The nephrology nurse is responsible for providing a bedside in-service and some system monitoring at the beginning of every shift or treatment.
3. The nephrology nurse will change the CRRT circuit as needed and is always available by phone to assist with system troubleshooting.
4. The ICU nurse is responsible for ongoing patient monitoring, CRRT system maintenance, treatment termination if emergently indicated, and documentation of all assessments and care provided.

C. Initiation of either the CRRT or SLEDD treatment.
1. Nephrology nurse.
   a. Notify ICU nurse of treatment orders and time treatment to be initiated; indicate supplies, medications, and equipment needed; verify consent is on chart.
   b. Set up the appropriate equipment, complete equipment calibration and safety checks, test system alarms. All equipment related to the treatment should be kept on one stand or machine if possible. This setup provides ease of coordination and documentation of monitoring and prevents inadvertently leaving an IV infusion (e.g., calcium or heparin) running upon treatment termination.
      (1) In a collaborative practice model, a supply basket or cart should be left at bedside for the nurses to use.
      (2) This should contain items that may be needed during the treatment but are not on the ICU supply cart or not close at hand.
      (3) The supply basket can contain a separate container identified for system discontinuation to assist the nurse by having all the items needed for the end of the treatment in one place.
      (4) The medications that are used in the initiation and discontinuation of treatment will need to be documented in/on the hospital's medical record, potentially including special labeling, scanning of identifying labels on the medication's packaging and on the patient, as well as on electronic or paper medication administration records.
      (5) The system support kit may include an extra cartridge or hemofilter or hemodialyzer and blood line tubing; IV tubing; extra normal saline; Y-connectors; 3-mL, 10-mL, and 20-mL syringes; arterial blood gas (ABG) syringes; needleless needles; standard needles; alcohol, betadine, or chlorhexidine gluconate (CHG) pads; plastic hemostats; extra tape; 2 x 2 gauze sponges; transparent dressings; recirculation tubes; eye protection wear; and transducer protectors if needed for the machine in use.
      (6) The discontinuation kit may include normal saline, IV tubing, female-female IV adaptor, sterile drape, sterile gloves, alcohol pads, catheter caps, 3 mL and 10 mL syringes, and a catheter lock solution.
   c. The CRRT circuit is usually flushed and primed with 1 to 2 liters of normal saline.
      (1) Sometimes 5,000 units of heparin are added to the final liter of saline.
      (2) Flushing and priming the circuit removes the air, flushes out sterilant, and may coat the membrane with heparin, if used.
   d. Pediatric blood prime.
      (1) When using a circuit volume that is ≥ 15% of the patient's circulating blood volume, a blood prime should be considered.
         (a) For infants (0 to 12 months), circulating blood volume is about 80 mL/kg.
         (b) For a child (1 to 12 years), about 75 mL/kg.

(c) For an adolescent (13 to 19 years), about 70 mL/kg.

(2) The circuit is first flushed and primed with saline.

(3) The volume of saline required for dilution of the mini (≤ 30 mL) packed red blood cells (PRBC) is calculated to achieve an HCT that matches the infant.

$$V_{saline} = \frac{V_{PRBC}(HCT_{PRBC} - HCT_{infant})}{HCT_{infant}}$$

(4) Connect both the mini PRBC and a 50 mL bag of normal saline to a volutrol. Fill the volutrol with the entire volume of the mini PRBC and the calculated volume of saline (V_{saline}) in the volutrol. Gently agitate the PRBC and saline mix.

(5) The mix is then primed into the SLEDD/CRRT circuit at a BFR of 20 mL/min.

(6) Prior to starting the treatment, the circuit should be recirculated with a calcium containing dialysis solution for several minutes to remove some of the citrate that is present in PRBC. Infusing the fully citrated blood product directly into the patient can result in a rapid drop in patient's ionized calcium level.

(7) The dialysis solution concentrate is changed to the ordered solution and a standard connection to the patient is performed.

(8) The BFR is started at 10 mL/min and slowly increased to the prescribed BFR.

(9) Typically, when a blood prime is used for initiating the SLEDD or CRRT circuit, the blood is not returned upon discontinuation of the treatment.

e. Prime, label, and connect calcium, citrate, and/or heparin IV lines to the circuit or patient as ordered.

f. Ensure a supply of replacement solutions, dialysis solutions, calcium, citrate, and/or heparin is available to last until the next scheduled check (30 to 60 minutes for SLEDD or 12 to 14 hours for CRRT).

g. Assess patient, vascular access catheter and system; review medications; document assessment and care on nephrology nursing progress record or EMR.

h. Cleanse both dialysis ports of the catheter. Using a syringe, aspirate two times the catheter fill volume of blood from each lumen of the dialysis ports of the catheter. Administer anticoagulant as ordered followed by saline flush as ordered. Wait 5 minutes.

i. Attach and secure the ends of the extracorporeal blood circuit to the patient's dialysis catheter. Initiate treatment per physician/APRN/PA order.

j. Review care of patient and documentation with ICU nurse using the bedside in-service checklist as a guide.

k. Monitor patient for a minimum of 15 minutes before leaving bedside.

l. Document treatment initiation and patient care on nephrology nursing progress record or EMR.

2. ICU nurse.

a. Draw baseline labs. Alternatively, the nephrology nurse can draw these labs from the dialysis catheter at the start of the treatment if no tests are ordered that will be impacted by the anticoagulant fill in the catheter such as a PTT.

b. Verify that a dialysis catheter has been inserted in the patient and placement verified by x-ray for subclavian or internal jugular placement. For a femoral line placement, check the cannulated limb for circulation, including pedal pulses.

c. Assess and document treatment initiation, patient's fluid and electrolyte balance, vital signs (VS), weight, BP, edema, lab values, lung and heart sounds, and overall condition.

d. Keep a 500 mL normal saline flush bag with gravity tubing for emergency termination at the bedside.

e. Receive in-service from nephrology nurse.

D. Maintenance of the CRRT treatment.

1. Nephrology nurse (Craig, 1998b).

a. Near the beginning of every ICU nursing shift and as needed (PRN), the nephrology nurse should do a bedside patient and system check followed by an in-service for the bedside nurse.

(1) This is not possible in some facilities, and a remote in-service between the ICU nurse and the nephrology nurse on-call occurs.

(2) The nephrology nurse must make this check at least once per day, and ideally once per shift to improve the consistency of delivery of CRRT to the patient.

(a) Assess patient, catheter, and system; review medications; document assessment and care on nephrology nursing progress record, entering a new note each day.

(b) Check the dialysis access catheter dressing and change per protocol.

(c) Note and implement changes in the CRRT orders. Refill supply basket, dialysate, replacement fluid, saline and heparin as needed.

(d) Verify calcium, citrate, or heparin pumps are operating as expected.

(e) Verify the air detector line is engaged.

(f) Review care of patient on CRRT and flowsheet documentation with the ICU nurse.

b. Every 2 to 3 days, or as needed, the nephrology nurse will change the CRRT filter and blood tubing.

c. Provide and document patient and family education and support.

2. ICU nurse: Every 1 to 2 hours and PRN.

a. Assess patient, catheter, and system. Monitor system for any changes or alarm conditions. Maintain MAP > 60 mmHg.

b. Document VS, BFR, I/O, equipment alarms, resolution of alarms, equipment pressures, and rates.

c. Assess patient and laboratory findings (e.g., hypocalcemia). Titrate and document calcium and citrate or heparin infusions.

d. For some treatment protocols, the IV pumps need to be cleared every hour so the I&O and fluid removal goals can be calculated and the new fluid removal target set on the appropriate screen. Some programs perform these functions once each shift.

e. Assess and document patient's fluid balance and overall condition. Consider weight, pulmonary artery wedge pressure (PAWP), VS, edema, laboratory values, and heart and lung sounds.

E. Termination of the CRRT treatment.

1. Nephrology nurse.

a. Assess patient condition and document on nephrology nursing note.

b. In some cases, the nephrology nurse will return blood to the patient with a saline flush. In other circumstances, the ICU nurse may return the blood.

c. Remove and dispose of tubing using standard precautions.

d. Disinfect equipment and return to appropriate storage area.

e. Document time and reason for termination of treatment.

2. ICU nurse.

a. Pediatric patients: consult with physician before returning blood. Blood return is usually contraindicated if blood prime was used.

b. In adult patients, return the blood to patient with normal saline flush.

c. For regional citrate anticoagulation, stop citrate and calcium infusions simultaneously.

d. Check a patient's ionized calcium value 20 to 30 minutes after CRRT termination.

e. Either the nephrology nurse or the ICU nurse can cap off the catheter with a normal saline flush and anticoagulant fill, depending on the circumstances. Label dressing with date, initials, capping solution, name, concentration, and volume used for catheter fill (e.g., "heparin 5,000 units/mL, arterial 1.8 mL, venous 1.9 mL" or "3% citrate, arterial 1.8 mL, venous 1.9 mL").

f. Document time and reason for termination of treatment.

F. Treatment overview for SLEDD.

1. When a SLEDD treatment is ordered by the nephrologist/APRN/PA, a nephrology nurse will set up the SLEDD system, assess the patient, initiate therapy, and document this care.

2. The nephrology nurse will provide the SLEDD bedside in-service to the ICU nurse.

3. The nephrology nurse will either stay and perform the treatment or return every 30 to 60 minutes to assess the patient and system and document the progress of the SLEDD treatment.

a. The nephrology nurse is available by pager for an immediate telephone response and/or a 5-minute bedside response time.

b. Every 30 to 60 minutes, the nephrology nurse will assess the patient, the catheter, and the system.

c. Document assessment and care in the medical record.

d. Provide and document patient and family education and support.

e. The ICU nurse will monitor the patient and the system; document any system alarms, the resolution of those alarms, and conditions; then document the information on the ICU nursing flowsheet.

4. The nephrology nurse terminates the SLEDD treatment and completes the documentation. The nephrology nurse reports the final patient assessment and UF volume to the ICU nurse.

X. Troubleshooting during CRRT and/or SLEDD treatments.

A. Hypotension.

1. For MAP < 60 mmHg, stop UF and administer a fluid bolus (not to be removed) as ordered by the intensivist or nephrologist.

a. For SLEDD, call the nephrology nurse to assess and determine changes to the UFR. Consider UF profiling to prevent hypotension. Patients using a linear decreasing UFR show a reduced incidence of hypotension.

b. For CRRT, call the nephrologist for changes to UFR.

(1) Lowering the dialysis solution temperature

to 35° to 36°C may increase vasoconstriction and minimize hypotension.

   (2) Assess volume status changes and evaluate the need for initiating or titrating vasopressors to maintain BP and MAP within established range depending on treatment goals.

B. Hemofilter/dialyzer clotting.
1. For rising TMP or VP, clotting should be suspected. Minimizing the time that the blood flow is stopped due to alarm conditions decreases the risk for clotting.
2. For SLEDD, call the nephrology nurse to assess and potentially terminate treatment.
3. For CRRT, notify the nephrologist and follow procedure for end of treatment.

C. Hypothermia.
1. During CRRT with unwarmed dialysis or replacement solutions, the patient's temperature may fall to < 35°C.
2. Warm patient by warming the dialysis or replacement solutions or by warming the blood with a blood warmer. Or warm the patient directly with a heating blanket until the patient is at desired temperature.

D. Hyperthermia.
1. The patient may be unable to elevate body temperature during exposure to large volumes of dialysis or replacement solutions at ≤ 37°C.
2. This may cloud the use of the patient's temperature as an indicator of infectious processes.

E. Patient bleeding.
1. Stop heparin infusion if being administered.
2. Notify physician for signs and symptoms of bleeding or for a hematocrit decrease > 5%.
3. Contact nephrologist to determine need for changes to anticoagulation orders.

F. Cardiopulmonary resuscitation (CPR).
1. Initiate CPR and follow Advanced Cardiac Life Support (ACLS) guidelines.
2. Turn off any UF, slow BFR, and maintain a patent system while ICU nurse initiates CPR. Call nephrology nurse and/or nephrologist/APRN/PA for assistance and instructions.
3. Use the dialysis access catheter lines for administering emergency meds if needed.
4. When patient has stabilized and has adequate IV sites for administration of medications, return blood to patient if possible, stop treatment, and clamp and cap lines.

G. Equipment alarms.
1. Refer to bedside in-service for most common alarm conditions.
2. Contact the nephrology nurse for less common alarm conditions.
3. Consult the operator's manual and/or contact the manufacturer's clinical resources for unusual or irresolvable alarm conditions.
   a. False positive blood leak alarm from air bubbles in dialysate.
   b. False positive from bilirubin or myoglobin in the effluent due to patient's disease state.
   c. Interference with the blood leak detector if patient has been treated with hydoxocobalamin or methylene blue (Sutter, 2012).
   d. Alarm may be generated by colorimetric or ultrasonic sensor monitor depending on the machine being used.

H. Serum electrolyte and solute imbalance.
1. Review the dialysis and/or the replacement solutions being used.
2. When necessary, the provider may prescribe a change to adapt solutions so patient can achieve desired serum electrolytes.
3. When the patient's lab values show a change in eletrolytes, follow standing orders to change the dialysis bath, or call the nephrologist/APRN/PA for orders if there are no standing orders or the event or condition warrants different and more careful consideration.

I. Procedure or test requiring patient to be transported out of the ICU.
1. If possible, work with ICU staff to schedule procedures during a time the patient is off SLEDD treatment or the CRRT system is scheduled for a change.
2. Alternatively, interrupt treatment as indicated and resume treatment when patient is available and as ordered by the nephrologist/APRN/PA.

J. Procedure in the ICU. If a procedure may cause patient agitation or disruption of dialysis circuit, contact nephrology nurse for additional monitoring of dialysis system during the procedure.

XI. Monitoring the system and the patient.

A. Therapy considerations.
1. Software, pumps, scales, and/or balance chambers manage the fluid balance under the control of the ICU nurse at the bedside.
2. The bedside nurse monitors patient intake and output volumes to allow for hourly adjustments of machine settings to maximize the accuracy and effectiveness of the therapy.

a. Intake must include all fluids administered including IV meds, total parenteral nutrition (TPN), tube feedings, flushes, blood products, and replacement solution if doing CVVH or CVVHDF.

b. Output must include all sources of loss including NG suction, emesis, urine, stool, Jackson-Pratt (J-P) drains, and wound-vac. Dressings can be weighed for output if they are frequently and heavily saturated. Insensible losses such as perspiration are difficult to measure so can be estimated or not included in the calculations.

c. Most practitioners monitor electrolytes and acid-base status every 6 to 8 hours. After 24 hours of a patient's condition remaining stable, this testing may decrease to every 12 hours (Tolwani, 2012).

B. Monitoring related to citrate anticoagulation.

1. During regional citrate anticoagulation, the patient and system-ionized calcium must be closely monitored and carefully differentiated. The citrate and calcium solutions are then titrated to achieve and maintain the desired ionized calcium range.

2. The patient ionized calcium sample, drawn from a stopcock on the arterial limb of the dialysis catheter, may be lower than the peripherally drawn sample due to the proximity of the citrate infusion to the sampling port (see Figure 7.10). To maximize the accuracy of the results, draw the patient's ionized calcium samples using the following steps.

a. Draw the system's ionized calcium sample before the patient's ionized calcium sample while maintaining the BFR.

b. Stop the citrate infusion.

c. Reduce or maintain the BFR at ≤ 50 mL/min.

d. Clamp the venous port (and the third port if present) on the CVC to prevent recirculation

e. Wait for an increased VP alarm, allowing time for patient's blood to enter the arterial line. Scrub the stopcock hub with alcohol, turn the stopcock off to the system, draw 1 mL blood to waste, and then draw the patient's ionized calcium sample from the stopcock on the arterial port of the CVC.

f. Flush stopcock with 1 mL of normal saline to clear the stopcock. Return system to standard position.

g. Turn stopcock off to syringe and unclamp all catheter ports.

h. Resume BFR and citrate infusion.

i. Send samples to stat laboratory (see Figure 7.10).

3. The ionized calcium is monitored every 30 to 60 minutes according to the facility's policy or after a change in BFR, DFR, ACD-A, or calcium infusion rate until the patient and system-ionized calcium are in the prescribed range. Monitoring continues every 2 to 6 hours and whenever there is a concern that the patient is becoming hypocalcemic based on the following signs and symptoms.

a. Circumoral tingling.

b. Muscle cramps.

c. Tetany.

d. Seizures.

e. Positive Chvostek or Trousseau sign.

f. Prolonged QT interval.

g. Decreased heart rate.

h. Cardiac arrhythmias.

i. Hypotension related to vasodilatation.

4. Most blood gas or STAT labs will provide an ionized calcium result in 15 to 30 minutes. The quick ionized calcium results aid in titrating the citrate and calcium solutions to maintain these levels in effective ranges.

5. The patient on regional citrate anticoagulation can develop alkalosis as citrate from the citrate/calcium complexes returned to the patient are metabolized to bicarbonate.

a. The dialysis solution bicarbonate should be lowered to physiologic concentrations and the flow rate increased to correct this state.

b. Look for other sources of bicarbonate that might explain changes, such as medications, TPN, and tube feeding formulations.

6. The composition of the dialysis solution or the replacement solution may need to be adjusted by reducing the sodium and bicarbonate content since citrate (delivered as tri-sodium citrate or citrate) is metabolized in the liver to bicarbonate.

7. The patient should be monitored for hypernatremia and metabolic alkalosis.

C. Monitoring the patient for phosphorus.

1. During KRT with higher clearance rates, phosphorus may become low. If this occurs, phosphorus needs to be replaced and/or treatment parameters evaluated to minimize removal of phosphorus from the patient.

a. Mild hypophosphatemia can be treated with oral supplements.

b. If the hypophosphatemia is severe and the patient is symptomatic, phosphorous should be replaced via IV administration.

c. Some units report adding oral Fleet® Phospho-soda solution to the dialysis solution in the bicarbonate concentrate to raise the phosphorus in the dialysis solution to 2.5 mg/dL (low physiologic).

d. In some cases, it may be added to replacement solutions.

2. Symptoms of hypophosphatemia include:
   a. Muscle weakness, including respiratory muscles, which might inhibit the ability to wean the patient from mechanical ventilation.
   b. Rhabdomyolysis.
   c. Paresthesias.
   d. Hemolysis.
   e. Platelet dysfunction.
   f. Cardiac failure.

D. Monitoring levels for magnesium.
   1. Magnesium is another element that may need to be replaced during CRRT.
   2. Repletion is done by IV infusion with the dose being dependent on the blood level.
   3. Symptoms of hypomagnesemia.
      a. Confusion.
      b. Irritability.
      c. Seizures.
      d. Muscle weakness.
      e. Lethargy.
      f. Arrhythmias.

XII. Effectiveness of CRRT – measuring the dose of dialysis.

A. The Acute Dialysis Quality Initiative Work Group in 2001 (http://www.adqi.org) recommended that delivered clearance should be monitored during all kidney replacement therapies (Ricci et al., 2006).

B. "Dosage" of CRRT is a measure of the quantity of blood that is purified of waste products and toxins using some means of blood purification to deliver that clearance.

C. Early studies supported the use of a calculated value of > 35 mL/kg/hr with the assumption that clearance is equal to the total effluent volume if there is no predilution (Luyckx & Bonventre, 2004; Ricci & Ronco, 2008).
   1. Predilution will reduce the effective effluent dose depending on the blood flow rate, the replacement solution rate, and the patient's hematocrit (Prowle et al., 2011).
   2. An adjustment in the prescribed dose needs to be made when using predilution to preserve outcomes.

D. The delivered dose is often significantly lower than the prescribed dose, so it is recommended that the prescribed effluent volume be increased by 25% to account for these changes (Macedo et al., 2012). Reasons for this discrepancy include:
   1. Interruptions of therapy for other procedures.
   2. Gradual clotting of the system leading to decreased surface area.

3. Anticoagulation being inhibited due to patient conditions.
   a. Type of anticoagulation being used.
   b. Sieving properties of the membrane.

E. Two major multicenter randomized controlled trials have been conducted, changing the current view of effective clearance.
   1. The Veterans Affairs/National Institutes of Health Acute Renal Failure Trial Network (ATN).
   2. The Randomized Evaluation of Normal vs. Augmented Level (RENAL) Replacement Therapy Study.
   3. These studies have provided evidence that there is no added benefit in terms of outcomes from effluent flow rates above 25 mL/kg/hr.
   4. These studies also provided evidence that doses of less than 20 mL/kg per hour may be harmful and therefore should be avoided.
   5. The prescribed dose was found to be typically 10% to 15% less than the delivered dose. This was described as most likely being due to treatment downtime and should be considered by the prescribing providers (Prowle et al., 2011).

F. The Kidney Disease Improving Global Guideline (KDIGO) group has published their evidence-based *Clinical Practice Guidelines for Acute Kidney Injury*.
   1. Recommendations in the guidelines are graded, with level 1 being a strong recommendation and level 2 being a suggestion or discretionary.
   2. Recommendations are further graded from A to D, with A representing a high quality of evidence and grade D as a very low evidence base (Khwaja, 2012).
   3. See Table 7.5 for a partial summary of recommendations relative to treatment of acute kidney injury (KDIGO, 2012).

G. It is important to include the CRRT program in the facility/unit's QAPI process. There are many targets that can be monitored related to these modalities. For example:
   1. Filter life.
   2. Prescribed vs. delivered dose.
   3. Hours of therapy.
   4. Interruptions of therapy and cause.
   5. Anticoagulation used and its effectiveness.
   6. Diagnoses being treated.
   7. Duration of therapy.
   8. Patient survival.
   9. Recovery of kidney function.
   10. Demographics of patient population.

XIII. Nutrition for patient on SLEDD/CRRT.

A. Inadequate nutrition increases morbidity and mortality.

B. These therapies enable full fluid volume and solute control even with TPN or tube feedings.

C. Minimize negative nitrogen balance in ICU patients.

D. Decrease the time the patient goes without feeding during the ICU stay.

E. Refer to Chapter 2 of this module for information on Nutrition in AKI.

XIV. Program selection and development for KRT in various ICU environments (Craig et al., 1996).

A. Program interest and viability. Determine the hospital's need for and ability to support a KRT program.

B. Patient population.
1. The ICU must have a sufficient number of patients with AKI requiring dialytic therapy.
2. The number of patient cases required to build a KRT program is based on the number of nurses that need to gain and maintain expertise on the therapy.
3. The more centralized these patient cases are (one ICU vs. multiple ICUs), the fewer bedside nurses need to be trained to provide the care of the patient on KRT. Because of the additional exposure with more frequent treatments, the bedside nurse will likely maintain expertise with minimal assistance from other experts, such as the nephrology nurses.
4. To maintain nursing expertise, the potential AKI cases in the ICU requiring kidney replacement therapy should be greater than 12 cases per year with an average of 5 to 7 days of CRRT therapy prescribed.

Table 7.5

Summary of KDIGO Clinical Practice Guidelines for AKI

5.1.1:	**Initiation of RRT:** When life-threatening changes in fluid, electrolyte and acid-base balance exist.	**Not Graded**
5.1.2:	Consider the broader clinical context, the presence of conditions that can be modified with KRT, and the trends of laboratory tests when making the decision to start KRT.	**Not Graded**
5.6.2:	**Type of KRT:** We suggest using CRRT, rather than standard intermittent KRT, for hemodynamically unstable patients	**2 B**
5.6.3:	We suggest using CRRT, rather than intermittent KRT, for AKI patients with acute brain injury or other causes of increased intracranial pressure or generalized brain edema.	**2 B**
5.4.1:	**Vascular Access:** We suggest initiating KRT in patients with AKI via an uncuffed, nontunneled dialysis catheter, rather than a tunneled catheter.	**2D**
5.4.2:	When choosing a vein for insertion of a dialysis catheter in patients with AKI, consider these preferences: First choice: RIJ, 2nd choice: femoral vein, 3rd choice: LIJ, last choice: subclavian vein with preference for the dominant side.	**Not Graded**
5.4.3:	We suggest using ultrasound guidance for dialysis catheter insertion.	**1 A**
5.4.4:	We recommend obtaining a chest radiograph promptly after placement and before first use of an IJ or SC dialysis catheter.	**1 B**
5.4.5:	We suggest not using topical antibiotics over the skin insertion site of a nontunneled dialysis catheter in ICU patients with AKI.	**2 C**
5.3.2.1:	**Anticoagulation:** For CRRT we suggest using regional citrate anticoagulation rather than heparin in patients who do not have contraindications to citrate.	**2 B**
5.3.2.3:	For patients who have contraindications for citrate, we suggest using either unfractionated or low-molecular weight heparin rather than other anticoagulants.	**2 C**
5.3.3.1:	We suggest using regional citrate anticoagulation, rather than no anticoagulation, during CRRT in a patient without contraindications for citrate.	**3 C**
5.3.3.2:	We suggest avoiding regional heparinization during CRRT in a patient with increased risk of bleeding.	**2 C**
5.8.1:	**Dose:** We recommend frequent assessment of the actual delivered dose in order to adjust the prescription.	**1 B**
5.8.4:	We recommend delivering an effluent volume of 20–25 mL/kg/hr for CRRT in AKI.	**1 A**
	This will usually require a higher prescription of effluent volume.	**Not Graded**
5.2.1:	**Discontinuation of therapy:** Discontinue RRT when it is no longer required, either because intrinsic kidney function has recovered to the point that it is adequate to meet patient needs, or because KRT is no longer consistent with the goals of care.	**Not Graded**

Source: KDIGO. Retrieved from http://kdigo.org/home/guidelines/acute-kidney-injury

5. The scenario of having a few AKI cases spread over many ICUs, perhaps even in different hospitals, increases the benefit of using the model of training the nephrology nurses as experts to support the ICU nurses with bedside in-services at the beginning of every ICU nursing shift. This minimizes the training effort while maximizing the benefit of having information at the time of implementation.

6. The pediatric patient population has great variability in patient size and treatment orders with more stringent monitoring requirements of hourly and cumulative fluid balance. An integrated fluid management system is essential to accurate fluid handling.

7. Burn patients may have large volumes of insensible fluid losses, requiring low to no ultrafiltration rates. Burn patients may have large dressing changes occurring over long time periods and possibly in a water tank. Consider nighttime SLEDD for more patient free time for these other essential interventions.

8. Choose a therapy that will effectively accomplish the goal of fluid removal and/or solute clearance for the identified patient population.

9. Choose a therapy that is relatively simple to learn for the healthcare providers that will be involved in its implementation.
   a. Keep It Super Simple (KISS) principle: The reality of patient care is that it is frequently fraught with complexities. Some of them are innate and others self-imposed, based on the knowledge of the importance of patient care outcomes.
   b. CRRT and SLEDD are no exception and although they are relatively complex, the KISS principle is a great reminder to not make it more complex than it must be (Craig, 1998b).
   c. Developing a SLEDD/CRRT workgroup with the KISS principle focus can move a program forward by addressing concerns, solving problems, and creating innovative solutions all in the spirit of simplicity like that intended by the original guru of CRRT, Peter Kramer.

C. Financial viability.
   1. Expenses.
      a. Equipment and supplies.
         (1) Some equipment and supplies are relatively inexpensive.
         (2) However, the cost of training to safely use that system may overwhelm that cost savings.
         (3) Equipment should be chosen that will safely deliver the desired therapy with minimal training effort.
      b. Training.
         (1) The largest KRT program expense will be the cost of training staff to establish and maintain competency.
         (2) A simpler KRT program will result in fewer training requirements and fewer dollars spent meeting those requirements.
         (3) Smaller hospitals may contract services from providers that own the equipment, generally service the equipment, and oversee the education of dialysis and ICU staff.
         (4) In the larger hospital setting, consider working collaboratively with the ICU's CNS/APRN, nurse manager and/or renal coordinator to establish an education program of the dialysis and critical care staff.
   2. Revenues are based on reimbursement for anticipated number of treatments.
   3. The daily cost of providing KRT and SLEDD is dependent on several factors (e.g., staffing, equipment, and supplies).

D. Program coordinator.
   1. The coordinator can be a CNS/APRN or other resource nurse, preferably with experience in both the nephrology and ICU environment.
   2. The program can be led by either a nephrology or ICU discipline, but a collaborative practice should be sought as the program is implemented.
   3. Develop expertise in the therapy of choice based on facility's needs and resources.
      a. Attend conferences, review the literature, and visit other working programs.
      b. The program must be designed to complement the existing patient population and the nursing, medical, and administrative resources.
   4. Evaluate and purchase equipment to best perform the therapy chosen.
   5. Develop documentation to support the delivery of KRT in the current facility.
   6. Establish and implement the training program as outlined in the education section above.
   7. Chair the CRRT/SLEDD workgroup.

E. KRT workgroup (see Figure 7.12).
   1. Determine the role each stakeholder will play.
   2. Hospital and/or dialysis unit (for contracted dialysis services) administration.
      a. Focus on financial viability, program liability, and ability and expense to train and maintain nursing resources.
      b. Determine who owns and maintains the SLEDD/CRRT equipment.
   3. Intensivists: Identify ICU patients with potential

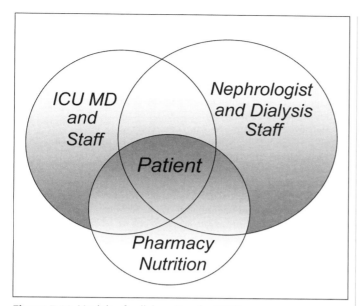

Figure 7.12. Models of collaboration for CRRT.

Courtesy of Maureen Craig, UC Davis Medical Center, Sacramento, California.

kidney replacement needs and consult nephrology.

4. Nephrologists (may be an APRN/PA).
   a. Develop CRRT and/or SLEDD order sets.
   b. Assess ICU patients requiring dialytic therapy for appropriateness of CRRT or SLEDD before considering IHD.
   c. Provide daily treatment orders reflecting assessment of the patient's changing condition and response to treatment.
5. Nephrology nurses.
   a. Develop outcome and patient care standards for patients on intermittent and continuous therapies.
   b. Provide training for nephrology and ICU nurses relevant to caring for patients on SLEDD and CRRT.
   c. Provide ICU nurse bedside in-service and treatment support during CRRT and/or SLEDD as outlined in the patient care standards.
6. ICU nurses.
   a. Receive training on providing SLEDD and CRRT as outlined in the patient care standards.
   b. Provide the appropriate therapy to the ICU patient with kidney replacement therapy needs.
7. Nursing unit managers: orchestrate getting adequate numbers of staff trained and then maintaining care providers' competency.
8. Pharmacists.
   a. Provide customized or stock anticoagulant, replacement, and/or dialysis solutions and information to support the use of each of these

solutions in CRRT or SLEDD, based on the type of modality and therapy, filter membrane, and equipment in use.
   b. Perform therapeutic drug monitoring of patient serum levels as indicated on patients receiving SLEDD and/or CRRT.
9. Dietitians or nutritionists.
   a. Provide guidance to the team on levels and types of nutrition that are available and effective for the KRT patient population.
   b. Monitor nitrogen balance, electrolyte changes, and fluid status. Suggest therapy adjustments when appropriate.
10. Pediatric ICU healthcare providers.
   a. Customize the existing adult KRT program to meet pediatric needs.
   b. Develop a new KRT program based on the existing pediatric patient population using the literature and other pediatric centers offering SLEDD and/or CRRT as resources.

F. Initiate the first treatment within 1 to 2 months of training the nursing staff.

G. Patient selection.
   1. The first few patients chosen for treatment may be those whose outcome is guarded at best.
   2. The goal should be to apply the KRT treatments to all patients in the intended population as soon as possible so care providers do not associate CRRT and SLEDD with only poor outcomes.

H. Follow the first several KRT cases with a debriefing and evaluation session chaired by the program coordinator and attended by all interested parties in the KRT workgroup.
   1. Continue to gather and evaluate ideas that evolve to improve the KRT program.
   2. Make program changes judiciously and disseminate the changes to all involved parties.
   3. Follow patient outcomes to evaluate various aspects of the program including:
      a. Patient selection.
      b. Patient outcomes based on diagnosis.
      c. Patient survival statistics including preservation of kidney function.
      d. Staff satisfaction including comfort level of providing this intense therapy.
      e. Staffing needs.
      f. Fiscal accountability of the program (Kellum et al., 2010).

References

Abra, G. (2010). *Disequilibrium syndrome.* Retrieved from http://renalfellow.blogspot.com/2010/10/disequilibrium-syndrome.html

Ahmad, S., & Tu, A. (2007). Heparin free slow low efficiency dialysis (SLED) using citrate dialysate (CD) is safe and effective. *Blood Purification 25*, 183-208.

Anderson, J.A.M., & Saenko, S.L. (2002). Heparin resistance. *British Journal of Anaesthesia, 88*(4), 467-469.

Baldwin, I., & Fealy, N.(2009). Clinical nursing for the application of continuous renal replacement therapy in the intensive care unit. *Seminars in Dialysis, 22*(2), 189-193.

Barenbrock,. M., Hausberg, M., Matzkies, F., de la Motte, S., & Schaefer, R.M. (2000). Effects of bicarbonate- and lactate-buffered replacement fluids on cardiovascular outcome in CVVH patients. *Kidney International, 58*, 1751-1757.

Bouchard, J.S., Soroko, S.B., Chertow, G.M., Himmelfarb, J., Ikizler, T.A., Paganini, E.P., ... Program to Improve Care in Acute Renal Disease (PICARD) Study Group. (2009). Fluid accumulation, survival and recovery of kidney function in critically ill patients with acute kidney injury. *Kidney International, 76*(4), 422-427.

Craig, M. (1998a). Applications in continuous venous to venous hemofiltration. Interactive case studies in the adult patient. *Critical Care Nursing Clinics of North America, 10*(2), 209-221.

Craig, M. (1998b). Continuous venous to venous hemofiltration: implementing and maintaining a program: Examples and alternatives. *Critical Care Nursing Clinics of North America, 10*(2), 219-233.

Craig, M.A., Depner, T.A., Chin, E., Tweedy, R.L., Hokana, L., & Newby-Lintz, M. (1996). Implementing a continuous renal replacement therapies program. *Advances in Renal Replacement Therapy, 3*(4), 348-350.

Cruz, D., Bobek, I., Lentini, P., Soni, S., Chionh, C., & Ronco, C. (2009). Machines for continuous renal replacement therapy. *Seminars in Dialysis, 22*(2) 123-132.

Culley, C.M., Bernardo, J.F., Gross, P.R., Guttendork, S., Whiteman, K.A., Kowiatek, J.G., & Skledar, S.D. (2006). Implementing a standardized safety procedure for continuous renal replacement therapy solutions. *American Journal of Health-System Pharmacy, 63*(8), 756-763.

Karkar, A. (2013). *Advances in hemodialysis techniques.* Retrieved from http://creativecommons.org/licenses/by/3.0

Kellum, J.A., Bellomo, R., & Ronco, C. (2010). *Continuous renal replacement therapy.* New York: Oxford University Press.

Khwaja, A. (2012). KDIGO clinical practice guidelines for acute kidney injury. *Nephron Clinical Practice, 120*(4), 179-184.

Kidney Disease: Improving Global Outcomes (KDIGO). (2012). *KDIGO Clinical practice guideline for acute kidney injury.* Retrieved from http://kdigo.org/home/guidelines/acute-kidney-injury

Lameire, N., VanBiesen, W., & Vanholder, R. (2005). Acute renal failure. *The Lancet, 365*(9457), 417-430.

Luyckx, V.A., & Bonventre, J.V. (2004). Dose of dialysis in acute renal failure. *Seminars in Dialysis, 17*(1), 30-36.

Macedo, E., Claure-Del Granado, R., & Mehta, R. (2012). Effluent volume and dialysis dose in CRRT: Time for reappraisal. *Nature Reviews Nephrology, 8*, 57-60.

Mehta, R.L. (2005). Continuous renal replacement therapy in the critically ill patient. *Kidney International, 67*, 781-795. doi:10.1111/j.1523-1755.2005.67140.x

NKF-K/DOQI. (2001). Clinical practice guidelines for vascular access: Update 2000. *American Journal of Kidney Diseases, 37*(Suppl. 1), S137-S181.

Oudemans-van Straaten, H.M., Kellum, J.A., & Bellomo, R. (2011). Clinical review: Anticoagulation for continuous renal replacement therapy – Heparin or citrate? *Critical Care, 15*(202). doi:10.1186/cc9358 Retrieved from http://ccforum.com/content/15/1/202

Prowle, J.R., Schneider, A., & Bellomo, R. (2011). Clinical review: Optimal dose of continuous renal replacement therapy in acute kidney injury. *Critical Care, 15*(207). doi:10.1186/cc9415 Retrieved from http://ccforum.com/content/15/2/207

Ricci., Z., Bellomo, R., & Ronco, C. (2006). Dose of dialysis in acute renal failure. *Clinical Journal of the American Society of Nephrology, 1*(3), 380-388. doi:10.2215/CJN.00520705

Ricci, Z. & Ronco, C. (2008). Dose and efficiency of renal replacement therapy: Continuous renal replacement therapy versus intermittent hemodialysis versus slow extended daily dialysis. *Critical Care Medicine, 36*(Suppl. 4), S229-S237. doi:10.1097/CCM.0b013e318168e467

Santoro, A., & Guadagni, G. (2010). Dialysis membrane: From convection to adsorption. *NDT Plus, 3*(Suppl. 1), i36-i39. doi:10.1093/ndtplus/sfq035

Sutter, M.E., Clarke, M.E., Cobb, J., Daubert, G.P., Aston, L.S., Poppenga, R.H., ... Albertson, T.E. (2012). Blood leak alarm interference by hydoxocobalamin is hemodialysis machine dependent. *Clinical Toxicology, 50*(10), 892-895.

Tolwani, A. (2012). Continuous renal-replacement therapy for acute kidney injury. *The New England Journal of Medicine, 367*(26), 2505-2514.

Vijayan, A. (2009). Vascular access for continuous renal replacement therapy. *Seminars in Dialysis, 22*(2), 133-136.

Weijmer, M.C., Vervloet, M.G. & ter Wee, P.M. (2004). Compared to tunnelled cuffed haemodialysis catheters, temporary untunnelled catheters are associated with more complicaions already within 2 weeks of use. *Nephrology Dialysis Transplantation, 19*, 670-677.

Appendix 7.1. Pediatric hemodialysis specification sheet

Courtesy of Lavjay Butani, Pediatric Nephrology, UC Davis Medical Center, Sacramento, California. Used with permission.

Pediatric Hemodialysis Specification Sheet

-Volutrol on all IV's
-Crying may increase patient blood pressure even though patient is volume depleted

Dialyzer	Prime (ml)	Surface Area (m²)
F3	28	0.4
F4	42	0.7
F5	63	1.0
F6	82	1.3
Polyflux 140 (high-flux)	94	1.4
F8	110	1.8

Blood Tubing	Prime (ml)	Pump Segment Diameter Set blood pump to coincide
Neonate (no arterial chamber)*	19 ml	2.6 mm
Husky Neonate (no arterial chamber)*	44 ml	4.8 mm
Pediatric	73 ml	6.35 mm
Adult	140 ml	8.0 mm

* When no arterial chamber is present, Arterial Pressure (AP) monitoring should be accomplished by using two 24" pressure-tubing lines. The first one is filled with normal saline and attached to a 3-way stopcock on the saline line of the blood tubing. The second pressure tubing line is filled with air and connects the first pressure tubing line to a transducer protector and then to the Arterial Pressure port on the Fresenius 2008K Hemodialysis System.

Suggested combinations based on Patient weight	Dialyzer	Tubing
Less than 13 kg	100 HG / F3	Neonate/Husky neonate
13kg-20 kg	F4 / F5	Husky neonate
20-40 kg	F6/Polyflux 140	Husky/Pediatric
Greater than 40 kg	F8/Polyflux 140	Pediatric/Adult

Blood Prime: Consider if the combined dialyzer / blood tubing volume is greater than **15%-20%** of the patient's total blood volume (TBV), i.e., patients less than 3 kg.

Estimate TBV using patient's weight.
Infant (0-1 year)   TBV = Weight x 80 ml/kg,
Child (1-12 years)   TBV = Weight x 75 ml/kg,
Adolescent (greater than 12 years)   TBV = Weight x 70 ml/kg.

Complete the Physician's Blood Order Form: 1. Select one Mini-Neonate type unit for anticipated blood loss. **2.**Select irradiated and CMV negative blood for infants less than 6mos. **3.**Indicate if patient is a transplant candidate and request *"Limited Donor Protocol"* blood in comments section for pediatric patients.

1. Fax both sides of this order form to Blood Bank at 734-8636
2. Prime the blood tubing circuit with normal saline.
3. Calculate $V_{saline} = \dfrac{V_{PRBC} (HCT_{PRBC} - HCT_{Infant})}{HCT_{Infant}} = $ _____**ml saline**

   Where V_{PRBC} is volume printed on PRBC unit and $HCT_{PRBC} = 74\%$.
4. Obtain "Leukoreduced" labeled "Limited Donor Protocol" Mini-PRBC from blood bank.
5. Mix Mini-PRBC with V_{saline} using a 150 ml volutrol.
6. Prime the blood tubing at BFR of 20ml/min from the volutrol of PRBC and saline mix.
7. Recirculate the blood primed circuit for two minutes with a dialysis bath that contains 2.5 mEq/L Calcium.
8. Change dialysate bath to ordered solution and perform standard connection to the patient.

Nephrologist Signature / Print Name:	Date/Time:
Nephrology Nurse Signature / Print Name:	Date/Time:

Appendix 7.2. CRRT bedside inservice checklist
Designed for use with the Prisma.

Courtesy of Dr. G. Corrigan, Western Nephrology Acute Dialysis, Denver, Colorado. Used with permission.

Date:_____   Patient Name:_____

List Modality on screen:_____ and modality prescribed for pt._____

Solute transport mechanism: Diffusion_____   Convection_____

Setting Flow Rates & Patient Removal rate:_____

Type of Dialysate:

PrismaSate:	**Type B:**	**Type C Citrate:**
Frangible broken	Calcium infusion Y / N	No Calcium in Dialysate or Replacement
Expiration Date & Time	Bicarb Sources	Low Na Dialysate
		Bicarb Sources

Dual Check of Solutions Documented on MAR: Y / N

Impact of Solutions on pt:

K_____   Ca_____   ICa_____   Post Filter ICa_____

pH_____   CO2_____   PO4_____   Mg_____

Table of Critical Lab Values & when to call the Nephrologist @ bedside: Y / N

Where & How to draw Post Filter Ionized Ca:_____No other labs drawn from system:_____

How to hang 2 1L bags of replacement solution & use of blue line clamps when Δ bags:_____

What to do if you run out of replacement or dialysate solutions:_____
Anticoagulaton:
Systemic Anticoagulation: Heparin_____   NS Flush_____

Regional Anticoagulation Citrate & How it works:_____ & Why we need Calcium:_____

I&O Sheet reviewed:

Citrate & Calcium included:_____   Finding Actual Fluid Removed on Tx History Screen:_____

Calculations reviewed:_____

Incorrect Weight Change Alarm and Alarm screen reviewed:_____

Effluent Bags: Date & Time: Y / N Δ q24hrs   Keep connections clean and capped _____

Catheter Issues: Are lines reversed Y / N Type of catheter: Temporary   Tunneled

How to reposition temporary catheters:_____   Site care of HD Catheters:_____

Machine & Emergency Procedures:
Emergency Rinseback:_____ NS for blood return with free flow IV tubing:_____

Blue line Clamps in room (2):_____ Diaphragm reposition procedure card on machine: Y / N

Prisma Status Lights Illuminated: Red_____   Yellow_____ Green_____

How to contact MD & Dialysis staff: _____   Gambro Help line # posted on machine:_____

_____   _____
Western Dialysis Staff Signature   Hospital Staff Signature

Appendix 7.3. CRRT bedside inservice checklist
Designed for use with the Fresenius 2008K.

Courtesy of Maureen Craig, UC Davis Medical Center, Sacramento, CA. Used with permission.

CRRT with Regional Citrate Bedside Inservice Checklist
(Given at the beginning of each shift when a patient is on CRRT)

Date:

The ICU RN should verbalize:	Neph RN	ICU RN
Reason for treatment, how CRRT works - fluid/solute balance, nutrition and medication changes		
Where the blood, fluid, and dialysate pathways are. Adult prime volume is ≈ 250 ml saline. See Pediatric Hemodialysis Specification Sheet for prime volume and pump segment diameter. Set CRRT machine to match		
How the R.O. works - purifies water		
How to respond to patient hypotension		
When and how to terminate CRRT and care for the catheter and access site (see CRRT Termination diagram)		
How to interpret patient and system ionized Calciums and adjust ACD-A and Calcium IV rates (see Regional Citrate diagram). When stopping ACD-A or Calcium drips, a new order set must be written.		
How to assess symptoms of hypocalcemia (seizures, Chvostek's sign, hypotention, prolonged Q-T interval) and hypercalcemia (lethargy, H/A, N/V) and associated changes in treatment		
When and how to contact the Nephrologist (clotted system or prescription changes) or Nephrology Nurse (equipment and documentation)		
How and why to trouble shoot equipment alarms (if not resolved or concerns exist, call Nephrology Nurse)		

Fresenius Alarm	Action - Slow response to alarms may lead to the blood circuit clotting	Neph RN	ICU RN
AP/VP	check lines for kinks, change transducer if wet, notify Neph MD if unable to achieve BFR		
Low TMP	increase rate and compensate with maintenance fluids, change transducer if wet		
Conductivity	Check wand connections, if concentrate jugs are empty, call Nephrology Nurse for refill. Concentrate jugs should be filled and tightly capped every 12-14 hours.		
Blood pump	check blood pump door is latched		
Air detector	raise venous chamber level with ^ arrow to 1cm of top, check lines below venous chamber are free of air, reset, replace transducer protector prn, check all blood line connections are tight		
No Water	check water tap is on (no hot water), hose connections are tight, RO plugged in and on, water pre filter "IN" pressure is at 20 PSI or more		
Blood leak	Hemastick dialysate, if + stop treatment without blood return, if - reset alarm		
Power failure	plug machine into red plate, turn machine on, select CRRT mode, confirm dialysate screen, select "Home" screen, touch "Tx Paused" button to turn it to "Tx Running" and confirm		
RO TDS	set TDS (Total Dissolved Solids) limit to 10 mg/L		

The ICU RN should demonstrate:	Neph RN	ICU RN
How to verify dialysate. How to verify and adjust ACD-A and Calcium solutions and rates. Zero Calcium dialyzing fluid must be used in tandem with ACD-A and IV Calcium solutions.		
How to draw/process patient and system ionized Calcium labs PRN (see Regional Citrate diagram).		
How to determine and set UF Rate (calculate Calcium and ACD-A fluid input into UF Rate). Nephrology Nurse will set up the Calcium and the ACD-A IV's on an IV pump on top of the Fresenius 2008K.		
How to reset "UF Removed" every hour for Pediatric treatments and every shift for Adult treatments.		
When and how to adjust BFR e.g. lab draws, frequent negative AP alarms (BFR should be > 20 ml/min) (If unable to achieve the prescribed BFR, notify the Nephrologist).		
How to assess clotting in the system		
How and when to adjust arterial and venous chamber levels		
How to complete ICU documentation (BFR, ACD-A, and Calcium rate, I/O's and system pressures). For Pediatric treatments refer to the "EMR Documentation Sheet."		

Inservice Provided by:_____   Inservice Received by:_____
                                   Signature/Print Name   Signature/Print Name

Craig, 1/30/2008

Appendix 7.4. SLEDD bedside inservice checklist
Designed for use with the Fresenius 2008K.

Courtesy of Maureen Craig, UC Davis Medical Center, Sacramento, CA. Used with permission.

Slow Extended Daily Dialysis (SLEDD) Bedside Inservice Checklist
(Given at the beginning of each treatment, when a patient is on SLEDD)

Date/Time:

The ICU RN should verbalize:	Neph RN	ICU RN
Reason for treatment, how SLEDD works - fluid/solute balance, medication adjustments		
Where the blood, fluid, and dialysate pathways are		
How to respond to patient hypotension - Stop UF, titrate vasopressors, give ordered fluids		
How to interpret Ionized Calcium and adjust ACD-A and calcium gluconate IV rate when on ACD-A anticoagulation. Follow ordered titration of drips.		
How to assess hypocalcemia (Chvostek's sign) and associated changes in treatment (increase IV calcium gluconate per orders) when on regional citrate anticoagulation		
When and how to contact the Nephrology Nurse		
How and why to trouble shoot equipment alarms (if not resolved, call Nephrology Nurse)		
Alarm Action - Slow response to alarms may lead to the blood circuit clotting	**Neph RN**	**ICU RN**
AP/VP check lines for kinks, when open press Areset@, change transducer if wet, notify Nephrology Nurse if unable to achieve BFR		
Other contact Nephrology Nurse		
The ICU RN should demonstrate:	**Neph RN**	**ICU RN**
How to assist in drawing and processing Ionized Calcium labs when on ACD-A anticoagulation		
How to assess for system clotting and procedure to return patient=s blood with a saline flush		

Inservice Provided by:_____   Inservice Received by:_____

Nephrology RN   ICU RN

Appendix 7.5. SLEDD/CRRT orders with regional citrate anticoagulation
Designed for use with the Fresenius 2008K.

Courtesy of Maureen Craig, UC Davis Medical Center, Sacramento, CA. Used with permission.

UNIVERSITY OF CALIFORNIA, DAVIS
MEDICAL CENTER
SACRAMENTO, CALIFORNIA

PHYSICIAN'S ORDERS

SLOW EXTENDED DAILY DIALYSIS (SLEDD) OR CONTINUOUS HEMODIALYSIS (CHD) ORDERS
WITH REGIONAL CITRATE ANTICOAGULATION

Date: _____ For Date: _____

Time: _____

Directions: Check (√) and complete those orders to be implemented (order renewal daily before noon).

For assistance, Monday – Friday 0700-1930 call x48730, other hours call operator for on-call nurse.

1. ☐ Priority: ☐ 1 ☐ 2 Dialysis type: ☐ SLEDD _____ (8) hours ☐ CHD (24 hours/day)

2. ☐ Monitor EKG (required)

3. ☐ Weigh daily at 0500 (CHD)

4. ☐ Ultrafiltration volume: _____ liters (SLEDD) Ultrafiltration Rate = Total patient input +/-_____ ml/hour(CHD)
   ☐ (Optional) Ultrafiltration Profile (linear-continuously-decreasing) (SLEDD) ⟍

5. ☐ Dialyzer: _____

6. ☐ Blood Flow Rate _____ (100-200) mL/min. Vascular Access: _____

7. ☐ Dialysate Flow Rate _____ (SLEDD 300 or CHD 200)ml/min.
   ☐ Dialysis solution temperature _____ (35-36)°C
   ☐ Dialysate: K+ _____ (0-4) mEq/L Na+ _____ (135) mEq/L Phos _____ (0-3) mg/dL
   Ca++ _____ (0) mEq/L HCO3 _____ (25-30) mEq/L

8. ☐ Support systolic blood pressure less than _____ mm Hg with 0.9% NaCl or _____ PRN. (SLEDD)

9. ☐ Call Nephrology if fluid bolus greater than 250mL/shift is given for BP support or if MAP falls below 60mmHg. (CHD)

10. ☐ (Optional) Replacement Fluid: Normal Saline(NS) _____ (1000-2000)mL/hour

11. ☐ (Optional) Replace patient Output (urine, stool, drains) mL for mL with normal saline.

Medications

12. ☐ Anticoagulant Citrate Dextrose (ACD-A) through dialyzer inflow (arterial) line _____ (150-250) mL/hour

13. ☐ Adjust ACD-A to maintain ionized calcium in the **extracorporeal outflow (venous)** blood at 0.35-0.50 mMol/L.

If **extracorporeal outflow** ionized calcium is:	Adjust ACD-A:
Less than 0.35	decrease by 25 mL/hour
0.35-0.50	no change
Greater than 0.50	increase by 25 mL/hour

14. ☐ Calcium gluconate 40mg/mL (20grams in 500 mL NS) at _____ (60-180) mL/hour in a patient IV line or in venous return line.

15. ☐ Adjust calcium gluconate to maintain **Patient** ionized calcium of 1.11 – 1.31 mMol/L

If **Patient** ionized calcium is:	Adjust calcium gluconate:
Less than 1.01	increase by 20 mL/hour, see order #19, and call Nephrologist
1.01-1.10	increase by 20 mL/hour
1.11-1.31	no change
Greater than 1.31	decrease by 20 mL/hour

16. ☐ Give calcium gluconate 1g in 50mL NS over 15mins for symptoms of hypocalcemia or for patient ionized calcium below 1.01 mMol/L.

Laboratory:

17. ☐ Draw pre treatment patient ionized calcium.
   ☐ Draw ionized calciums from both system and patient 60 minutes after start and 60 minutes after prescribed BFR, DFR, ACD-A, or calcium gluconate infusion rate change, then every 2-3 hours for SLEDD or every 4-6 hours for CHD when rates are stable.
   ☐ Draw ionized calciums if patient is symptomatic of hypo or hyper-calcemia.
   ☐ Draw patient ionized calcium 20 minutes after discontinuing treatment.

18. ☐ CMP, ☐ CBC, ☐ Pre BUN, ☐ Post BUN, ☐ Hepatitis B surface Antigen, ☐ Hepatitis C Antibody

Treatment Termination:

19. ☐ Return blood with a _____ (250)mL normal saline flush.
   ☐ Do not return blood.

20. Pulsatile flush to each limb of catheter with 10 mL (adult) or 5 mL (pediatric) normal saline. Fill Arterial and Venous lumen of dialysis catheter (volume printed on catheter A _____ mL, V _____ mL) with:
   ☐ Heparin 5000 units/mL (adult standard).
   ☐ Heparin 1000 units/mL (pediatric standard).
   ☐ ACD-A from pharmacy.

Nephrologist (Signature/Print Name): _____ P.I.: _____ Pager: _____

Nephrology Nurse (Signature/Print Name): _____ Date/Time: _____

ICU Nurse (Signature/Print Name): _____ Date/Time: _____

AC6504 (9/07) **SLEDD OR CHD WITH REGIONAL CITRATE ANTICOAGULATION** MR#10/071142

Appendix 7.6. CRRT orders with heparin or no anticoagulation
Designed for use with the Fresenius 2008K.

Courtesy of Maureen Craig, UC Davis Medical Center, Sacramento, CA. Used with permission.

UNIVERSITY OF CALIFORNIA, DAVIS
MEDICAL CENTER
SACRAMENTO, CALIFORNIA

PHYSICIAN'S ORDERS

CONTINUOUS RENAL REPLACEMENT THERAPY ORDERS
WITH HEPARIN ANTICOAGULATION

Directions: Check (√) and complete orders to be implemented (order renewal daily before noon).	
For assistance, Monday – Friday 0700-1930 call x48730, other hours call operator for on-call nurse.	
Date:	For, Date:
Time:	

1. ☐ Weigh daily at 0500
2. ☐ Blood Flow Rate (BFR) _____ (100-200) mL/minute.
3. ☐ Hemofilter _____
4. ☐ Ultrafiltration Rate = Total patient input +/-_____mL/hour
5. ☐ Dialysate Flow Rate_____ (100-300) mL/minute.
   ☐ Dialysis solution temperature_____ (35-36)°C
6. ☐ Dialysate: K^+_____(3-4) mEq/L Na^+ _____ (140) mEq/L   Phos_____(2-3) mg/dL
   Ca^{++}_____(2.5) mEq/L HCO_3_____(30) mEq/L
7. ☐ Call Nephrology if fluid bolus greater than 250mL/shift is ordered for blood pressure support or if MAP is less than 60mmHg.
8. ☐ (Optional) Replacement Fluid: Normal Saline (NS)_____(1000-2000mL/hour)
9. ☐ (Optional) Replace patient Output (urine, stool, drains) mL for mL with Replacement Fluid.

Medications

10. ☐ Prime hemofilter with 5000 units heparin in normal saline.
11. ☐ Heparin bolus: _____units (10-30 units/kg) IV.
    ☐ Based on goal APTT (see below), repeat bolus _____units (5-15 units/kg) IV to maximum of 80 units/kg heparin.
12. ☐ Heparin infusion: Initial rate_____units/hour (10-25 units/kg/hour)IV . Concentration: 1000 units/mL
13. ☐ Maintain goal APTT (see below) by repeat bolus and /or infusion adjustment per primary MD.

Laboratory:

14. ☐ Goal APTT: _____-_____ (45-65) seconds.
    ☐ Check APTT BID, After each heparin bolus, Four hours after all heparin dosing changes, and Immediately after blood product administration.
15. ☐ Pre treatment draw: APTT, INR, CBC, CMP, Magnesium, and ionized Calcium.
16. ☐ Draw: CBC, BMP, Magnesium, Phosphorus, and Calcium every 12 hours x 2 then daily.

Treatment Termination:

17. ☐ Return blood with a _____ml normal saline flush.
    ☐ Do not return blood.
18. Pulsatile flush to each limb of catheter with 10 mL (adult) or 5 mL (pediatric) normal saline. Fill Arterial and Venous lumen of dialysis catheter (volume printed on catheter A_____mL, V_____mL) with:
    ☐ Heparin 5000 units/mL (adult standard).
    ☐ Heparin 1000 units/mL (pediatric standard).
    ☐ ACD-A from pharmacy.

Nephrologist (Signature/Print Name):	P.I.:	Pager:
Nephrology Nurse (Signature/Print Name):	Date/Time:	
ICU Nurse (Signature/Print Name):	Date/Time:	

AM2555 (9/07)	**CRRT ORDERS WITH HEPARIN ANTICOAGULATION**	MR# 10/96/371

Appendix 7.7. Pediatric CRRT orders with regional citrate anticoagulation
Designed for use with the Fresenius 2008K.

Courtesy of Maureen Craig, UC Davis Medical Center, Sacramento, CA. Used with permission.

UNIVERSITY OF CALIFORNIA, DAVIS
MEDICAL CENTER
SACRAMENTO, CALIFORNIA

PHYSICIAN'S ORDERS

PEDIATRIC CONTINUOUS RENAL REPLACEMENT THERAPY (CRRT) ORDERS
WITH REGIONAL CITRATE ANTICOAGULATION

Directions: Check the appropriate boxes and complete those orders to be implemented (order renewal daily before noon).

For assistance, Monday-Friday 8-5 call x48730, other hours call operator for on-call Nephrology Nurse.

Date: _____ For Date: _____

Time: _____

Fluid/ Solute Balance:

1. ☐ Daily Weights (kg). Admission Weight (kg): _____
2. ☐ Dialyzer _____ (See Pediatric Specification Sheet).
3. ☐ Blood Tubing: ☐ Neonate, ☐ Husky, ☐ Pediatric, ☐ Adult **(See Pediatric Specification Sheet to set Pump Segment Diameter)**.
4. ☐ Prime circuit with: ☐ Saline, ☐ 5% Albumin, ☐ PRBC & normal saline for a HCT of ____ % (Sign Pediatric Specification Sheet).
5. ☐ Blood Flow Rate (BFR) _____ (20-200) ml/min (5-10 ml/kg/min) (consider reducing to decrease clearance).
6. ☐ Pediatric UFR = _____ ml/hr (0.5-1 ml/kg/hr) + Total Intake rate – patient's previous hour Output.
7. ☐ Dialysate Flow Rate (DFR) _____ (100) ml/min at _____ (36°-38°) C.
   ☐ (Optional) Dialysate Flow Co-current to Blood Flow (consider when needing to decrease clearance).
8. ☐ Dialysate: K⁺ _____ (3-4) mEq/L   Na⁺ _____ (135) mEq/L   PO₄⁻³ _____ (2.5) mg/dL
   Ca⁺² ___0___ (0)mEq/L   HCO₃⁻ _____ (25-30) mEq/L   Mg⁺² _____ (2 - 2.5) mEq/L
   (1 mEq/L Mg⁺² = 1.2 mg/dL Mg)
9. ☐ (Optional) Replacement Fluid: Infuse normal saline at _____ (10% of BFR) ml/hour.
10. ☐ Call Nephrology if fluid bolus greater than 60ml/Kg/shift is ordered for BP support.

Medications:

11. ☐ Anticoagulant Citrate Dextrose (ACD-A) _____ ml/hour (BFR x 2, in ml/hour, i.e., BFR of 150 ml/min, ACD-A 300 ml/hr) Rx.
12. ☐ Adjust ACD-A to maintain the System (venous port) ionized Calcium 0.25-0.35 mMol/L.

For System (venous port) ionized Calcium (mMol/L)	Patient less than 5Kg Adjust ACD-A infusion	Patient 5-20 Kg Adjust ACD-A infusion	Patient more than 20 Kg Adjust ACD-A infusion
Less than 0.25	Decrease by 2.5 ml/hour	Decrease by 5 ml/hour	Decrease by 10 ml/hour
0.25-0.35	**No Change**	**No Change**	**No Change**
0.36-0.45	Increase by 2.5 ml/hour	Increase by 5 ml/hour	Increase by 10 ml/hour
Greater than 0.45	Increase by 5 ml/hour	Increase by 10 ml/hour	Increase by 20 ml/hour
Notify Nephrologist ASAP if ACD-A infusion is greater than 300 ml/hour			

13. ☐ Calcium Chloride (8 g/L 0.9% saline) _____ ml/hour (2/3 of BFR in ml/hour, i.e., BFR of 150 ml/min, CaCl 100 ml/hour) Rx.
14. ☐ Adjust Calcium Chloride to maintain the Patient (arterial) ionized Calcium 1.2 – 1.4 mMol/L

For Patient Ionized Calcium (mMol/L)	Patient less than 5Kg Adjust Calcium infusion	Patient 5-20 Kg Adjust Calcium infusion	Patient greater than 20 Kg Adjust Calcium infusion
Less than 0.9	**Notify PICU MD. Increase calcium infusion by 10%. Hold ACD-A for 1 hour, and then restart at 30% of previous ACD-A rate.**		
0.90-1.00	Increase by 5 ml/hour	Increase by 10 ml/hour	Increase by 20 ml/hour
1.01-1.19	Increase by 2.5 ml/hour	Increase by 5 ml/hour	Increase by 10 ml/hour
1.20-1.40	**No Change**	**No Change**	**No Change**
1.41-1.60	Decrease by 2.5 ml/hour	Decrease by 5 ml/hour	Decrease by 10 ml/hour
Greater than 1.60	**Notify PICU MD**	**Notify PICU MD**	**Notify PICU MD**
Notify Nephrologist ASAP if Calcium infusion is greater than 200 ml/hour			

Laboratory:

15. ☐ Pretreatment draw: Patient ionized Calcium, CBC, BMP, Calcium, Magnesium, Phosphorus, and Albumin.
16. ☐ Every six hours x 2, then every 12 hours draw: CBC, BMP, Calcium, Magnesium, Phosphorus, and _____.
17. ☐ 30 minutes after treatment initiation or blood product administration draw Patient and System ionized Calcium.
18. ☐ 30-60 minutes after a change in BFR, DFR, ACD-A or Calcium infusion rate draw Patient and System ionized Calcium.
19. ☐ Every four hours draw Patient and System ionized Calcium.
20. ☐ For patient symptoms of hypocalcemia or hypercalcemia draw Patient ionized Calcium and System ionized Calcium.

Treatment Termination:

21. ☐ Return blood with a _____ ml normal saline flush (see Pediatric Specification Sheet for standard volume = circuit volume).
    ☐ (Optional) Do not return blood.
22. ☐ Pulsatile flush to each limb of catheter with 5 ml normal saline. Fill Arterial and Venous lumen of dialysis catheter (volume printed on catheter A_____mL, V_____mL) with:
    ☐ Heparin 1000 units/ml (standard).
    ☐ ACD-A from pharmacy.
    ☐ _____
23. ☐ 20 minutes after treatment termination draw Patient ionized Calcium, notify PICU MD if not in range of 1.20-1.40mMol/L.
24. ☐ Notify Nephrologist of treatment termination.

Nephrologist signature / print name: _____ P.I.: _____ Pager: _____

Nephrology Nurse signature / print name: _____ Date/Time: _____

ICU Nurse signature / print name: _____ Date / Time: _____

A5804-1 (10/07)   **PEDIATRIC CRRT ORDERS WITH REGIONAL CITRATE ANTICOAGULATION**   MR#02/05371

Appendix 7.8. Pediatric CRRT orders with heparin or no anticoagulation

Courtesy of Maureen Craig, UC Davis Medical Center, Sacramento, CA. Used with permission.

UNIVERSITY OF CALIFORNIA, DAVIS
MEDICAL CENTER
SACRAMENTO, CALIFORNIA

PHYSICIAN'S ORDERS

PEDIATRIC CONTINUOUS RENAL REPLACEMENT THERAPY (CRRT) ORDERS
WITH HEPARIN OR NO ANTICOAGULATION

Date:	For Date:
Time:	

Directions: Check the appropriate boxes and complete those orders to be implemented (order renewal daily before noon).
For assistance, Monday-Friday 8-5 call x48730, other hours call operator for on-call Nephrology Nurse.

Fluid/Solute Balance:

1. □   Daily Weights (kg).   Admission Weight (kg):
2. □   Dialyzer _____ (See Pediatric Specification Sheet).
3. □   Blood Tubing: □ Neonate, □ Husky, □ Pediatric, □ Adult **(See Pediatric Specification Sheet to set Pump Segment Diameter)**.
4. □   Prime circuit with: □ Saline, □ 5% Albumin, □ PRBC & normal saline for a HCT of _____% (See Pediatric Specification Sheet).
5. □   Blood Flow Rate (BFR) _____ (50-200) ml/min (consider 5-10 ml/kg/min).
6. □   Pediatric UFR = _____ ml/hr (0.5-1ml/kg/hr) + Total Intake rate – patient's previous hour Output.
7. □   Dialysate Flow Rate (DFR) _____(100) ml/min at _____ (36°-38°) C.
   □   (Optional) Dialysate Flow Co-current to Blood Flow (consider when needing to decrease clearance).
8. □   Dialysate: K^+ _____ (3-4) mEq/L Na^+ _____ (135-140) mEq/L PO_4^{-3} _____ (2.5) mg/dL
                Ca^{+2} _____ (2.5)mEq/L HCO_3^- _____ (30) mEq/L Mg^{+2} _____ (2 - 2.5) mEq/L
                                                        (1 mEq/L Mg^{+2} = 1.2 mg/dL Mg)
9. □   (Optional) Replacement Fluid: Infuse normal saline at _____(10% of BFR) ml/hr.
10. □   Call Nephrology if fluid bolus greater than 60ml/Kg/shift is ordered for BP support.

Medications:

11. □   No Anticoagulation
12. □   Flush circuit with _____ (25-100) ml normal saline every 15-30 minutes.
13. □   Heparin bolus _____ units IV (25-50 units/kg/dose) and rebolus _____ units IV (10 units/kg) to achieve range.
14. □   Heparin (100 units/ml) infusion _____ units/hr IV (10-20 units/kg/hr).
15. □   Adjust Heparin infusion to achieve a PTT in the range of 45-65.

PTT	Bolus (units/kg)	Hold (minutes)	Rate Change (units/kg/hr)
Less than 34	25	0	Increase by 2
35-44	0	0	Increase by 1
45-65	**0**	**0**	**No Change**
66-75	0	0	Decrease by 1
76-100	0	30	Decrease by 2
Greater than100	0	60 Notify PICU MD	Decrease by 2

Laboratory:

16. □   Pretreatment draw: BMP, Calcium, Magnesium, Phosphorus, Albumin, CBC, INR, PTT, Fibrinogen, FDP, and D-dimer.
17. □   Every 12 hours draw: BMP, Calcium, Magnesium, Phosphorus, CBC, PTT, and _____.
18. □   Check PTT 5 minutes after a heparin bolus, 4 hours after an heparin infusion change, and after blood product administration.
19. □   Call PICU attending for a decrease in platelet count ≥ 50% from baseline at start of CRRT therapy.

Treatment Termination:

20. □   Return blood with a _____ml normal saline flush (see Pediatric Specification Sheet for standard volume = circuit volume).
   □   (Optional) Do not return blood.
21.   Pulsatile flush to each limb of catheter with 5 ml normal saline. Fill Arterial and Venous lumen of dialysis catheter (volume printed on catheter A_____mL, V_____mL) with:
   □   Heparin 1000 units/ml (standard).
   □   ACD-A from Rx.
   □   _____
22. □   Notify Nephrologist of treatment termination.

Nephrologist signature / print name:		P.I.:	Pager:
Nephrology Nurse signature / print name:		Date/Time:	
ICU Nurse signature / print name:		Date / Time:	

A5805-1 (9/07)   **PEDIATRIC CRRT ORDERS WITH HEPARIN OR NO ANTICOAGULATION**   MR#020/05964

Appendix 7.9 CRRT orders with regional citrate (page 1 of 2)

Courtesy of Jina Bogle, DCI Acute Program, Omaha, Nebraska. Used with permission.

ACUTE HEMODIALYSIS SERVICES **CITRATE CRRT ORDERS**	Addressograph

Allergies: _____   Page 1 of 2

1. ☐ Consent for CRRT by Dr. _____.   ☐ Consent for vascular access by Dr. _____.
2. **Therapy type:**
    ☐ SCUF (ultrafiltration only)   ☐ CVVHD (using dialysate)
    ☐ CVVH (using replacement solution)   ☐ CVVHDF (using dialysate and replacement solution)
3. Blood Flow Rate: 100 ml/min
4. Hemofilter: M100 (AN69)
5. **Fluid Balance:**
    ☐ Start-up CRRT Weight: _____   ☐ Desired Net Negative Ultrafiltration _____ ml/hr
    ☐ Daily Weight & Hourly I & O   ☐ Desired Net Positive Fluid Gain _____ ml/hr
    ☐ Zero Balance Ultrafiltration   ☐ 24-hour Fluid Balance Goal _____ liters
                                                       ☐ Other _____
6. **Lock Hemodialysis Catheter when not in use with:**
    ☐ Heparin 5000 units/ml: Red lumen __ ml Blue lumen _____ ml
    ☐ Heparin 1000 units/ml: Red lumen __ ml Blue lumen _____ ml
    ☐ Heparin 100 units/ml: 3rd Infusion lumen _____ ml
    ☐ For catheter thrombosis instill Alteplase Cathflo® 2 mg/2 ml: Red lumen _____ ml
       Blue lumen _____ ml   Infusion lumen _____ ml PRN for patency/thrombosis
7. ☐ For Heparin Induced Thrombocytopenia patients, lock catheter with Anticoagulant Citrate
       Dextrose Formula A 2% / 5 ml syringe, PRN for patency: Red lumen _____ ml Blue lumen _____ ml
       Infusion lumen _____ ml
8. ☐ Change circuit every 72 hr. If system fails between 2200 & 0600, restart: ☐ in AM   ☐ ASAP
9. **IV Replacement/Substitution Fluid:**
    ☐ A. 1 liter of 0.45% Sodium Chloride (1/2 strength Normal Saline) with 75 mEq Sodium Bicarbonate at _____ ml/hr
    ☐ B. 1 liter of 0.9% Sodium Chloride (Normal saline) at _____ ml/hr
    ☐ C. 1 liter of 0.45% Sodium Chloride (1/2 strength Normal Saline) at _____ ml/hr
    ☐ D. Other: _____ ml/hr
10. **Dialysate:**
    ☐ A. Dialysate flow rate _____ ml/hr (0-2500 liter/hr)
    ☐ B. Normocarb® base solution (total volume 3246.5 ml) (Normocarb 240 ml, Sterile Water 3 L, Dextrose 50% 6.5 ml)
          Total Anions 141.5 mEq/L   Total Cations 141.5 mEq/L

Components	Sterile Water	Na+	Mg	Cl	HCO$_3$	Ca^{2+}	KCl	Dextrose
Concentration mEq/L	3 Liters	140	1.5	106.5	35.0	0	0	0.1%

POTASSIUM MUST BE ADDED TO ALL ORDERS!
    ☐ C. To customize dialysate, check desired additives to 3246 ml base solution (Pharmacy to add/mix).
          ☐ Potassium Chloride 3.2 mEq (provides 1 mEq KCl/liter)
          ☐ Potassium Chloride 6.5 mEq (provides 2 mEq KCl/liter)
          ☐ Potassium Chloride 9.7 mEq (provides 3 mEq KCl/liter)
          ☐ Potassium Chloride 13 mEq (provides 4 mEq KCl/liter)
          ☐ Potassium Chloride 16.2 mEq (provides 5 mEq KCl/liter)
    ☐ D. Other _____
11. **Circuit Management:**
    ☐ Stop Citrate and Calcium infusions if:
       - Filter clots / termination of therapy
       - Machine alarms that stop blood pump
       - Stop for 1 minute only during NS flush or when returning blood
    ☐ Hang 1000 ml 0.9% Sodium Chloride to flush circuit (pharmacy to provide). Flush circuit with 100 ml 0.9% Sodium
       Chloride PRN to check circuit patency, add flush volume to patient fluid removal and follow instructions per circuit
       management.

Acute Unit\CRRT Forms\Citrate CRRT Orders\6-07

Appendix 7.9 CRRT orders with regional citrate (page 2 of 2)

Courtesy of Jina Bogle, DCI Acute Program, Omaha, Nebraska. Used with permission.

ACUTE HEMODIALYSIS SERVICES **CITRATE CRRT ORDERS**	Addressograph
Allergies:	Page 2 of 2

12. **Anticoagulation:**
☐ CRRT Regional Citrate Anticoagulation infusion
    1. ☐ 1 liter Anticoagulant Citrate Dextrose Solution Formula A ACD(A) Citrate Solution 2% IV rate 150 ml/hr via CRRT access bloodline
    2. ☐ 1 liter D5W + 6 grams Calcium Chloride IV rate 60 ml/hr via central line.
    3.

Citrate Titration Table	
Post-Filter ionized Calcium (mmol/L)	Citrate Infusion Adjustment
Less than 0.25	↓ Rate by 10 ml/hr
0.25 – 0.35 (optimal range)	NO ADJUSTMENT
0.36 – 0.45	↑ Rate by 10 ml/hr
Greater than 0.45	↑ Rate by 20 ml/hr

        Safety Parameters – Notify Nephrologist if the following occur:
        1. Citrate Rate greater than 200 ml/hr
        2. Systemic ionized Calcium less than 0.75 mmol/liter
        3. Serum Na^+ greater than 150 mEq/liter consider changing replacement solution to 0.45% Sodium Chloride.
        4. If the patient is hypotensive consider holding the citrate protocol for ½ hour until BP stable
    4.

Calcium Titration Scale	
Systemic (Patient) ionized Calcium (mmol/L)	Calcium Infusion Adjustment
Greater than 1.3	↓ Rate by 10 ml/hr
1.1 – 1.3 (optimal range)	NO ADJUSTMENT
0.9 – 1.0	↑ Rate by 10 ml/hr
Less than 0.9	↑ Rate by 20 ml/hr

    5. ➢ Serum Bicarb greater than 26 mEq/liter – Call Nephrologist to adjust replacement rate. If no replacement solution ordered, add NS as a replacement solution rate @ 200-400 ml/hr and decrease the dialysate rate by this amount. This will remove the excess bicarb in the ultrafiltered fluid and replace it with Normal Saline And reduce the Bicarbonate from the dialysate **OR**
        ➢ Alternatively the amount of replacement can be calculated as follows:
        = <u>bicarb current – desired bicarb) x 0.3 x patient weight (kg)</u>
           Time between the bicarb samples (hours) x current bicarb
        i.e. <u>(26-24) x 0.3 x 78</u> = <u>0.30 liter/hr</u> = 300 ml/hr replacement solution rate
              6 x 26

13. **Labs 1 hour after initiation and every 6 hours thereafter while on CRRT:**
☐ Post filter (Prisma) ionized Ca^{2+} (draw from blue sample port)
☐ Systemic ionized Ca^{2+} (draw from patient [true] arterial line or peripherally)
☐ For lab draws via central line, stop Citrate/Calcium Chloride infusions x 1 minute, waste 10 ml prior to draw
Labs 1 hour after initiation and every 12 hours thereafter while on CRRT:
☐ CBC
☐ Renal Function Panel: Alb, Ca^{2+}, CO_2, Cl^-, Creatinine, BUN, Glucose, Phosphorus, K^+, NA^+
☐ Mg^{2+}
☐ ABG
Miscellaneous Labs:
☐ Hepatic Function Panel (Alb, Total Bilirubin, Direct Bilirubin, Alk Phos, Total Protein, AST, ALT) at initiation of therapy
☐ Lactic acid at initiation of therapy
☐ If Platelet trend decreases at day 4 of therapy, draw Heparin Induced Antibody
☐ Other _____

Date/Time: _____ Nephrologist: _____ Noted by: _____
For initial notification call DCI-Acute (402) 449-5355 or (after-hours) Answering Service (402) 231-1032.

Acute Unit\CRRT Forms\Citrate CRRT Orders\6-07

Appendix 7.10. CRRT orders with heparin or regional citrate anticoagulation (page 1 of 2)

Courtesy of Jina Bogle, DCI Acute Program, Omaha, Nebraska. Used with permission.

STAT: Place an "**X**" in the box if STAT.   Please rule off unused lines after order sent to Pharmacy.

DATE / TIME	ORDERS	DATE	PROGRESS NOTES
	Rev: 01/06 **PPO.430**		
	Page 1 of 2		
	CONTINUOUS RENAL REPLACEMENT THERAPY (CRRT)		
	Date: _____ Procedure: ☐ SCUF ☐ CVVHD		
	☐ CVVH ☐ CVVHDF		
	Filter: ☐ M100		
	BFR: ☐ 150mL per min. OR _____mL per min		
	☐ Daily Wts.		
	Desired net fluid loss _____mL per hour		
	Replacement Solution		
	☐ Pre-Filter		
	Rate: ☐ 1200mL per hour OR _____mL per hour		
	Type A: ☐ 1L 0.9NaCl + 5mL 10% CaCl2		
	Type B: ☐ 1L 0.45NaCl + 75mL 8.4% NaHCO₃		
	Type C: ☐ PrismaSate® 5L (KO/Ca3.5)		
	add KCL _____ mEq/L and Glucose ___.___ mg/dL		
	Type D: ☐ Other_____		
	Mode: ☐ Simultaneous ("Y" connector)		
	(May use with type A / B)		
	☐ Sequential (alternate every L)		
	Dialysate Solution		
	Rate: ☐ 1200mL per hour OR _____mL per hour		
	Type A: ☐ PrismaSate® Formula (Bicarb with KO/Ca3.5)		
	Sodium 140 mEq per L		
	Calcium 3.5 mEq per L		
	Magnesium 1 mEq per L		
	Potassium 0 or _____ mEq per L		
	Chloride 109.5 mEq per L		
	Lactate 3 mEq per L		
	Bicarbonate 32 mEq per L		
	Glucose 0 or _____ mg per dL		
	(suggest 1gm per L=100 mg per dL, 2gm per L=200 mg per dL)		
	Type B: ☐ No Lactate Formula (made in pharmacy)		
	Na (variable) _____ mEq per L (suggest 140 mEq per L)		
	Bicarb (variable) _____mEq per L (suggest 35 mEq per L)		
	Cl (variable) _____mEq per L (CL = Na – Bicarb)		
	K (variable) _____ mEq per L		
	Magnesium sulfate 2 mEq per L		
	Dextrose (variable) _____ mg per dL		
	(suggest 1gm per L=100 mg per dL, 2gm per L=200 mg per dL)		
	Zero Calcium		
	Type C: ☐ Formula for use with Citrate ONLY		
	Na 117 mEq per L		
	K (variable) _____ mEq per L		
	Magnesium sulfate 1.5 mEq per L		
	Cl (variable) _____mEq per L (CL = Na + K)		
	Dextrose (variable) _____ mg per dL		
	(suggest 1gm per L=100mg per dL, 2 gm per L=200mg per dLl)		
	Zero Calcium		

DRUG ORDERS: UNLESS INITIALED PBO (PRESCRIBED BRAND ONLY) ANOTHER BRAND OF A GENERICALLY EQUIVALENT PRODUCT IDENTICAL IN CONTENT OF ACTIVE INGREDIENT(S) MAY BE ADMINISTERED

PHYSICIAN'S ORDERS AND PROGRESS NOTES INSTRUCTIONS

1. Attach patient's label or complete required information before placing in chart.
2. Rule off unused lines.
3. If STAT order, please rule off unused lines after order sent to Pharmacy.

PATIENT LABEL
Patient Name:
DOB:
Date of Procedure:
Diagnosis:
Patient Room#/Unit _____

Appendix 7.10. CRRT orders with heparin or regional citrate anticoagulation (page 2 of 2)

Courtesy of Jina Bogle, DCI Acute Program, Omaha, Nebraska. Used with permission.

☐ **STAT:** Place an "X" in the box if STAT. Please rule off unused lines after order sent to Pharmacy.

DATE / TIME	ORDERS	DATE	PROGRESS NOTES

ORDERS

Rev: 01/06   PPO.430
       Page 2 of 2
CONTINUOUS RENAL REPLACEMENT THERAPY (CRRT)

Anticoagulation   Current Weight _____ kg

1.   Select dose (check one box only)
☐ Heparin: Bolus 5,000 units then start 10 units/kg/hour infusion
☐ Tight Heparin: Bolus 1,000 units then start 5 units/kg/hour infusion

2.   Select method of administration (check one box only)
☐ Heparin via syringe on Prisma pump. Pharmacy to prepare 500 units/mL, 20mL syringe.
     Use for heparin doses of 250 units/hour or greater
☐ Heparin drip via pump (25,000 units/500 mL D5W bag)
     Use for heparin doses less than 250 units/hour
     Select heparin protocol to use: (See other orders)
       ☐ Neuro Protocol (goal aPTT 51-70)
       ☐ Cardiac Protocol (goal aPTT 70-90)
☐ No Heparin: Flush with 0.9% NS 100 mL every hour

☐ Citrate Regional Anticoagulation
     Initiate 4% sodium citrate solution at 180 mL/hour pre-hemofilter using a pump. (Infusion will be connected to access port and be directed toward filter.)
***Citrate infusion should not exceed 210 mL/hr unless ordered by MD.**
     Pharmacy will prepare a solution of Calcium Chloride 8.2 gm/L (82 mL of 10% calcium chloride in 0.9% NS 1L). Initiate Calcium Chloride infusion at 60 mL/hr via a central venous catheter.
     CAUTION: Both IV pumps-Citrate/Calcium Chloride must be stopped when Prisma pump is stopped.
☐ Do not use algorithm. Adjust per specific MD orders only.
☐ Use algorithm in table at right to adjust citrate infusion using post-filter ionized calcium.
CAUTION: Infuse to Prisma circuit ONLY. NOT for IV infusion.

Labs

☐ Chem. Panel, Phos, Mg Baseline and every _____ hours.
     (labs can only be drawn pre replacement fluid or arterial line)
☐ PT, aPTT Baseline and every _____ hours.
☐ CBC   Baseline and every _____ hours.
☐ Lactate Baseline and every _____ hours.
☐ Post filter ICa every 6 hours X 24 hours, then per MD order with use of Citrate ONLY
☐ Serum ICa every 6 hours x 24 hours, then per MD order.

Filter to be replaced every 72 hours or earlier if indicated.

_____
Physician Signature   Date/Time

_____
Nurse Signature   Date/Time

PROGRESS NOTES

Citrate Anticoagulation for Continuous Renal Replacement Therapy (CRRT)

Purpose
To provide an alternative to heparin-based anticoagulation for patients requiring CRRT who are also at risk for serious hemorrhage or in whom heparin is otherwise contraindicated (e.g. HIT). Such conditions include, but are not limited to (HIT), post-surgical bleeding and traumatic bleeding.

Policy
1. Citrate anticoagulation requires a physician order.
2. Citrate should not be employed for CVVH, but is reserved for methods in which there is dialysate flow (i.e. CVVHD or CVVHDF). This is to ensure adequate removal of the citrate complex.
3. An adequate supply of 4% sodium citrate will be dispensed by the hospital pharmacy in a pre-mixed 250 mL bag.
4. Initiate citrate solution at 180 mL per hour pre-hemofilter, or other rate ordered by physician. (Infusion will be connected to access port and be directed toward filter.)
     CAUTION: FOR INFUSION TO PRISMA CIRCUIT ONLY. IV pump must be stopped when PRISMA pump is stopped.
5. Pharmacy will prepare a solution of 8.2 gm per L Ca++ (82 mL of 10% $CaCl_2$ inj., U.S.P.) in 1000 mL 0.9% saline. Initiate $CaCl_2$ infusion at 60 mL per hour via central venous catheter.
     CAUTION: IV pump must be stopped when PRISMA pump is stopped.
6. In the event of premature clotting of the hemofilter, checking the post-filter ionized calcium (ICa) level will permit adjustment of the citrate infusion. Ideally, the post-filter ionized calcium (ICa) should be maintained between 0.25-0.35 mmol per L to reduce the risk of clotting.
7. Measurement of post-filter ionized calcium and adjustment of the citrate infusion will be done by physician order. In general, the citrate infusion should not exceed 210 mL / hour *unless* ordered by a physician.
8. Adjust citrate infusion by following algorithm:

Post-filter ionized Ca++		Change in 4% Sodium Citrate Infusion rate
mg/dL	mmol/L	
>2.00	>0.50	↑ rate by 30mL per hour
1.60-1.99	0.40-0.50	↑ rate by 20 mL per hour
1.41-1.59	0.36-0.39	↑ rate by 10 mL per hour
1.00-1.40	0.25-0.35	No change
<1.00	<0.25	↓ rate by 10 mL per hour

*4% Sodium Citrate – Do not exceed 210 mL per hour unless ordered by physician.
*Ideally, the post filter ionized calcium should be maintained between 0.25-0.35 mmol per L to reduce risk of clotting.
9. Potential complications of citrate anticoagulation include metabolic alkalosis, hypernatremia, hyper- or hypocalcemia, and bleeding.

DRUG ORDERS: UNLESS INITIALED PBO (PRESCRIBED BRAND ONLY) ANOTHER BRAND OF A GENERICALLY EQUIVALENT PRODUCT IDENTICAL IN CONTENT OF ACTIVE INGREDIENT(S) MAY BE ADMINISTERED

PHYSICIAN'S ORDERS AND PROGRESS NOTES INSTRUCTIONS
1. Attach patient's label or complete required information before placing in chart.
2. Rule off unused lines.
3. If STAT order, please rule off unused lines after order sent to Pharmacy.

PATIENT LABEL
Patient Name:
DOB:
Date of Procedure:
Diagnosis:
Patient Room#/Unit _____

Appendix 7.11. Pediatric CRRT orders with regional citrate anticoagulation (page 1 of 2)

Courtesy of Helen Currier, Texas Children's Hospital, Houston, Texas. Used with permission..

RENAL DIALYSIS: Continuous Renal Replacement Therapy (CRRT) - Acute

Orders need renewal in 3 days. For 24-hour assistance Monday-Friday 8-5 call x 6-0851, other hours call operator x 4-2099 to page the on-call dialysis nurse.

ACCESS:

□ Catheter site:_____   size:_____F_____cm

□ triple lumen   □ dual lumen   □ single lumen   □ uncuffed   □ cuffed

packing volume: arterial port _____mL; venous port _____mL; pigtail (triple lumen only) _____mL

CIRCUIT SET-UP AND PRIMING (* Dialysis nurse responsibility):

1.*   Please □ initiate or □ restart CRRT using □ PRISMA® machine □ PRISMAFLEX® machine.
Extracorporeal blood volume is _____mL, which equals _____% of patient's blood volume.

2.*   Set PRISMA /PRISMAFLEX® to CVVHDF mode.

3.*   Discard prime: □ Yes   □ No
If prime not discarded, use one of the following:
□ 5% Albumin
□ 5% Albumin mixed with PRBC to final Hct 40%
□ 50 ml PRBC, 50 mL (50 mEq) 8.4% $NaHCO_3$ and 4 mL (400 mg) 10% calcium gluconate. PRBC and $NaHCO_3$ mixed via blood transfusion y-set during manual CRRT prime. Calcium gluconate should be infused separately into venous limb of CRRT circuit during initiation.
□ 0.9% Saline with 50 mL 8.4% $NaHCO_3$ and _____mL 10% calcium gluconate (50 mg/kg, maximum 2 g). $NaHCO_3$ should be infused into CRRT circuit over 2 minutes during initiation. Calcium gluconate should be infused separately into venous limb of CRRT circuit during initiation.

4.*   Warm blood in CRRT circuit with blood warmer (35-36° C) as needed.

CRRT MACHINE SETTINGS

5.   Set Blood Pump flow rate (Qb) at _____ mL/min
(2-8 mL/kg/min; minimum 20 mL/min; maximum 400 mL/min/1.73m^2)

6.   □ No Replacement Fluid   □ Begin Replacement Fluid (□ Pre   □ Post) with _____at rate ____ mL/hr
(*For PRISMAFLEX®, always use post-replacement fluid of 50 mL/hr minimum*).

7.   Set Patient Removal flow rate (UFR=ultrafiltration rate) at _____ mL/hr
Keep total UFR rate <10% of Blood Pump flow rate.

Remember to account for ACD-A rate and CaCl₂ infusion rate in Patient Removal rate if given by separate IV pump.

8.   Increase UFR mL for mL during administration of the following blood products:
□ PRBC   □ FFP   □ Albumin   □ Platelets

9.   Call Renal Service to adjust UFR, if patient has other new peripheral or central IV fluids added or an increase or decrease in existing IV fluid rates of more than 10 mL/hr.

Appendix 7.11. Pediatric CRRT orders with regional citrate anticoagulation (page 2 of 2)

Courtesy of Helen Currier, Texas Children's Hospital, Houston, Texas. Used with permission..

DIALYSIS FLUID (DIALYSATE)

10. Normocarb® 240 mL in 3 L of sterile water (final volume 3.24 L)
     Other additives:
     - Potassium chloride _____ mEq/L (max conc: 4 mEq/L)
     - Potassium phosphate _____ mmol/L (2-3 mmol phos/L) (Each mmol Kphos =1.4 mmol K and 2 mmol phos)
     - Dextrose   □ None   □ 6 mL D$_{50}$W (~90 mg/dl)   □ 12 mL D$_{50}$W (~ 180mg/dl)
     - Other: _____

11. Set Initial Dialysate flow rate (Qd) at _____mL/hr (2000 mL/1.73M^2/hr)

CITRATE REGIONAL ANTICOAGULATION

Baseline Monitoring

12. Prior to initial set-up, check Chem-7, ionized calcium, total calcium, phosphorus, magnesium, total serum protein, glucose, CBC with diff & platelets, serum HbSAg and HbSAb if not already done.

Initial Citrate anticoagulation

13. Order from pharmacy: □ ACD-A 1000 ml   □ 8000 mg calcium chloride in 1000 ml NS
14. Start IV ACD-A at _____ mL/hr (rate=1.5min/hr X Qb) into arterial limb of CRRT circuit
15. Infuse IV calcium chloride 8000 mg/L NS in □ central line other than CRRT circuit or □ pigtail of triple lumen access or □ venous limb of catheter via stopcock. Run at _____ mL/hr (rate = 0.4 min/hr X Qb)

Citrate anticoagulation monitoring and adjustments

Optimal range: CRRT circuit ionized calcium (0.2-0.4 mmol/L); patient ionized calcium (1.1-1.3 mmol/L)

16. Check the CRRT circuit ionized calcium (draw from venous port) and patient's ionized calcium and total calcium (draw from site other than CRRT circuit) 10 minutes after initiation of therapy, then again 2 hours after initiation of therapy and every 6 hours thereafter (10 AM, 2PM, 10 PM, 2 AM).

17. Re-check CRRT circuit ionized calcium and patient's ionized calcium 1 hour after any change in anticoagulation orders.

PROBLEMS/TROUBLE SHOOTING

18. Notify Renal Service for
     - Patient ionized calcium less than 1.0 mmol/L or greater than 1.5 mmol/L
     - Circuit ionized calcium less than 0.2 mmol/L or greater than 0.4 mmol/L
     - Patient's total calcium less than _____ or greater than _____
     - Hourly UFR greater or less than_____ mL for 2 hours (+/- 30 mL per hour from prescribed UFR)
     - Access pressure less than _____ (Default @ -250 mmHg)
     - Filter pressure greater than _____ (Default @ 300 mmHg)
     - Return pressure greater than _____ (Default @ 350 mmHg)
     - Patient BP less than _____/_____ or greater than _____/_____

19. Notify the Renal Dialysis Nurse if the CRRT circuit clots.

Noted by:_____RN (Renal Dialysis nurse) Noted by:_____RN (ICU nurse)

_____MD   Pager #_____

Format update November18, 2005

Appendix 7.12. Nephrology nursing flowsheet for IHD, SLEDD, or CRRT

Courtesy of Maureen Craig, UC Davis Medical Center, Sacramento, CA. Used with permission.

Use Patient Plate

**UNIVERSITY OF CALIFORNIA DAVIS
MEDICAL CENTER
SACRAMENTO, CALIFORNIA
RENAL SERVICES PROGRAM**

Page _____ of _____   **DIALYSIS PROGRESS RECORD**

Date:

Prescription: Routine _____   Emergent _____   Treatment # _____   Location _____

Prescription:
- Treatment Type — IHD/PUF/CRRT / Extended Daily Dialysis
- Nephrologist
- Duration — Hours
- UF goal — L
- Dialyzer
- Blood Flow Rate — mls/min
- Dialysate Rate — mls/min

Dialysate Solution
- K / Ca — mEq/L
- Na / Bicarb — / mEq/L
- Phosphorus — mg/dL
- Na Model — step / Linear / Exponential / Off
- Na level — mEq/L

Anticoagulation
- Heparin Load — units
- Heparin Rate — units/hr
- ACD-A — ml/hr
- Ca G — ml/hr
- Labs

Machine, Water & Dialysate
- Chlorine/Chloramine — - / + / NA
- Machine #
- R.O. #
- Conductivity / (K/Phoenix) — / mS/L
- Temp / pH (Phoenix) — C/
- PHT / Alarm Test — Pass / No Pass

Assess / care	Pre Dialysis	Post Dialysis	Assess / care	Pre Dialysis	Post Dialysis
Temp / Fever Chills	/ Yes No	/ Yes No	N/V / Cramping	Yes / No	Yes / No
HR/Rhythm/CP	Reg / Irrg Y/N	Reg / Irrg Y/N	Access /Needle Size	R / L ___ Gauge	Held / Site Care
BP lying/sit/stand			Access Type / Care	Cath/Cuff/Graft/Fistula	
Edema			Bruit-Thrill Lidocaine	Y/N/NA	Y/N/NA
Neurologic	A & O x 3 / lethargic unresponsive / confused	A & O x 3 / lethargic unresponsive / confused	Access S / S Infection	None/Red/Swollen/Warm	None/Red/Swollen/Warm
Respiratory	Clear/Rales/Whz/SOB	Clear/Rales/Whz/SOB	Pressors / Hypotension	Yes / No	Yes / No
Vent /Rate	yes / no /min	yes / no /min	Isolation status	Blood Processed:	
O2/O2 Sat	%	%	Filter: Clear/Streaked/Clotted		
			Lab Date/Time:	Report to:	

Patient Education

Time	BP	HR	BFR ml/min.	AP/VP mm Hg	TMP/UFR	ACD-A mLs Heparin units	CaG ml/hr	Fluid Out	Fluid In	Patient/ System ICa	Pain 1-10	RBV	Hct	Keen	Kt/V	CVP	Comments/Meds/Rate changes	Initials
Post																		
	Totals							Net Fluid						Volume: ____ L				

Signature: _____   Initials _____

Print Name: _____

Signature: _____   Initials _____

Print Name: _____

∨ ∧ ++ ∨∧∨

| AR5353 (12/05) | **DIALYSIS PROGRESS RECORD** | MR 11/03860 |

Appendix 7.13. Nephrology nursing flowsheet for CRRT

Courtesy of Western Nephrology Acute Dialysis, Denver, Colorado. Used with permission.

PROCEDURE: ☐ SCUF   ☐ CVVHD

        ☐ CVVH   ☐ CVVHDF

Primary Dx _____

PHYSICIAN CRRT ORDER

Filter   ☐ M100

Blood Flow Rate _____

Dialysate Flow Rate _____

Replacement Flow Rate _____

Heparin Bolus _____

      Continuous _____

Citrate _____

Calcium Chloride _____

Net Fluid Removal _____

Dialysate Solution _____

Replacement Solution _____

ACCESS

Type _____

Redness _____

Edema _____

Bruising _____

Drainage _____

Insertion Date _____

Insert by _____

Dressing Changed: _____

Date Setup due
to be Changed _____

MACHINE CHECKLIST

	Previous	Time	Time
Dr. Ordered Net Loss			
Access			
Filter			
Effluent			
Return			
Blood Flow Rate			
Dialysate Flow Rate			
Replacement Flow Rate			
Heparin			
Citrate			
Calcium			
Machine #			
Lot #			

Western Acute Dialysis

CRRT Record

Date: Date CRRT Initiated

Hospital:

Patient Name:

	Prev	Time	Time
BP			
MAP			
HR			
TEMP			
WT			
Hgb/HcT			
PLT			
PTT			
PT/INR			
Na			
K			
Cl			
CO2			
BUN			
CR			
Glucose			
Mg			
Ionized Ca			
Serum Ca			
Lactate			

Date   Time   Nursing Notes

Setup _____   Technical Assist _____   Nursing Visit _____

Staff Signature _____   Physician Signature _____

Western Acute Dialysis CRRT Record   PATIENT LABEL

Appendix 7.14. ICU Nursing Kardex for CRRT with regional citrate

Courtesy of Jina Bogle, DCI Acute Program, Omaha, Nebraska. Used with permission.

ADDRESSOGRAPH

Citrate Kardex for CRRT

Diagnosis: _____ Allergies: _____
Recent Surgery: _____
CRRT Start Date: _____
Therapy Mode: _____ **CODE STATUS:** _____

CIRCUIT MANAGEMENT

Stop Citrate and Calcium drips if:
- **filter clots / termination of therapy**
- **machine alarms that stop the blood pump**
- **during NS flush or returning blood for any reason**

Therapy Prescription:
Net Fluid Removal: _____
Replacement Solution: _____
_____
_____

Replacement Flowrate: _____ ml/hr
Dialysate Solution: _____
_____

Dialysate Flow: _____ ml/hr
Blood Flow Rate: _____ ml/min

Lab draws from Circuit:
- During SCUF or CVVDH, draw labs from <u>any</u> red port.
- During CVVH or CVVHDF, draw labs from access red port.
- When anticoagulating, draw coags from blue port.
- When not anticoagulating, draw coags from access port.

Ca⁺⁺ Labs 1° before initiation & q6hr thereafter:
- Prisma Post-Filter ionized Ca⁺⁺ (blue sample port)
- Systemic ionized Ca⁺⁺ (pt. (true) art. line or peripherally)
- Labs draws via central line, stop citrate/CaCl infusion x1min, waste 10ml prior to draw
- **ALL IONIZED Ca⁺⁺ to RUN STAT IN LAB—results obtained within 15 min.**
- CBC
- CMP, Phos, Mg
- Miscellaneous: (check)
  ☐ Liver panel @ initiation of Tx
  ☐ Lactic acid @ initiation of Tx
  ☐ ABG in AM
  ☐ Heparin Induced Antibody PRN

Vascular Access:
CXR Verified   Y or N
Access Physician: _____
Date: _____
Type: _____
Location: _____
Prep: _____
Dressing: _____

Anticoagulation:
☐ 1L ACD(A) Citrate 2% rate @ _____ ml/hr via CRRT access blood line
☐ 1L D5W + 6 grams CaCl IV rate @ _____ ml/hr via central line

Citrate Titration Table

Prisma Post-Filter ionized Ca⁺⁺ (mmol/L)	Citrate Infusion Adjustment
< 0.25	↓ Rate by 10 ml/hr
0.25 – 0.35 (optimal range)	NO ADJUSTMENT
0.36 – 0.45	↑ Rate by 10 ml/hr
> 0.45	↑ Rate by 20 ml/hr

Safety Parameters – **Notify Nephrologist** if the following occur:
1. Citrate Rate > 200 ml/hr
2. Replacement Rate > 1000 ml/hr
3. Systemic ionized Ca⁺⁺ < 0.75 mmol/l (compare to total Ca⁺⁺). Consider holding citrate for 3 hours and resuming infusion at 150 ml/hr.
4. Serum Na+ > 150 mEq/L consider changing replacement solution to 0.45% NaCl.
5. Serum Bicarb is > 26 mEq/L

Calcium Titration Table

Systemic (Patient) ionized Ca⁺⁺ (mmol/L)	Calcium Infusion Adjustment
> 1.3	↓ Rate by 10 ml/hr
1.1 – 1.3 (optimal range)	NO ADJUSTMENT
0.9 – 1.0	↑ Rate by 10 ml/hr
< 0.9	↑ Rate by 20 ml/hr

Dialysis Catheter Loads:
☐ Heparin 5,000 units/ml ☐ Heparin 1,000 units/ml ☐ 0.9% NS
☐ Citrate 2% ACA-A Sol. ☐ Cathflo 2 mg/ml
Arterial/Red or Proximal Port _____ Volume ml
Blue/Venous or Distal Port _____ Volume ml

☐ Heparin 100 units/ml   ☐ 0.9% NS   ☐ Citrate 2% ACA-A Sol.
☐ Cathflo 2 mg/ml
INF/infusions/3ʳᵈ Port _____ Volume ml

Acute Unit/CRRT Forms/Citrate Kardex/6-07

Appendix 7.15. ICU nursing flowsheet for CRRT

Courtesy of Western Nephrology Acute Dialysis, Denver, Colorado. Used with permission.

Previous Wt. _____
Current Wt. _____

24 Hour Flow Sheet for CRRT

Today's Date _____

Time	1900	2000	2100	2200	Total	2300	2400	0100	0200	Total	0300	0400	0500	0600	12 HR	24 HR
A. Intake															A	
IV's (CITRATE AND CALCIUM MUST BE INCLUDED)																
Saline Flush																
Extended Bolus Amt.																
Other															Total Intake	
Total intake																
B. Output															B	
Urine																
Other																
Gastric															Total Output	
Total Output																
C. Intake minus output															C	
D. Dr. ordered fluid removal															D	
E. Line C + D = E (Removal goal)															E	
F. Adjust from previous hour (difference from machine)															F	
If too much removed, subtract from goal																
If too little removed, add to goal																
G. Machine set to remove this hour															G	
H. Actual fluid removed (from machine)															H	
Difference between (G-H)					4 hr					4 hr				4 hr		
I. Net Fluid Removal (H-C)															I	
J. Flow Rates															J	
Blood																
Dialysate																
Replacement																
K. Pressures															K	
Access																
Filter																
Effluent																
Return																
TMPa																
△ P Filter																
L. Anticoagulant															L	
Heparin continuous																
Heparin bolus																
Citrate infusion rate																
CaCl$_2$ infusion rate																

Nurse Signature: _____

6/7/2007

CHAPTER **8**
Therapeutic Apheresis

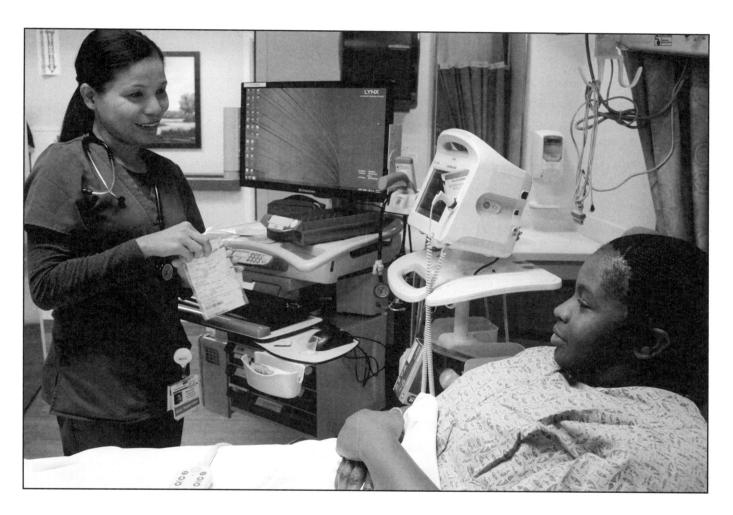

Chapter Editor
Helen F. Williams, MSN, BSN, RN, CNN

Author
Regina Rohe, BS, RN, HP(ASCP)

CHAPTER **8**

Therapeutic Apheresis

This offering for **1.6 contact hours** is provided by the American Nephrology Nurses' Association (ANNA).

American Nephrology Nurses' Association is accredited as a provider of continuing nursing education by the American Nurses Credentialing Center Commission on Accreditation.

ANNA is a provider approved by the California Board of Registered Nursing, provider number CEP 00910.

This CNE offering meets the continuing nursing education requirements for certification and recertification by the Nephrology Nursing Certification Commission (NNCC).

To be awarded contact hours for this activity, read this chapter in its entirety. Then complete the CNE evaluation found at **www.annanurse.org/corecne** and submit it; or print it, complete it, and mail it in. Contact hours are not awarded until the evaluation for the activity is complete.

Example of reference for Chapter 8 in APA format. One author for entire chapter.

Rohe, R. (2015). Therapeutic apheresis. In C.S. Counts (Ed.), *Core curriculum for nephrology nursing: Module 4. Acute kidney injury* (6th ed., pp. 211-234). Pitman, NJ: American Nephrology Nurses' Association.

Interpreted: Chapter author. (Date). Title of chapter. In …

Cover photo by Counts/Morganello.

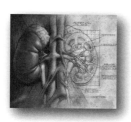

CHAPTER 8

Therapeutic Apheresis

Purpose

The purposes of this chapter are to present the history of apheresis technology; facilitate cognitive understanding of the concepts, principles, and clinical application of therapeutic apheresis (TA); explain therapeutic plasma exchange (TPE); and present information for nephrology nurses to help them provide effective care for patients receiving TPE treatment.

Objectives

Upon completion of this chapter, the learner will be able to:
1. Define the terms used in therapeutic apheresis.
2. List the six major categories of apheresis treatments.
3. List two methods of plasma separation.
4. Describe the anticoagulation options available for each type of plasma separation method.
5. State one resource for a current listing of clinical applications of therapeutic apheresis procedures.

Significant Dates in the History of Apheresis Technology

00 BC Bloodletting, leeches, and manual phlebotomy all thought to be useful in removing toxins and treating diseases.

1877 Manual continuous flow centrifugation instrument was designed by a Swiss physician, Carl Gustav Patrik DeLaval, and used throughout Europe for cream separation.

1881 DeLaval device patented for use in the United States.

1914 Plasma exchange procedure done on uremic dogs, which consisted of phlebotomy, separation by centrifuge, and the removal of plasma cells while returning RBCs and saline through a separate intravenous (IV) line.

1940s Dr. Edwin Cohn adapted a cream separator to separate plasma from whole blood for use on injured soldiers during World War II.

1950s Dr. Cohn, while at the Harvard Medical School, invented the "Cohn Fractionator," which was successful in separating blood into all of its components.

1952 Human plasma was made commercially available.

1959 Plastic containers were introduced, increasing storage time and cutting down on cost of producing and distributing plasma.

1960s Engineers and physicians at the National Cancer Institute and International Business Machines designed an automatic continuous flow blood cell separator called "model 2990." This machine does not have a completely disposable unit, and the separation bowl must be washed and sanitized by hand.

1970s Celltifuge® (Aminco Corporation, Silver Spring, Maryland) marketed a completely disposable continuous flow blood cell separator that was adapted for use in TPE treatments.

    1. 1972 – IBM 2997 introduced to U.S. market.

    2. 1976 – CS3000, the first centrifugal machine with microprocessors, was introduced by Baxter-Fenwal. Inc.

1982   Century TPE System® (Gambro BCT, Lakewood, Colorado) introduced the first plasma membrane exchange system.

1987   UVAR-XTS Photopheresis device (Therakos, division of Johnson & Johnson, Raritan, NJ) approved for photopheresis treatment of Cutaneous T-cell Lymphoma.

1987   COBE Spectra® (Gambro BCT, Lakewood, Colorado) introduced a continuous-flow centrifugation device used for plasma exchange, cytapheresis, and other clinical applications.

1987   Prosorba Protein A column® (IMRE, Seattle, WA), the first immunoadsorption device, was approved by the Food and Drug Administration (FDA) for idiopathic thrombocytopenia purpura (ITP) and later approved for refractory rheumatoid arthritis (RA).

      1. The manufacture of this column was discontinued in 2007.

      2. A similar Protein A column, the Excorim (Excorim AB, Lund, Sweden), was introduced to the European market.

1994   AS 104® (Fresenius Hemocare Bad Homburg, Germany) was FDA approved as another continuous flow centrifugation device for use in the US.

1996   Liposorber® system (Kaneka Pharma, Osaka, Japan) introduces a plasma column for reducing low density lipids (LDL) in patients with familial hypercholesterolemia.

1997   Heparin-induced Extracorporeal Lipoprotein Precipitation (HELP®) system (B. Braun Medical Inc, Melsungen, Germany) was FDA approved for LDL removal from plasma.

2005   Spectra Optia® (CaridianBCT, Lakewood, Colorado) introduced a continuous flow centrifugation device in the European market, and in the United States in 2009.

      1. Initially approved by the FDA for use in the United States for plasma exchange only.

      2. 2012 – Approved by the FDA for white blood cell collection in the United States.

      3. Used outside the United States for both plasmapheresis and cytapheresis procedures.

      4. 2013 – Approved by FDA for red blood cell exchange in United States.

2006   Com.Tec® (Fresenius Hemocare Bad Homburg, Germany) FDA approved as a continuous flow, centrifugation device for plasmapheresis only. Used outside of the United States for plasmapheresis and cytapheresis procedures.

2009   CellEx™ introduced by Therakos, approved by FDA for Extracorporeal Photopheresis (ECP). Used continuous flow design. Approved for use in Europe in 2008 and in Canada in 2009.

2011   Amicus™ cell separator (Fenwal, Inc., Lake Zurich, IL) approved by FDA for plasma exchange in United States

2011   NxStage® (Nxstage Medical, Inc., Lawrence, MA) dialysis device approved by FDA for plasma exchange with membrane separator and a disposable set specifically for TPE.

2012   Prismaflex® (Gambro, Lund Sweden) dialysis device approved by FDA for plasma exchange with membrane separator set – "TPE 2000."

(Corbin et al., 2010)

I. Definition of terms.

A. Aperesis: derived from a Greek word meaning to remove or to separate a part from its whole. It has become synonymous with *hemapheresis* as an umbrella term encompassing all blood separation procedures.

    1. Therapeutic apheresis (TA) is used to describe apheresis procedures used in the treatment of patients with specific diseases or syndromes.

    2. It differs from donor apheresis, which describes apheresis procedures used in blood banking to collect blood products for transfusion or fractionation.

B. Plasmapheresis is the separation of plasma from whole blood.

    1. Plasma exchange (PE) and therapeutic plasma exchange (TPE) are terms used interchangeably to describe the separation and removal of plasma,

along with the reinfusion of the remaining blood components and an equal amount of either plasma or other replacement fluid for the treatment of a variety of diseases or conditions.

2. Plasmapheresis is also employed in cascade or secondary filtration, where the separated plasma is then passed through a second filter or column to remove a specific plasma constituent. The filtered plasma is then returned to the patient.

C. Leukapheresis: separation and removal of white blood cells (leukocytes) from whole blood.
   1. Therapeutic leukapheresis can be employed to remove excess white blood cells (WBCs) for patients with leukemia.
   2. Therapeutic leukapheresis can also be used to collect WBCs from patients with a variety of conditions that benefit from ex-vivo manipulation and subsequent reinfusion (i.e., stem cell collection).
   3. Leukapheresis is an integral part of extracorporeal photopheresis (ECP).

D. Thrombocytapheresis or plateletpheresis: separation and removal of platelets from whole blood. Used therapeutically to deplete platelets from patients with thrombocytosis.

E. Erythrocytapheresis: separation and removal of red blood cells from whole blood. This term is used to describe both red blood cell depletion and red blood cell exchange procedures.
   1. Also referred to as red blood cell exchange or RBCX. This procedure replaces removed red blood cells (RBCs) with donated RBCs.
   2. RBCX is used most often for patients in sickle cell disease crisis, but it is also used in certain life-threatening cases of *Plasmodium falciparum* malaria and Babesiosis; it has also been used in cases of severe carbon monoxide poisoning (Zengin et al., 2013).
   3. Red blood cell depletion procedures are most often used for patients with disorders producing erythrocytosis (i.e., polycythemia vera).

F. Cytapheresis: separation and removal of a particular cellular component.

G. Extracorporeal photopheresis (ECP): separation of buffy coat from whole blood, injection of cell product with 8-methoxypsoralen, exposure of cells to UVA light, and then reinfusion of cells into patient (Scarisbrick, 2009).

H. Low density lipoprotein cholesterol apheresis (LDL apheresis): removal of apolipoprotein B-containing lipoproteins from either whole blood or separated plasma (Winters, 2011).

II. Devices used in therapeutic plasmapheresis (Burgstaler, 2010a; 2010b).

A. Centrifugation devices.
   1. Continuous flow devices.
      a. COBE Spectra®.
         (1) Can perform TPE as either a single-needle or a dual-needle procedure.
         (2) Using the single-needle option lengthens the time to perform the treatment and is only used when the patient does not have vascular access to support two needles.
      b. Spectra Optia®.
         (1) Replacement for the COBE Spectra®.
         (2) Uses different disposable sets from COBE Spectra®.
      c. AS 104® (Fresenius-Kabi, Bad Homburg, Germany). No longer manufactured but disposable sets still available for TPE and platelet depletion.
      d. COM.TEC® – replacement for AS104®.
         (1) Single-needle option is not available in the United States.
         (2) Uses same disposable sets as AS104®.
      e. Amicus® cell separator used in United States for plasmapheresis and MNC collection procedures.
      f. All of these devices use the continuous flow technology but differ in device-specific ways.
         (1) These machines replaced the centrifuge bowl used in intermittent device machines with a spinning separation channel that uses centrifugal forces to separate the various elements of the blood according to their specific gravity.
         (2) Based on specific gravity, the heaviest elements, erythrocytes, pack along the outer wall of the channel while the lighter plasma moves to the inner wall.
         (3) The "buffy coat," a layer that consists of all the white blood cells and platelets, forms between the erythrocytes and plasma (see Table 8.1).
      g. Advantages of using continuous centrifugal flow devices compared to membrane separation devices (Kiprov, Sanchez, & Pusey, 2014).
         (1) Lower blood flow rates.
         (2) Smaller extracorporeal blood volume.
         (3) More efficient separation leads to faster treatment times.
      h. Disadvantages.
         (1) Loss of platelets during TPE procedures.
         (2) Requires citrate anticoagulation. Continuous flow centrifugation treatments are primarily performed for patients in acute care settings and in hospital outpatient departments.

Table 8.1

Specific Gravity of Blood Components

Component	Specific Gravity (g/mL)
Plasma	1.025–1.029
Platelets	1.040
B-lymphocytes	1.050–1.060
T-lymphocytes	1.050–1.061
Blasts/promyelocytes	1.058–1.066
Monocytes	1.065–1.066
Myelocytes/basophils	1.070
Reticulocytes	1.078
Metamyelocytes	1.080
Bands and segmented neutrophils	1.087–.092
Erythrocytes	1.078–1.114

Zielinski, I (2002). Principles of apheresis. In C. Andrzejewski, P. Golden, B. Kong (et al.) (Eds.), *Principles of apheresis technology* (3rd ed., p. 36). Vancouver, BC: American Society for Apheresis. Used with permission.

2. Intermittent flow devices.
   a. A predetermined volume of whole blood is drawn from an access site into a spinning bowl-shaped device. When full, the desired blood component is siphoned off and the remaining components are returned to the patient, along with replacement fluid, if necessary, through the same venous access. This cycle is repeated several times until the desired amount of collected component is achieved.
   b. Intermittent devices, or discontinuous flow devices, are used almost exclusively for donor apheresis procedures with the exception of ECP procedures.
   c. The Haemonetics MCS® LN 9000 (Haemonetics, Braintree, Massachusetts) is occasionally used in the United States for TPE and is an intermittent flow centrifugal system.
   d. UVAR-XTS® cell separator (Therakos, Raritan, NJ), used only for extracorporeal photopheresis (ECP), is an intermittent flow device.
   e. Advantages of intermittent flow devices.
      (1) Single-needle vascular access option.
      (2) Variable extracorporeal blood volumes, depending on the bowl sizes available.
   f. Disadvantages of intermittent flow procedures.
      (1) Limited blood flow rates of approximately 30 to 60 mL/min.
      (2) The extended length of time needed to

process adequate amounts of whole blood in batches or cycles.
      (3) Hemodynamic instability in patients that can result from several cycles of whole blood volume depletion and reinfusion that is required with this type of device.
      (4) This potential for instability is a major reason intermittent flow devices are not the technology of choice for TPE.

B. Membrane filtration.
   1. Membrane filters separate plasma components according to their size.
   2. Membrane filtration used for plasma exchange is the result of technological advances made with hemodialysis membranes.
   3. Membrane filtration therapies focus on the ability of solute and fluid to move across a semipermeable membrane, which is customarily encased in plastic using either a hollow fiber or parallel plate design.
   4. The membrane filtration device works by pressure gradients across the membrane.
   5. Plasma separation filters.
      a. The hollow fiber filter is composed of a bundle of parallel single fibers, which resembles a straw with numerous holes in it, encased in a plastic cylinder.
      b. The patient's whole blood enters the filter under pressure, and as it flows through, plasma is squeezed out through the holes in the "straw."
      c. A more concentrated cell suspension exits at the other end.
      d. Whole blood enters the bottom port, cells go up and exit from the top port, and plasma withdraws from a side port.
      e. An additional side port is used to monitor pressures.
      f. The Plasmaflo® membrane (Asahi Medical Co. Ltd., Tokyo, Japan) is a filter made by a company that manufactures hemodialyzers. The membrane has a sieving coefficient (ratio of concentration in filtrate to blood) between 0.8 and 0.9 for albumin, IgG, IgA, IgM, C3, C4, fibrinogen, cholesterol, and triglycerides at blood flow of 100 mL per minute and a transmembrane pressure (TMP) of 40 mmHg (Kiprov, Burgstaler, & Sanchez, 2014).
      g. Plasauto®, Cascadeflo®, Plasorba®, and Immusorba® (Asahi Medical Co. Ltd., Tokyo, Japan) are all membrane filters produced by this same manufacturer.
         (1) These filters are not currently FDA approved in the United States but are widely used abroad.
         (2) Other filters or columns can be used in conjunction with the Plasmaflo® to remove

pathogenic substances from the separated plasma for a variety of diseases.

6. Two devices are FDA approved for plasma exchange with membrane separators.
   a. NxStage® (Nxstage Medical, Inc., Lawrence, MA) uses Plasmaflo® separator.
   b. Prismaflex® (Gambro, Lund, Sweden) uses Prismaflex 2000™ membrane separator.

7. Plasma membrane separators used in membrane filtration are capable of removing plasma and all of its dissolved elements. "The pore size of the membrane separator is 0.6 microns" (Zielinski, 2002). The other elements of a patient's whole blood are larger and therefore do not pass through the porous walls of the membrane (see Table 8.2).

8. Clearance of proteins will depend on where the fraction of a particular protein is located (i.e., intravascular or extravascular). When antibody subclasses are the target for removal, it is important to note that approximately 76% of IgM is found in the intravascular space while only 45% of IgG is intravascular (Weinstein, 2010).

9. Advantages of using membrane filtration technology.
   a. The equipment is often similar to the dialysis equipment nephrology nurses are familiar with.
      (1) Familiarity with membrane technology has led nephrology nurses into the care of patients for whom TPE is prescribed.
      (2) Similarity in the equipment is a common reason for establishing TPE programs in dialysis units.
   b. Since the membrane pore size does not allow cellular components to exit the patient's circulation, there is no platelet loss in waste plasma.
      (1) May be preferred equipment for patients with thrombocytopenia.
      (2) Many adsorption columns used for cascade procedures require that the plasma be free of cellular material.

Table 8.2

Size of Blood Components

Component	Diameter in Microns
Platelet	3 microns
Erythrocyte	7 microns
Lymphocyte	10 microns
Granulocyte	13 microns

Zielinski, I (2002). Principles of apheresis. In C. Andrzejewski, P. Golden, B. Kong (et al.) (Eds.), *Principles of apheresis technology* (3rd ed., p. 36). Vancouver, BC: American Society for Apheresis. Used with permission.

10. Disadvantages of using membrane separation devices.
    a. The primary disadvantage of using membrane separation devices is that it can only be used for plasma exchange since the membrane pore size is too small to allow for passage of any of the other blood components.
    b. Membrane separators are not as efficient at removing plasma as centrifugal devices because the red blood cells within the separator are damaged, causing hemolysis, if the hematocrit exiting the separator is too high. In comparison with centrifuge devices, more whole blood must be processed to extract the same amount of plasma, making procedures longer and blood flow rates higher.
    c. Higher blood flow rates require the use of central venous access catheters, whereas peripheral venous access can often be used with centrifugal devices.
    d. Higher blood flow rates can mean higher infusion rates of citrate anticoagulant, if used.
    e. Angiotensin-converting enzyme (ACE) inhibitor medications can cause significant adverse reactions in patients undergoing apheresis with membrane separators. Those medications should be held for 48 to 72 hours prior to initiating procedures with that technology.
    f. Membrane separators available in the United States are not recommended for treating patients with hyperviscosity due to paraproteinemia (such as Waldenstrom macroglobulinemia or cyroglobulinemia) because these devices "are not efficient in removing very large macromolecules" (Kiprov, Burgstaler, & Sanchez, 2014).

C. Secondary filtration devices.
   1. LDL apheresis devices available in the United States (Winters, 2011). There are two devices that use cascade or secondary filtration that are approved by the FDA for use in the United States for LDL removal. They are approved to treat patients with familial hypercholesterolemia (FH).
      a. The Liposorber LA-15® system on the MA03 apheresis device (Kaneka Pharma America LLC, New York, NY).
         (1) Uses a hollow fiber plasma separator and two dextran sulfate LDL adsorption columns.
         (2) Unlimited amount of plasma can be treated because columns are regenerated when saturated during the procedure.
         (3) Device-specific disposables.
         (4) Columns cannot be reused for subsequent treatments.

b. Heparin-Induced Extracorporeal Precipitation HELP® system on the Plasmat® Secura and Plasmat® Futura (B. Braun Medical, Bethlehem, PA).
   (1) Uses a hollow-fiber membrane plasma separator.
   (2) Removes LDL from separated plasma via a heparin-induced precipitation filter.
   (3) Device-specific disposables.
   (4) Filters cannot be reused.
c. Treatment specifics.
   (1) Heparin is used as the anticoagulant with both devices.
   (2) Patients requiring this therapy must continue treatment every 2 weeks for the duration of their lives.
   (3) No replacement fluid is required.
   (4) Treatment time is approximately 3 to 4 hours.
   (5) The volume of plasma processed through these LDL removal devices varies from patient to patient.
d. Indications for treatment of FH patients in the United States.
   (1) Heterozygous FH patients: LDL-C levels of ≥ 200 mg/dL who have a documented history of coronary heart disease (CHD).
   (2) Heterozygous patients: LDL-C levels of ≥ 300 mg/dL without CHD but refractory to cholesterol lowering medications.
   (3) Homozygous patients: LDL-C levels of ≥ 500 mg/dL.
e. Criteria for treatment of FH patients outside the United States have been developed by:
   (1) German Federal Committee of Physicians and Health Insurance Funds.
   (2) International Panel on Management of FH.
   (3) HEART-UK.
2. There are four additional LDL removal apheresis systems available outside the United States (Winters, 2011).
a. Plasmaselect system (Plasmaselect, Teterow, Germany).
   (1) Passes separated plasma through two columns containing sheep polyclonal antihuman apo B linked to Sepharose®.
   (2) Columns can be regenerated and reused, lowering cost per procedure.
   (3) Unlimited volume of plasma can be treated.
   (4) System exposes the patient to animal proteins.
b. Liposorba® D (Kaneka, Osaka, Japan) uses columns of dextran sulfate bound to cellulose.
   (1) Whole blood is passed through column – no plasma separation needed.
   (2) Columns cannot be regenerated, limiting volume treated.
   (3) Columns come in several sizes to treat larger volumes.
c. DALI system – Polyacrylamide Direct Perfusion (Fresenius-Kabi G, Bad Hömburg, Germany).
   (1) Whole blood is passed through the column – no plasma separation needed.
   (2) Columns cannot be regenerated; come in 750 mL and 1000 mL sizes. The patient's blood volume dictates which column to use.
d. Double filtration plasmapheresis (DFPP).
   (1) Passes separated plasma through a plasma fractionator (PF) with a pore size of 15 nm.
   (2) Requires a plasma heater in the system to prevent cryogel formation.
   (3) Used extensively worldwide (Winters, 2011).

III. Extracorporeal photopheresis (ECP). Originally termed *extracorporeal photochemotherapy* (Ward, 2011).

A. Method of collecting, altering, and reinfusing a patient's white blood cells (WBCs) to cause down-regulation of T-lymphocyte activity.
   1. ECP machines collect buffy coat in a storage bag while returning the remaining blood components to the patient.
   2. After collection is complete, 8-methoxypsoralen is injected into the collection bag and mixed with the cells.
   3. The cells are then exposed to ultraviolet A (UVA) light. Photoactivated psoralens cause cross-linking of DNA in cell nuclei. This damage induces lymphocytes to undergo programmed cell death (apoptosis) (Ward, 2011, p. 277).
   4. The cells are then reinfused into the patient resulting in down-regulation of active T-cell clones.

B. Used in diseases that are mediated by cytotoxic T-lymphocytes.
   1. Originally used in cutaneous T-cell lymphoma (CTCL) (Edelson et al., 1987).
      a. CTCL is the only FDA approved indication for ECP in the United States.
      b. It is used off-label for conditions listed below.
   2. Also used in graft vs. host disease (GvHD) following allogeneic stem cell transplant, including pediatric patients undergoing transplant (Chan, 2006; Kanold et al., 2005). Although use of ECP for GvHD and heart transplant rejection is not approved by the FDA, it is reimbursed by the Centers for Medicare and Medicaid Services (CMS).
   3. Used to treat cellular rejection of solid organ transplants (heart, lung, liver, kidney).

4. Also being tried for certain diseases with suspected cell-mediated autoimmunity, such as pemphigus vulgaris and Crohn's disease (Bladon & Taylor, 1999; Scarisbrick, 2009; Ward, 2011).

IV. Clinical applications of therapeutic apheresis.

A. Indications for treatment. Guidelines for indications of therapeutic apheresis (TA) were developed by the American Medical Association (AMA) in 1985. These guidelines have been further refined by the American Society for Apheresis (ASFA) and are updated regularly as new evidence appears in the literature. For the most current listing of diseases and their categories, see http://www.apheresis.org for the *Journal of Clinical Apheresis*, Vol. 28, Issue 3, 2013, "Special Issue: Clinical Applications of Therapeutic Apheresis: An Evidence Based Approach, 6th edition. As per the latest edition of the guidelines, published in 2013, the indications for TA treatment are divided into four categories (Schwartz et al., 2013).
   1. Category I. Disorders for which apheresis is accepted as first-line therapy, either as a primary stand-alone treatment or in conjunction with other modes of treatment.
      a. Example: Plasma exchange in Guillian-Barre syndrome as first-line stand-alone therapy.
      b. Example: Plasma exchange in myasthenia gravis as first line in conjunction with immuno-suppression and cholinesterase inhibition.
   2. Category II. Disorders for which apheresis is accepted as second-line therapy, either as a stand-alone treatment or in conjunction with other modes of treatment.
      a. Example: Plasma exchange as stand-alone secondary treatment for acute disseminated encephalomyelitis after high-dose IV corticosteroid failure.
      b. Example: ECP added to corticosteroids for unresponsive chronic graft-vs.-host-disease.
   3. Category III. Optimum role of apheresis therapy is not established.
      a. Decision making should be individualized.
      b. Example: Plasma exchange in patients with sepsis and multiorgan system failure.
   4. Category IV. Disorders in which published evidence demonstrates or suggests apheresis to be ineffective or harmful.
      a. IRB approval is desirable if apheresis treatment is undertaken in these circumstances.
      b. Example: Plasma exchange for active rheumatoid arthritis.

B. Role of plasmapheresis in renal disorders (Kiprov, Sanchez, & Pusey, 2014).
   1. Thrombotic thrombocytopenic purpura (TTP) and hemolytic uremic syndrome (HUS) both lead to microangiopathy. (See Chapter 2 for more complete description of TTP/HUS.)
      a. HUS primarily affects kidneys, while TTP frequently affects the central nervous system.
      b. In severe TTP, TPE should begin as soon as possible and continue until platelet count is normalized, hemolysis ceases, and lactate dehydrogenase (LDH) is below 400 IU/L (Kiprov, Sanchez, & Pusey, 2014).
   2. Antiglomerular basement nembrane (GBM) disease.
      a. Early use of TPE is indicated since response to therapy is highest when serum creatinine is low (< 500 µmol/L).
      b. In dialysis-dependent patients, TPE is usually reserved for patients with pulmonary hemorrhage. Kidney function is unlikely to recover (Kiprov, Sanchez, & Pusey, 2014).
   3. Antineutrophil cytoplasm antibody (ANCA)-associated vasculitis.
      a. Small vessel vasculitis affecting kidneys with pauci-immune rapidly progressive glomerulonephritis (RPGN).
      b. Include granulomatosis with polyangiitis, microscopic polyangiitis, and eosinophilic granulomatosis with polyangiitis.
   4. Multiple myeloma.
      a. Can lead to kidney impairment, especially light chain cast nephropathy.
      b. TPE can be used in combination with chemotherapy.
   5. Systemic lupus erythematosus (SLE) – in lupus nephritis.
      a. TPE removes circulating autoantibodies and immune complexes.
      b. May be used in life-threatening crescentic nephritis, pulmonary hemorrhage, cerebral lupus, or catastrophic antiphospholipid syndrome.
   6. Henoch-Schönlein purpura (HSP) and IgA nephropathy.
      a. Have similar features to ANCA-associated vasculitis.
      b. TPE used in combination with immunosuppressive medication.
   7. Hyperviscosity syndromes.
      a. Can be seen with Waldenstrom macroglobulinemia, cyroglobulinemia, and myeloma.
      b. Leads to ischemic dysfunction of organs due to red blood cell aggregation.
      c. TPE used to reduce viscosity and improve blood flow.

Table 8.3

Prominent Indications for TPE

Indication	Disease/Syndrome
Auto-antibody	TTP, myasthenia gravis (MG), Guillain-Barre syndrome (GBS), neuromyelitis optic (NMO), anti-GBM, Goodpasture syndrome, ANCA-associated glomerulonephritis, Wegener's granulomatosis, antiphospholipid crisis, etc.
Probable auto-antibody	Chronic inflammatory demyelinating polyradiculoneuropathy (CIDP), multiple sclerosis (MS), etc.
Antigen-antibody complexes	Hepatitis C vasculitis, systemic lupus erythematosus, etc.
Allo-antibody	Transplant sensitization, transplant rejection (humoral), transfusion reactions, etc.
Paraprotiens	Wandenstrom's hyperviscosity, light-chain neuropathy, light-chain glomerulopathy, myeloma cast nephropathy, etc.
Non-Ig proteins	Focal segmental glomerulosclerosis (FSGS)
Endogenous toxins	Hypercholesterolemia, liver failure, systemic inflammatory response syndrome (SIRS), etc.
Exogenous poisons	Amantia (mushroom), drugs, etc.

Source: Ward, D.M. (2011). Conventional apheresis therapies: A review. *Journal of Clinical Apheresis, 26,* 230-238. Used with permission from Wiley.

8. Cryoglobulinemia.
   a. Often associated with hepatitis C.
   b. TPE removes large immune complexes.
9. Focal segmental glomerulosclerosis (FSGS).
   a. Recurrent in kidney transplants – may be caused by circulating factor which increases glomerular permeability.
   b. TPE is used after a kidney transplant to improve graft survival. (Kiprov, Sanchez, & Pusey, 2014).

C. Role of TPE in kidney transplantation. TPE is aimed at removal of donor specific antibodies (DSA) and is used to improve access to transplantation as well as the graft survival for recipients who are negatively cross-matched with the donor organ (George et al., 2011).
   1. Pretransplant. TPE is used to desensitize the patient by removing DSA, usually anti-HLA antibodies, to prevent hyperacute rejection.
      a. Successful treatment results in conversion from positive to negative crossmatch.
      b. Can also be used to reduce anti-ABO antibodies in cases of blood type incompatibility.
      c. Immunoadsorption columns can also be used to remove anti-ABO antibodies, where available.
   2. Posttransplant. TPE used to "remove pathogenic antibodies presumed to contribute to antibody

mediated rejection (AMR)" in conjunction with other therapies, such as IV gammaglobulin and immunosuppressing medication regimens, aimed at reducing the production of these antibodies (George et al., 2011).

D. Prominent indications for TPE (see Table 8.3) (Ward, 2011).

V. Total plasma exchange considerations.

A. Importance of estimating total blood volume (TBV) and plasma volume (PV) (Tronier et al., 2010).
   1. These calculations are used to determine the dose or volume of plasma to be exchanged in TPE procedures.
   2. Typically, 1.0 to 1.5 times the patient's PV is exchanged.
   3. The physician may decide to increase or decrease PV exchanged for a variety of clinical reasons.
   4. The larger the amount of plasma exchanged, the longer the procedure will take, exposing the patient to more citrate anticoagulant, possible side effects, and potential adverse events.
   5. TBV is used as an endpoint in platelet depletion procedures and white blood cell depletion and collection procedures. Typically, 2.0 TBVs are processed for these procedures.

6. TBV and the hematocrit (Hct) are used to calculate the patient's red blood cell volume when performing RBCX procedures.

7. *Important to note*: TBV is used by many machines to calculate the maximum citrate infusion rate delivered to the patient during TA procedures.

B. Calculation of estimated TBV and PV (Tronier et al., 2010).

1. Centrifuge devices have software installed to calculate TBV and PV, but those calculations are dependent upon the correct input of the patient's gender, height, weight, and hematocrit.

2. The following formulas are based on actual patient weight. In very obese or edematous patients, the weight may need to be adjusted to the ideal body weight.

3. Formulas for estimated TBV.
   a. Estimated TBV by age and weight.
      (1) Patient ≥ 12 years: TBV = Weight (kg) x 70 mL for males.
      (2) Patient ≥ 12 years: TBV = Weight (kg) x 65 mL for females.
      (3) Patient 3 months–12 years: TBV = Weight (kg) x 70 to 75mL.
      (4) Patient 0–3 months: TBV = Weight (kg) x 80 to 90 mL.
      (5) Premature infant: TBV = Weight (kg) x 90 to 105 mL.
   b. Nadler's formula is for adults only and is based on patient height in inches, actual patient weight in pounds and gender.
      (1) Males: TBV (mL) = (0.006012 x Height^3 [in]) + (14.6 x Weight [lb]) + 604.
      (2) Females: TBV (mL) = (0.005835 x Height^3 [in]) + (15 x Weight [lb]) + 183.

4. Formula for calculating PV (Tronier et al., 2010).
   a. PV (mL) = TBV (mL) x (100 – Hct)
   b. Example: Patient = 70 kg, Hct = 42%
      TBV = 70 kg x 70 mL= 4900 mL
      PV = 4900 mL x (100 – 42) = 2842 mL or 2.8 L.

5. The volume of plasma exchanged during the TPE treatment is selected based on the desired percent of disease mediator removed. Because the plasma is continuously removed and replaced throughout the procedure, the larger the plasma volume processed, the less efficient is the removal of the patient's original plasma. For removal rates of intravascular plasma constituents per PV multiples removed, see Table 8.4 (Tronier et al., 2010).
   a. Recirculation in the TPE circuit, redistribution between intravascular and extravascular spaces, and other factors may result in less than calculated clearances (Weinstein, 2010).
   b. Typically, 1.0 to 1.5 PV is exchanged.

Table 8.4

Removal Rates of Intravascular Plasma

Plasma Volumes Exchanged	% Disease Mediator Removed
0.5	39
1.0	63
1.5	78
2.0	86
2.5	92

Source: Tronier, W., Goodfellow, E., & Larson, K. (2010). Apheresis math and useful physical constants. In Linz, W. (Ed.), *Principles of apheresis technology* (4th ed., pp. 101-106). Vancouver, B.C.: American Society for Apheresis. Used with permission.

c. Some rebound effect may be observed within 24 to 48 hours after a TPE treatment (Dau, 1995; Weinstein, 2010).

C. Treatment considerations for TPE.
1. Diagnosis.
   a. Proper diagnosis is critical to the successful incorporation of TPE into the treatment regimen. Refer to the ASFA guidelines as mentioned in Sec. V(A) (Schwartz et al., 2013).
   b. Physician must determine if the patient's diagnosis warrants TPE therapy and if the patient can tolerate the procedure (Chhibber & King, 2010).
   c. The timing of the initial TPE treatment course, the length of the treatment course, the target treatment parameters, the appropriate replacement fluids, and the optimal vascular access option are all decisions that must be made by the ordering physician based on the patient's diagnosis and clinical picture.

2. Amount of plasma to be removed in TPE procedures (TPE dose).
   a. TPE is a treatment prescribed by volume, not by time. Typically, it is ordered as a multiple of the patient's PV or as a set volume (e.g., 3,500 mL).
   b. As noted in Table 8.4 , the efficiency of plasma component removal decreases dramatically beyond one PV exchange.
   c. Additionally, there is no evidence that demonstrates any clinical benefit to performing TPE more than once in 24 hours.

d. In plasmapheresis procedures other than TPE, the volume of plasma processed will depend on the procedure and the device used.

3. Frequency of treatments.

   a. The schedule for treatment is dictated by the patient's disease and may change depending on the patient's response to therapy.

   b. The physician, in deciding the number and frequency of TPE treatments, is guided by the American Society for Apheresis (ASFA) *Clinical Applications of Therapeutic Apheresis Guidelines* for the particular disease being treated (Schwartz et al., 2013).

4. Replacement fluids for TPE.

   a. 5% albumin.
      (1) The preferred replacement fluid for patients without coagulation problems.
      (2) Blood volume expander, containing plasma proteins but not clotting factors or immunoglobulins (Kiprov, Sanchez, & Pusey, 2014).
      (3) When using citrate anticoagulant, calcium replacement may be added to albumin replacement fluid to supplement the patient's calcium bound by citrate. There is no risk of clot formation.
      (4) Incidence of reactions and disease transmission are rare compared to fresh frozen plasma (FFP) and cryoprecipitate reduced plasma (CRP). It can be used whenever the replacement of clotting factors is not necessary.
      (5) If only 25% albumin is available, care must be taken that the only diluent used is 0.9% sodium chloride solution, since mixing with any other solution can cause hemolysis when infused into patients in large quantities.
      (6) Can be stored at room temperature (Kiprov, Sanchez, & Pusey, 2014).

   b. Fresh frozen plasma (FFP).
      (1) FFP is the fluid portion of whole blood and contains all of the coagulation factors and plasma proteins present in whole blood, including immunoglobulins and complement (Kiprov, Sanchez, & Pusey, 2014).
      (2) FFP is used in diseases and situations requiring the immediate replacement of clotting factors such as reduced fibrinogen levels, preoperatively, and before and after solid organ biopsy.
      (3) FFP is used as replacement fluid in TTP because the patient has a deficiency of effective von Willebrand Factor (vWF) cleaving metaloprotease (ADAMTS13) that is replaced with FFP (Weinstein, 2010).

      (4) FFP is preserved with citrate to prevent clotting. Using FFP as a replacement fluid increases the amount of citrate delivered to the patient during TPE. Adjustment to the rate of citrate infusion from the blood circuit is necessary to prevent citrate toxicity.
      (5) Calcium replacement should not be added directly to FFP, as it will bind with the citrate and allow fibrin clots to form within the FFP.
      (6) Must be ABO compatible with patient (Kiprov, Sanchez, & Pusey, 2014).

   c. Cryoprecipitate-reduced plasma (CRP) (Smith, 2010).
      (1) Also termed "cryo-poor plasma" and "cryoprecipitate-poor plasma." CRP is that fraction of plasma remaining after the removal of cryoprecipitable proteins.
      (2) The fibrinogen, factor VIII, factor XIII, fibronectin, and large multimers of vWF have been removed (Tronier et al., 2010).
      (3) In patients unresponsive to TPE with FFP, the physician may decide either to switch to CRP alone or a combination of FFP and CRP as replacement fluids (Smith, 2010).

   d. Normal saline.
      (1) Normal saline is used to prime disposable circuits and may be administered to wash or clear the plasma separation membrane of proteins, to treat hypotension with a fluid bolus, and to assist with reinfusion of the patient's blood at the end of treatment.
      (2) Normal saline is used as an adjunct with other replacement fluids but not used as the primary replacement fluid since it does not provide any of the components of plasma.

   e. Other solutions.
      (1) A combination of any of these replacement fluids can be ordered depending on the patient's medical condition, fluid status, and/or response to treatment.
      (2) In situations where patients are, or chronically become, hypotensive early in a TPE treatment, a bolus of normal saline or a small amount of 25% albumin may be administered before the procedure to maintain hemodynamic stability during TPE.

5. Anticoagulation. An anticoagulation solution is routinely used during TPE procedures with centrifugal devices to prevent clotting in the extracorporeal circuit.

   a. Anticoagulant citrate dextrose, Formula A (ACD-A®).
      (1) ACD-A® is a citrate-based anticoagulant that contains dextrose, 2.2 g/dL of sodium citrate, and 0.73 g/dL of citric acid.

(2) Citrate works as an anticoagulant by binding to calcium and thereby blocking the clotting cascade.

(3) Citrate is metabolized to bicarbonate by the mitochondria of the liver, kidneys, and muscle (Winters et al., 2011).

(4) ACD-A® is prescribed as a ratio infusion of whole blood to anticoagulant. For example: the COBE Spectra® has a default ratio of 10:1 for TPE procedures, which means for every 10 revolutions of the inlet flow pump, the anticoagulant (AC) pump will turn once.

(5) During TPE, approximately 80% to 90% of the citrate anticoagulant solution added to the extracorporeal circuit goes into the plasma waste bag, depending on the device used. The patient receives only 10% to 20% of the total amount of citrate added to the extracorporeal circuit.

(6) Patients with active bleeding problems, low platelet and HCT values, or liver or kidney dysfunction may need a higher anticoagulant ratio to reduce the exposure to citrate.

(7) Approximately 14% of the total volume of each unit of FFP used as replacement fluid is citrate. The citrate infusion rate to the patient can be managed by lowering the whole blood flow rate when using FFP as a replacement fluid to reduce the citrate delivered to the patient from the extracorporeal circuit (Kiprov, Sanchez, & Pusey, 2014).

(8) Citrate can temporarily lower the ionized calcium level causing symptoms as mild as perioral paresthesia and as severe as tetany, seizures, and cardiac dysfunction, necessitating IV calcium replacement.

(9) Patients with liver or kidney disease may have impaired citrate metabolism and are at an increased risk for citrate toxicity. Lowering the citrate infusion rate to the patient is done by lowering the whole blood pump flow rate.

b. Heparin (used with membrane filtration) in adult TPE treatments.

(1) At the start of a TPE treatment with membrane filtration, a heparin bolus is often administered prefilter.

(a) Heparinization requirements vary according to the patient's platelet count.

(b) Patients with significant kidney dysfunction and/or qualitative and possibly quantitative platelet defects may benefit from a small heparin bolus.

(c) Patients who have platelet counts > 0.5 million/mm^3 may require additional heparin.

(2) After the initial heparin bolus, the blood flow through a plasma membrane separation device is established between 100 and 150 mL/min and a heparin infusion may be started to maintain continuing anticoagulation. Orders may include the following.

(a) Continuous infusion dosage/hour.

(b) ACT goals.

(c) ACT threshold for increasing heparin infusion dose/hour.

(d) Threshold for ceasing heparin infusion.

(e) Frequency of monitoring ACT levels.

(f) When to stop heparin infusion prior to treatment termination.

(3) With centrifugal instruments that normally use only citrate as an anticoagulant, some heparin in combination with citrate may be used in certain situations, either given as a bolus or added to the citrate infusion bag.

(a) Patients acutely sensitive to citrate or unable to quickly metabolize citrate due to liver and/or kidney failure.

(b) Some pediatric patients.

(c) When added to the citrate infusion bag, the ratio of citrate to whole blood is increased to deliver less citrate.

6. Fluid balance considerations.

a. Apheresis instruments differ in the manner that they calculate fluid balance. Some machines, i.e., COBE SPECTRA® and AS104®, do not include the rinseback volume or saline boluses in the calculation, while most newer instruments, such as the Spectra Optia® and COM.TEC®, do. It is important to know how fluid balance is managed by the specific instrument being used in order to enter the appropriate fluid balance parameter for each patient and procedure.

b. The patient's condition determines the fluid balance parameters ordered for each TPE treatment.

c. Adjustments to a patient's fluid balance of more than ± 5% should be avoided because the fluid being removed/replaced contains large amounts of plasma proteins.

d. Unlike hemodialysis or ultrafiltration, which removes water and electrolytes, removal of a large quantity of plasma protein can seriously compromise the ability of a patient to maintain sufficient intravascular oncotic pressure to support blood pressure.

7. Medication considerations.

a. Premedications are often recommended before

infusing large quantities of FFP or CRP as plasma replacement fluid, and prior to infusing packed red blood cells during RBCX.
(1) Used to prevent or mitigate transfusion reactions.
(2) To treat the signs and symptoms of transfusion reactions.
(3) The medications can include (Kiprov, Sanchez, & Pusey, 2014):
  (a) Diphenhydramine hydrochloride, an antihistamine, given either IV or orally.
  (b) Hydrocortisone IV or methylprednisolone IV.
  (c) H2 antagonists such as cimetidine or IV.
  (d) Prednisone, given orally.
  (e) Acetaminophen, given orally.
  (f) "In patients with persistent moderate-to-severe allergic reactions despite premedication, a continuous infusion of 50 to 100 mg of diphenhydramine in 100 to 250 mL of saline during TA might be considered" (Chhibber & King, 2010).
  (g) Premedications are usually not needed when using albumin as the replacement fluid.
b. Medications used to prevent and treat citrate toxicity during TPE procedures include:
  (1) 10% calcium gluconate. It is the preferred medication since it is one third the strength of calcium chloride and does not need dilution before administering.
  (2) It can be added directly to the 5% albumin bottles but not directly to the bags of FFP/CRP.
  (3) When using FFP/CRP, the 10% calcium gluconate can be given in small increments through a port, via a stopcock, or preferably, as a slow, continuous infusion piggybacked at the point on the tubing set close to reinfusion.
  (4) Calcium chloride, 10%, can be used with caution when calcium gluconate is not available.
    (a) "It has three times as much calcium per unit of volume calcium gluconate" (Chhibber & King, 2010).
    (b) Can cause tissue damage if extravasation occurs (Winters et al., 2011). Therefore, it should not be administered via a peripheral IV line, but only via a central line (Chhibber & King, 2010).
  (5) "Frequent monitoring of ionized calcium is recommended for patients with severe liver failure" (Chhibber & King, 2010).
c. Evaluation of patient's current medications for

potential removal during TPE. Focus is on the timing of administration of medications and whether dose adjustment may be needed (Ibrihim & Balogun, 2013).
(1) Few clinical studies have been done to assess specific medication removal during plasma exchange. Many factors affect drug removal including the volume of exchange, the frequency of exchange, and the length of the procedure (Crookston & Novak, 2010).
  (a) "If a drug exerts its desired effect quickly, then removal by TPE may not be as clinically important, i.e., rituximab. However, waiting as long as possible after administration of this type of drug is advised" (Crookston & Novak, 2010).
  (b) Caution should be taken when performing TPE on patients undergoing chemotherapy. No data is available on the ways TPE might affect the course of treatment (Crookston & Novak, 2010).
(2) If a medication has a low volume of distribution and a high affinity for plasma proteins, then the medication is more likely to be partially removed by TPE and should be administered after plasma exchange. Drug infusion and the extravascular distribution phase should be complete before initiating TPE.
(3) Medications distributed outside of the plasma.
  (a) Many of the medications routinely given to dialysis and apheresis patients are not bound to plasma proteins and have a higher volume of distribution, meaning that the medications migrate into the extravascular tissues and cells.
  (b) Any medication that is within a blood cell will not be eliminated with the plasma and little is removed by TPE. Example: Tacrolimus.
(4) Frequency of administration.
  (a) The frequency of medication administration can influence how quickly a medication is distributed in the plasma volume and how effectively it is removed during TPE.
  (b) Medications taken once a day should be taken after a TPE procedure.
  (c) Medications taken at more frequent intervals have a better chance of being distributed into the extravascular tissues and are less likely to be removed during TPE.

(5) Some medications recommended for administration after TPE.
  (a) Prednisone, cyclosporine, cyclophosphamide, azathioprine, IV gammaglobulin (IVIG), thymoglobulin, basiliximab, heparin, lepirudin, digoxin, and propranolol.
  (b) Data suggests that the dosing of these medications need not be adjusted (Chhibber & King, 2010).
  (c) IV antibiotics should be administered after TPE when possible (Kintzel et al., 2003).
(6) Patients taking angiotensin-converting enzyme (ACE) inhibitors within a 24-hour period before TPE, especially when using a membrane separation device, can develop bradykinin reactions, exhibiting hypotensive, bradycardic episodes with accompanying symptoms of flushing, nausea, and vomiting. ACE inhibitors must be held for 24 to 72 hours before TPE with membrane separators.

8. Laboratory data.
  a. Specific lab test samples should be collected shortly before the initiation of TPE and/or 2 to 4 hours after the procedure is terminated.
  b. Lab tests are ordered according to the patient's diagnosis and medical condition.
    (1) All patients require a CBC prior to TPE procedures. A pretreatment HCT is needed for several reasons.
      (a) It is needed to calculate an accurate PV.
      (b) It is required for the automatic setting of plasma pump flow rates on certain instruments that control interface levels without optical interface detectors.
      (c) It is used to determine if the citrate-to-whole-blood ratio can be adjusted. Patients with low Hct and platelet levels need less citrate for effective anticoagulation.
      (d) It is needed to ensure that the patient can tolerate a small decrease in red cell volume that occurs when the patient's blood is in the extracorporeal circuit. A drop in red cell volume of > 15% can result in hypoxia. In this case, the circuit can be primed with packed RBCs to offset the decrease in intra-procedure Hct (Chhibber & King, 2010).
    (2) Chemistry panel results, especially calcium, potassium, and magnesium, allow clinicians the opportunity to correct deficiencies prior to treatment initiation.
      (a) Calcium levels in particular are helpful when determining if and how much calcium replacement may be needed during the procedure.
      (b) Citrate anticoagulation and plasma removal can affect serum calcium, potassium, and magnesium levels; these electrolytes are reduced during PE when the replacement fluid is other than FFP or CRP.
    (3) Coagulation panel data is needed to assess the patient's risk of bleeding and/or anticoagulation therapy status.
    (4) Metabolic panel data is needed to assess the patient's hepatic and kidney function. This is particularly important when evaluating the patient's ability to metabolize citrate anticoagulant.
    (5) Some disease specific labs tests include:
      (a) For TTP – ADAMTS13, lactate dehydrogenase (LDH), and reticulocytes.
      (b) For myasthenia gravis (MG) – anti-acetylcholine receptor antibodies.
      (c) For Goodpasture syndrome – Anti-GBM antibodies (Chhibber & King, 2010).

9. Assessment of pretreatment vital signs.
  a. An elevated temperature may indicate a systemic infection or one related to central line placement. Determining the cause of fever pretreatment can prevent untoward and adverse events.
    (1) Using an infected central catheter can circulate local pathogens throughout a patient's vascular system and cause sepsis that can be dangerous, difficult, and costly to treat.
    (2) TPE can cause immunosuppression as a result of the removal of antibodies, placing the patient at risk for opportunistic infections.
    (3) Physician orders should indicate the threshold of change from the baseline vital signs that require physician notification during TPE.
    (4) The physician should always be notified preprocedure if the patient is febrile.
  b. Pretreatment blood pressure (BP) must be high enough to tolerate the expected BP drop at the start of the TA procedure due to volume shifts.
    (1) A bolus of normal saline or a small amount of 25% or 5% albumin may be infused to increase the patient's blood pressure to an acceptable starting range.
    (2) Physician orders should include a limited number and/or volume of normal saline boluses for patient hypotension.

(3) Some apheresis instruments have the option of either diverting or infusing the prime saline at the beginning of the procedure. For unstable or hypotensive patients, the option to infuse the prime saline should be considered.

c. Respiratory assessment should be performed prior to a TA procedure to determine the patient's ability to adequately oxygenate and to check for signs of fluid overload. As the procedure begins, the patient's hematocrit will lower slightly as red blood cells enter and remain in the extracorporeal circuit.

(1) Monitor respiratory response to the lowered Hct throughout the procedure.

(2) Critically ill or unstable patients may require oxygen prior to treatment to boost oxygen saturation levels and prevent respiratory distress.

(3) Patients with certain neurological syndromes may be particularly prone to respiratory insufficiency or failure and should be closely observed during TPE. These patients include those diagnosed with MG and GBS.

d. Heart rate and rhythm should be evaluated for preexisting arrhythmias, including tachycardia and bradycardia, so that these conditions are not confused with adverse events that may be caused by the procedure. Special attention should be given to patients with a history of cardiovascular disease as citrate toxicity can decrease cardiac output.

VI. Procedure considerations.

A. Initial patient assessment.
1. Before installing the disposable set, it is important to ensure that the vascular access is adequate and usable.
   a. Ensure that the central venous catheter has been medically cleared for use, is properly positioned, and is patent and functioning well.
   b. If peripheral veins are to be used, perform a visual assessment of all suitable vascular options.
2. A complete body systems assessment should be performed with the patient's diagnosis used to focus on specific system-related abnormalities, such as kidney, integument, cardiac, and neuromuscular.
3. The patient's and family's knowledge of the disease state, planned therapy, and planned course of therapy should be evaluated and appropriate education provided.
4. Evaluate, document, and monitor the patient's emotional and cognitive response to treatment,

including pain assessment from the catheter site, as well as any pain caused by the patient's medical condition.

5. Document the patient's weight and vital signs. Included in the assessment of a critically ill patient also may be hemodynamic parameters, such as central venous pressure, pulmonary capillary wedge pressure, and cardiac output.

6. The most recent laboratory data should be reviewed, as discussed above.

7. Fluid balance assessment.
   a. If either volume deficit or excess is present, it may require hydration or ultrafiltration before commencing TA.
   b. TPE is best delivered as an isovolemic procedure. If more plasma is removed than replaced, the patient may become hypoalbuminemic, which can lead to undesirable extravascular fluid shifts.
   c. Administration of extra fluid during TPE to support blood pressure usually does not present problems unless the patient has kidney dysfunction.

8. Review pertinent diagnostic tests or exams before starting TA (e.g., pulmonary function test, electrocardiogram, peripheral nerve studies, and neuromuscular reflexes).

9 All current medications should be reviewed, including PRN and IV medications.
   a. IV medications, with the exception of calcium replacement, are not routinely administered just before and during TPE because they may be removed by plasma exchange. These can include antibiotics and pain medications.
   b. Confer with the patient's physician, primary care nurse, and pharmacist about scheduling specific medications in relation to TPE.
   c. TA procedures other than TPE do not remove medications.

B. Vascular access (see Module 3, Chapter 3, for additional information on vascular access).
1. Peripheral veins.
   a. Ideally, bilateral antecubital veins are used for blood access and return.
      (1) At times, other veins in the patient's forearms may be used.
      (2) The access, or draw needle, cannot be smaller than 17 gauge.
      (3) Most needles used for peripheral vein cannulation are 15- or 17-gauge steel needles with a back-eye for smooth blood flow.
      (4) The return line needle or catheter, if using a smaller vein in the arm, can be slightly smaller, but anything smaller than a

19-gauge needle can cause lysis of red blood cells (RBC).

(5) The needles must be able to sustain minimum blood flow rates of 40 to 50 mL/min and substantial positive or negative pressure for several hours.

    (a) Using peripheral veins in the feet and legs are contraindicated due to the high risk of blood clots.

    (b) Arteries are very rarely accessed due to the risk of complications secondary to infiltration and thrombosis.

    (c) Risks associated with inserting peripheral catheters.

        i. Hematoma.

        ii. Uncontrolled bleeding.

        iii. Infection at the insertion site.

        iv. Thrombi or emboli formation during the treatment that can travel and cause ischemic damage to other organs.

    (d) When antecubital veins are used, pressure is held for several minutes after the needle is removed and a gauze pad secured over the site.

(6) Using either topical or injectable local anesthesia at the venipuncture sites adds comfort and reduces anxiety for patients and can aid in reducing anxiety-induced vaso-vagal reactions.

(7) Patients with peripheral neuropathy or vasculitis are poor candidates for peripheral access. Pain and the lack of adequate venous blood vessels make catheters a better choice.

2. Nontunneled central venous catheter (CVC).

  a. A double lumen, nontunneled CVC placed in the internal jugular, subclavian, or femoral vein may be used short term, but should be monitored closely for signs of infection.

    (1) Follow manufacturer's recommendation or facility policy for care and maintenance of catheter.

    (2) A femoral vein catheter is difficult to keep clean and is susceptible to kinking and infection. However, for patients presenting with dangerously low platelet counts, femoral catheters can be safer to insert than either subclavian or jugular catheters because bleeding at the insertion site can be managed more effectively with direct pressure.

    (3) Often CVC are removed because of kinking or clotting problems that inhibit adequate blood flow.

    (4) Double lumen dialysis catheters with a

third, smaller, lumen for use as a central IV line are also available, but their use is discouraged because of the additional risk of infection that the third lumen poses.

  b. Peripherally inserted central catheter (PICC) and "power PICC" lines are too small and flexible for use during a TPE procedure.

3. Tunneled CVC.

  a. Long-term catheters are tunneled beneath the skin to increase patient comfort and reduce complications.

    (1) The double lumen tunneled catheter has a cuff. As the tissue grows into the cuff, it produces a barrier that prevents bacteria from invading the tunnel.

    (2) A tunneled CVC may be inserted into a jugular or subclavian vein and tunneled into the upper chest near the collarbone.

  b. The tunneled, cuffed catheters are usually composed of silicone or polyurethane composites. These composites are softer than polyurethane but are stronger than silicone to allow larger lumen sizes able to withstand higher pressures from blood flow.

  c. Double lumen implanted ports can also be used for patients requiring long-term, chronic apheresis. However, some ports may require declotting prior to each use.

  d. Check with the individual catheter manufacturer to determine safe durations for each access device.

4. Sites for placement (Chhibber & King, 2010).

  a. The CVC may be placed in the internal jugular, femoral, or subclavian veins.

  b. The internal jugular is the vein of choice. However, circumstances may dictate that another vein be cannulated.

  c. Patients needing both hemodialysis and apheresis on a long-term basis benefit from early placement of an arteriovenous (AV) graft or fistula.

5. CVC complications.

  a. Hemothorax, pneumothorax, and/or air embolisms can result from improper insertion of a CVC.

  b. Puncture of the femoral vein during insertion of a CVC may lead to a retroperitoneal hemorrhage.

  c. Bleeding at the insertion site may occur with any CVC.

    (1) Pressure applied at the CVC exit site to stop bleeding can kink the tubing and make the catheter unusable.

    (2) Special care should be taken when using sand bags to apply pressure to these fragile catheter insertion sites.

(3) For an internal jugular or a subclavian vein catheter, position the patient with the head of the bed (HOB) elevated at least 45 degrees for the first 24 hours after catheter placement to decrease bleeding from intravascular pressure at the site.

(4) An ice pack can be applied to the exit site to help stop oozing after line placement.

(5) Patients with coagulopathy disorders may need platelet infusions due to the amount of oozing from the CVC site.

d. An infected catheter can suspend or delay TPE treatments until the patient has completed a course of antibiotics and is able to receive a new vascular access device.

6. Arteriovenous (AV) fistula or graft.

a. The patient with maintenance TPE needs may benefit from a more permanent vascular access, i.e., AV fistula/graft.

b. A native AV fistula or synthetic graft may be cannulated with the access needle pointing either with or against the direction of blood flow and the return needle pointing with the direction of blood flow in the vascular access.

c. The needles ideally are placed at least 2 inches apart to reduce recirculation of blood.

d. When accessing a fistula/graft, the nurse must avoid aneurysms, curves, and flat spots; the tip of the needle should be at least 1.5 inches away from the anastomosis.

e. Complications include thrombosis, infection, aneurysms, venous hypertension, and local bleeding.

f. When removing the needles from this type of access, gentle pressure will stop bleeding while not occluding blood flow.

g. After hemostasis occurs, a dressing is secured over the needle site.

C. Intraprocedure monitoring and patient care.

1. Vital signs and cardiac and equipment monitoring.

a. After the extracorporeal circuit is established, the patient's vital signs are measured within the first few minutes of treatment to assess the patient's response to the initiation of TPE.

b. Vital signs are monitored and documented every 15 to 30 minutes or as necessary during the treatment.

c. Pump flow rates, citrate infusion rate to the patient, or other anticoagulation parameters such as ACT results, cumulative volumes, and system pressure readings should be monitored and documented every 15 to 30 minutes or per institution protocol.

d. When using a centrifugal device, the extracorporeal circuit is established with a blood flow rate that should not exceed the citrate infusion rate recommended by the device manufacturer and the threshold of patient symptoms of citrate tolerance.

e. Blood flow rates for a membrane separation device are usually set at approximately 100 to 150 mL/min.

(1) At these flow rates, the nurse expects a relatively low resistance throughout the system, as expressed by the return line pressure sensor.

(2) Pressure is monitored on both the access and return line.

(3) Audible alarms indicate pressures outside the pressure window that require intervention by the nurse.

(4) Pressure thresholds vary, depending on the TPE equipment used.

f. The initial access blood pump speed should be documented.

(1) The pump speed can be increased by 5 to 10 mL/min every 15 minutes if the patient remains stable and there is adequate blood flow.

(2) The maximum speed is determined by the device, the rate the anticoagulant is infused into the patient, the type of replacement fluid infused, the equipment manufacturer's recommendations, and/or the physician's prescription and institutional protocol.

g. Membrane separation equipment.

(1) The plasma filtrate pressure should be documented.

(2) The plasma pump controls plasma removal.

(3) The plasma flow rate varies depending upon what device or filter is used for the treatment. Often the plasma flow rate will run about 30% to 40% of the whole blood flow rate.

(4) The plasma flow rate is also dependent on the patient's HCT.

(a) The higher the HCT (i.e., > 40%), the less plasma the patient has for exchange and the shorter the treatment will be.

(b) For a very low HCT (i.e., < 30%), the plasma exchange may take longer.

(5) During TPE with membrane filtration, monitor the patient's ACT every 20 to 30 minutes. Adjust heparin to maintain ACT in desired, prescribed range.

2. Maintaining vascular access.

a. It is important to maintain blood flow from the patient to prevent positive and negative system pressure alarms.

(1) If alarms occur, the machine will pause and the reason for restricted flow should be corrected.

(2) Flushing the access or return line with saline may correct the problem, but frequent flushing dilutes the blood volume and gives the patient additional fluid.

b. Access and return pressure changes, when using a central line, can be caused by a thrombus or a fibrin sheath around the tip of the catheter.
   (1) If a clot is present, infusion into the port may be possible, but aspiration may be compromised, leading to an increased chance of recirculation (Chhibber & King, 2010).
   (2) This can result in a less efficient plasma exchange.

c. The fistula needles, whether using the antecubital vein or a fistula/graft, should be taped securely in place to prevent unintended removal or infiltration by patient movement.
   (1) Needle infiltration can lead to the permanent damage or loss of the blood vessel or graft.
   (2) The insertion sites should always be visible to the nurse to ensure prompt action if an infiltration occurs or the needle is accidentally removed completely from the access.

d. The patient should not feel constant pain at the insertion sites. "Buzzing" sensation of the vein is common and can indicate venospasm. This may be alleviated by:
   (1) Having the patient squeeze and release a soft object in the hand.
   (2) Repositioning the needle of the accessed extremity to ensure proper alignment within the blood vessel.

e. Keeping the extremity warm can dilate the vein, allowing good blood flow.

3. Fluid shifts.
   a. TPE may involve significant changes to the intravascular volume and hemodynamic changes may occur.
      (1) At the start of the TPE treatment, some instruments, such as the Cobe Spectra®, divert the prime saline into a waste bag leaving the patient with an initial fluid volume deficit of approximately 150 mL, which some patients cannot tolerate.
      (2) Those same devices often provide an option to allow the infusion of the saline prime to prevent this deficit.
      (3) The decision to waste or administer the prime should be defined in the treatment order.
      (4) It is important to know the options for prime saline delivery for the particular equipment being used.

b. Patients with heart disease and/or kidney failure are at a greater risk for hypervolemia.
   (1) In this situation, it may be advantageous to leave the patient isovolemic by decreasing the fluid balance slightly to accommodate the additional fluid administered during the blood reinfusion at the end of the procedure.
   (2) The TPE machine is designed to remove pathogens and proteins, not to perform ultrafiltration. Therefore, fluid volume removal is not routinely ordered as part of the TPE procedure.

c. The concepts of blood component rebound and equilibration should be understood in order to prevent TPE treatments from being scheduled too closely together.
   (1) Equilibration occurs as the body attempts to restore a normal, physiologic distribution of a particular substance in the intravascular and extravascular space.
   (2) For example, fibrinogen is restored to its pre-apheresis level in approximately 72 hours. If a patient's fibrinogen is critically low and TPE treatments are scheduled closer than 72 hours, the fibrinogen will not be able to replenish completely, leaving the patient at risk for bleeding.

4. Diagnosis related care.
   a. The nurse must take into account the neurologic and psychological status of the patient and provide patient care in light of this assessment.
      (1) A patient with TPE or a neurologic disorder may have an altered mental status. Patients may pull at, or dislodge, the vascular access.
      (2) It may be difficult for the patient to lie in bed for the length of time it takes to complete the TPE treatment.
      (3) In rare cases, the patient may need to be physically and/or chemically restrained while the treatment is taking place.

   b. Patients with cyroglobulinemia or cold-agglutinin disease cannot tolerate reduced blood temperatures. For these patients, and any patient receiving FFP as a replacement fluid, a blood warmer is added to the circuit.

   c. Certain medications and foods can affect the color of the plasma in the waste bag.
      (1) Patients with high lipid levels may have opaque plasma, making it difficult for automated interface detectors and hemolysis detectors to function properly.
      (2) Patients receiving antineoplastic medications may have green-tinged plasma.

(3) Patients with disease-causing hemolysis can present with very dark-colored plasma, resembling cola or tea.

d. It is customary to hold TPE treatments for uncontrolled bleeding at the biopsy site. If TPE is necessary, adding FFP to the replacement fluid near the end of the procedure can replace lost clotting factors.

e. TPE treatments typically precede rather than follow hemodialysis. The patient may present with a relatively low intravascular volume after hemodialysis related to ultrafiltration requirements. The patient's relatively low intravascular volume makes it difficult to maintain adequate blood pressure during the TPE treatment.

f. Patients with liver or kidney disease may have impaired citrate metabolism and are at increased risk of citrate toxicity. The patients usually require more calcium replacement during a treatment.

g. Some hyperviscosity syndromes can cause significant hypotension near the end of the treatment due to the sudden change in oncotic pressure. Occasionally, they may require extra fluid boluses to safely complete the treatment.

h. Patients receiving apheresis must have serial laboratory assessments done to document improvement or decline in his/her condition in response to the apheresis treatments.

D. TPE treatment termination.
1. Reinfusion/rinseback of cells in extracorporeal circuit.
   a. Once the PV has been exchanged, the cells in the disposable circuit should be reinfused with a normal saline rinseback. The entire circuit, including the blood warmer tubing, is flushed with normal saline to avoid loss of red cell volume.
   b. In certain situations, rinseback/reinfusion is avoided, such as when the procedure is terminated because the patient is expressing signs of moderate-to-severe citrate toxicity. During rinseback, the patient receives more citrate as the red blood cells are returned from the centrifuge. Patients experiencing citrate toxicity should not be given the rinseback, or rinseback should be deferred until symptoms have subsided.
2. Disconnection from apheresis devices.
   a. The patient's access and return lines must be disconnected prior to removing the disposable circuit set from the apheresis equipment. A failure to do so can result in excess fluid or citrate, or even air, entering the patient's circulation.
   b. After disconnection, the patient should slowly

go from a lying or sitting position to a standing position to allow for blood pressure equilibration and to avoid orthostatic hypotension, syncope and/or falling.

3. Care of vascular access.
   a. Peripheral access.
      (1) The needle sites must be held until hemostasis occurs.
      (2) Adequate pressure is held to prevent bleeding, but not occlusion of intravascular blood flow.
      (3) A dressing is then secured over the site.
      (4) Patients should be instructed to resume direct pressure at the site if bleeding recurs spontaneously after the nurse has left.
   b. Central venous catheter (CVC).
      (1) Flush each port with normal saline.
      (2) Fill with heparin or other anticoagulant. The lumen volume is usually printed on the catheter.
      (3) The concentration of the heparin fill is dictated by facility policy and varies from 1,000 to 5,000 units/mL.
      (4) The exit-site dressing on the catheter should be clean and dry at all times to prevent infection.
      (5) Document catheter and exit-site assessment and care, including pain at site.
      (6) Educate the patient regarding catheter care and infection prevention (e.g., have the patient verbalize signs and symptoms of CVC infection).
      (7) The CVC should be labeled to clarify the catheter must only be used for TPE and/or hemodialysis.

4. Disposing of the TPE circuit.
   a. The patient's plasma is collected in a closed collection container, and it must be handled using standard precautions for biohazardous waste disposal.
   b. Disposable supplies are discarded in contaminated/biohazard waste receptacles with care to remove any needles that may be part of the system.
   c. Needles must be disposed of in an appropriate sharps container.
   d. The machine is cleaned and stored in an area where it will not obstruct patient care or safety.

E. Adverse events (see Table 8.5).
1. Reaction categories (Kiprov et al., 2001).
   a. Mild reactions can be considered those reactions that can normally be anticipated and/or treated successfully without discontinuation of the procedure. Signs and symptoms include:

(1) Hypotension.
(2) Paresthesia.
(3) Hyperventilation.
(4) Nausea.
(5) Lightheadedness.
(6) Mild allergic reactions such as uticaria.
b. Moderate reactions may be classified as mild reactions that persist for > 20 minutes,

requiring intervention such as treatment pause, and/or medication.
c. Severe reactions include the moderate reactions along with any or all of the following.
(1) Respiratory insufficiency.
(2) Convulsions.
(3) Rigidity or tremor of the extremities.
(4) Cardiopulmonary arrest.

Table 8.5

Adverse Events

Problem	Signs & Symptoms	Potential Cause	Treatment	Rationale
Allergic reaction (Mild)	Urticaria Itching Rhinitis Cough	Allergy to iodine	Cleanse skin with an alternative antimicrobial	Decrease amount of allergic substance to the patient
		Allergy to FFP	Pause procedure, consider Benadryl, continue procedure if symptoms subside	Decrease generation of allergic substances
		Allergy to albumin	Change albumin to Dextran 40 or HES and/or saline after consult with physician	Decrease amount of allergic substance to the patient
Allergic reaction/ Anaphylactic (Moderate/ Severe)	Widespread urticaria Itching Rhinitis Cough Tongue swelling Wheezing	Allergy to FFP	Stop procedure Change unit of FFP Consider Benadryl Consider short-acting steroid Consult with physician	Decrease amount of allergic substance to the patient May require further medical attention
Air embolus (rare)	Chest Pain SOB Shock Pallor Confusion Cold sweats Death	Air entering venous system via tubing Requires > 15–25 mL in adults	Stop procedure and put patient on left side and Trendelenburg Consult with physician	Minimize effect on circulation Symptomatic treatment of SOB May require further medical treatment
Anxiety/ Apprehension	Restlessness Pallor Perspiration	Psychological (fear of procedure)	Reassure patient Be alert for signs of anxiety	Treat early symptoms Reverse possible causes Prevent further reaction
		Hypovolemia	Pause treatment Open IV lines to NS Consult with physician	Treat early symptoms Reverse possible causes Prevent further reaction
		Hypotension	Pause treatment Trendelenburg Open IV lines to NS Consult with physician	Treat early symptoms Reverse possible causes Prevent further reaction
		Allergic reaction	Consider drugs Consult with physician	Decrease generation of allergic substances
		Citrate toxicity	Decrease blood flow rates of blood return Warm with blanket or use blood warmer	Allow citrate to be metabolized Provide warmth to increase metabolism
		Hyperventilation	Have patient breathe into paper bag	Decrease respiratory alkalosis

Table continues

Table 8.5 (page 2 of 3) ——————— **Adverse Events**

Problem	Signs & Symptoms	Potential Cause	Treatment	Rationale
Arrhythmia	Pulse rate < 60 or > 100 Irregular pulse Both may cause: hypotension, dizziness, anxiety, perspiration, nausea or citrate toxicity	Vasovagal reaction Hypovolemia Hypotension Citrate toxicity Anaphylaxis	Stop procedure Identify cause Consult with physician	Maintain perfusion May require further medical attention
Cardiac arrest	Cessation of pulse and respiration	Citrate toxicity (rare) Severe hypotension or convulsion Related to primary disease	Stop procedure and initiate emergency resuscitation Initiate a CODE or call for emergency services Consult with physician	Must maintain oxygen perfusion
Chills/Tingling	Feeling cold especially in extremities, nose, and ears Vibratory or tingling sensation of face and extremities	Cold blood return	Use blood warmer or warm blankets	Some replacement fluids are below room temperature
		Anxiety	Educate and reassure patient frequently	Patients who know what to expect have less fear of procedure
		Citrate effect	Slow blood return: consider administering oral calcium (TUMS) in adult patient	Allow citrate to be metabolized Source of non-prescription calcium
		Hyperventilation	Use paper bag for hyperventilation	Decrease respiratory alkalosis
Citrate toxicity (mild)	Circumoral paresthesia Chills Coldness Vibratory or tingling sensation in face and extremities	Decrease in circulating ionized calcium	Slow or stop procedure until symptoms subside	Allow citrate to be metabolized
			Cover with blanket or use blood warmer	Provide warmth to increase metabolism
			Consider TUMS in adult patient	Source of nonprescription calcium
Citrate toxicity (moderate to severe)	Heaviness in chest Nausea/vomiting Muscle cramps Cardiac arrhythmias (irregular pulse) Tetany Cardiac arrest	Decrease in circulating ionized calcium	Stop procedure Consult with physician Consider IV calcium gluconate Treat arrhythmias Call CODE or emergency services	Allow citrate to be metabolized Replace calcium Further medical attention may be necessary
Congestive heart failure	SOB Chest pain Shock Pallor Confusion Death	Fluid overload	Raise HOB Reduce fluid infusion to KVO to maintain patent IV access Consult with physician Initiate CODE or emergency services if patient loses consciousness	Prevent additional fluids from building around the heart Prevent exacerbation of CHF Allow for injection of medication if necessary May require further medical attention

Table continues

Table 8.5 (page 3 of 3) ———— **Adverse Events**

Problem	Signs & Symptoms	Potential Cause	Treatment	Rationale
Fever	Temperature increase > 1°C during procedure May be accompanied by rigors	Incompatible blood transfusion Bacteremia: infected catheter Primary disease	Stop procedure and obtain blood sample as needed for lab Consult with physician	Stop infusion with potentially incompatible blood Obtain sample for workup and cultures May require further medical attention
Hemolysis	PINK or RED plasma Fever/chills Chest or back pain	Lysis of red blood cells May be caused by faulty disposable set May be caused by incompatible blood transfusion	Discontinue procedure immediately Consult with physician Notify manager	Do not return any additional hemolyzed cells to the patient Determination should be made as quickly as possible to determine cause in order to take appropriate corrective action Manager to notify manufacturer if equipment is suspected of being faulty
Hypotension	Restlessness Lightheadedness Dizziness Nausea/vomiting SOB	Vasovagal reaction Hypovolemia Citrate toxicity Anaphylaxis	Stop procedure Trendelenburg Consider saline infusion Rinseback blood if possible Consult with physician	Expand blood volume, restore blood pressure, and normalize circulation May require further medical attention
Hypovolemia	Decrease in BP Increase in pulse Pallor Dizziness Weakness Syncope	Volume loss usually greater than 15% of patients estimated blood volume	Stop treatment Trendelenburg Rinseback blood Consider saline infusion Consult with physician	Stop volume loss Increase venous return Replacement of lost volume May require further medical treatment
Nausea/Vomiting	May be accompanied by lightheadedness, hyperventilation, bradycardia, tachycardia, and/or hypotension	Hypotension Vasovagal reaction Hypovolemia Severe allergic reaction Citrate toxicity	As per potential cause	As per potential cause
Vasovagal reaction (mild)	Decrease in BP and pulse Pallor Dizziness Weakness Lightheadedness Hyperventilation Nausea Sweating	Anxiety Fear Pain Rapid blood removal from circulation Fatigue Hunger	Stop procedure Trendelenburg Open IVs to saline Instruct patient on procedure and reassure frequently throughout procedure Apply cold compress to forehead or back of neck For hyperventilation, have patient breathe into a paper bag Consult with physician	Increase venous return If patients have good understanding of procedure, their fears are more likely to be alleviated. The more comfortable patients are, the less likely they will have this type of reaction Decrease respiratory alkalosis
Vasovagal reaction (moderate to severe)	Bradycardia Hypotension Syncope	Anxiety Fear Pain Rapid blood removal from circulation Fatigue Hunger	Stop procedure Trendelenburg Open IVs to saline Consult with physician If pulse < 40 may require atropine with physician order	Improve perfusion May require further medical attention

References

Bladon, J., & Taylor, P.C. (1999). Extracorporeal photopheresis induces apoptosis in the lymphocytes of cutaneous T-cell lymphoma and graft-versus-host disease patients. *British Journal of Haematology, 107*(4), 707-711.

Burgstaler, E.A. (2010a). Apheresis instrumentation. In W. Linz, K. Crookston, D. Duvall, B. Kong, H. Jones, & S. Sabin (Eds.), *Principles of apheresis technology* (4th ed., pp. 13-26). Vancouver, B.C.: American Society for Apheresis.

Burgstaler, E.A. (2010b). Current instrumentation for apheresis. In B. McLeod, R. Weinstein, J. Winters, & Z. Szczepiorkowski (Eds.), *Apheresis: Principles and practice* (3rd ed., pp. 71-109). Bethesda, MD: AABB Press.

Chan, K.W. (2006). Extracorporeal photopheresis in children with graft-versus-host disease. *Journal of Clinical Apheresis, 21*(1), 60-64.

Chhibber, V., & King, K.E. (2010). Management of the therapeutic apheresis patient. In B. McLeod, R. Weinstein, J. Winters, & Z. Szczepiorkowski (Eds.), *Apheresis: Principles and practice* (3rd ed., pp. 229-249). Bethesda, MD: AABB Press.

Corbin, F., Cullis, H.M., Freireich, E.J., Ito, Y., Kellog, R.M., Latham, A., & McLeod, B.C. (2010). Development of apheresis instrumentation. In B. McLeod, R. Weinstein, J. Winters, & Z. Szczepiorkowski (Eds.), *Apheresis: Principles and practice* (3rd ed., pp. 1-25). Bethesda, MD: AABB Press.

Crookston, K.P., & Novak, D.J. (2010). Physiology of apheresis. In B. McLeod, R. Weinstein, J. Winters, & Z. Szczepiorkowski (Eds.), *Apheresis: Principles and practice* (3rd ed., pp. 45-69). Bethesda, MD: AABB Press.

Dau, P.C. (1995). Immunologic rebound. *Journal of Clinical Apheresis, 10,* 210-217.

Edelson, R., Berger, C., Gasparro, F., Jegasothy, B., Heald, P., Wintroub, B., … Laroche, L. (1987). Treatment of cutaneous T-cell lymphoma by extracorporeal photochemotherapy: Preliminary results. *The New England Journal of Medicine, 316,* 297-303.

George, S.M., Balogun, R.A., & Sanoff, S.L. (2011). Therapeutic apheresis before and after kidney transplantation. *Journal of Clinical Apheresis, 26,* 252-260.

Ibrahim, R.B., & Balogun, R.S. (2013). Medications and therapeutic apheresis procedures: Are we doing our best? *Journal of Clinical Apheresis, 28*(1), 73-77.

Kanold, J., Messina, C., Halle, P., Locatelli, F., Lanino, E., Cesaro, S., Demeocq, F., & Pediatric Diseases Working Group of the European Group for Blood and Marrow Transplantation (EBMT). (2005). Update on extracorporeal photochemotherapy for graft-versus-host-disease treatment. *Bone Marrow Transplantation, 35*(Suppl. 1), S69-S71.

Kintzel, P.E., Eastlund, T., & Calis, K.A. (2003). Extracorporeal removal of antimicrobials during plasmapheresis. *Journal of Clinical Apheresis, 18,* 194-205.

Kiprov, D., Golden, P. Rohe, R., Smith, S., & Weaver, R. (2001). Adverse reactions associated with mobile therapeutic apheresis-analysis of 17,940 procedures. *Journal of Clinical Apheresis, 15,* 19-21.

Kiprov, D.D., Burgstaler, E.A., & Sanchez, A. (2014). Apheresis instrumentation. In W. Linz (Ed.), *Principles of apheresis technology* (5th ed.) Vancouver, B.C.: American Society for Apheresis.

Kiprov, D.D., Sanchez, A., & Pusey, C. (2014). Therapeutic apheresis. In J.T. Daugirdas, T.S. Ing, & P.G. Blake (Eds.), *Handbook of dialysis* (5th ed., pp 333-359). Philadelphia: Lipppincott.

Morelli, A.E., & Larregina, A.T. (2010). Apoptotic cell-based therapies against transplant ejection: Role of recipient's dendritic cells. *Apoptosis, 15*(9), 1083-1097.

Scarisbrick, J. (2009). Extracorporeal photopheresis: What is it and when should it be used? *Clinical and Experimental Dermatology, 34*(7), 757-760.

Schwartz, J., Winters, J., Padmanabhan, A., Balogun, R., Delaney, M., Linenberger, M., … Shaz, B.H. (2013). Guidelines on the use of therapeutic apheresis in clinical practice-evidence based approach from the Writing Committee of the American Society for Apheresis: The sixth special issue. *Journal of Clinical Apheresis, 28*(3), 145-158.

Smith, J.W. (2010). Automated donations: Plasma, red cells, and multicomponent donor procedures. In B. McLeod, R. Weinstein, J. Winters, & Z. Szczepiorkowski (Eds.), *Apheresis: Principles and practice* (3rd ed., pp. 269-293). Bethesda, MD: AABB Press.

Tronier, W., Goodfellow, E., & Larson, K. (2010). Apheresis math and useful physical constants. In Linz, W. (Ed.), *Principles of apheresis technology* (4th ed., pp. 101-106). Vancouver, B.C.: American Society for Apheresis.

Ward, D.M. (2011). Conventional apheresis therapies: A review. *Journal of Clinical Apheresis, 26,* 230-238.

Weinstein, R. (2010). Basic principles of therapeutic blood exchange. In B. McLeod, R. Weinstein, J. Winters, & Z. Szczepiorkowski (Eds.), *Apheresis: Principles and practice* (3rd ed., pp. 269-293). Bethesda, MD: AABB Press.

Winters, J. (2011). Lipid apheresis, indications, and principles. *Journal of Clinical Apheresis, 26,* 269-275.

Winters, J.L., Crookston, K.P., Eder, A.F., King, K.E., Kiss, J.E., McLeod, B.C., & Sarode, R.S. (Eds.) (2011). *Therapeutic apheresis A physician's handbook* (3rd ed.). Bethesda, MD: AABB.

Zengin, S., Yilmaz, M., Al, B., Yildirim, C., Yavuz, E., & Akcali, A. (2013). Therapeutic red cell exchange for severe carbon monoxide poisoning. *Journal of Clinical Apheresis, 28*(5), 337-340.

Zielinski, I.D. (2002). Principles of apheresis. In C. Andrzejewski, P. Golden, B. Kong, A. Koo, J. Smith, & I. Zielinski (Eds.), *Principles of apheresis technology* (3rd ed., pp. 35-40), Vancouver, B.C.: American Society for Apheresis.

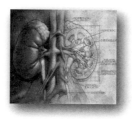

SELF-ASSESSMENT QUESTIONS FOR MODULE 4

These questions apply to all chapters in Module 4 and can be used for self-testing. They are not considered part of the official CNE process.

Chapter 1

1. The nephrology nurses' role in the acute care setting includes all of the following except
   a. delivering direct patient care using a variety of modalities of treatment.
   b. communicating with hospital care providers before, during, and after the dialysis treatment to ensure continuity of care.
   c. providing education on usual indications for dialysis including fluid overload, hyperkalemia, metabolic acidosis, and complications of uremia (e.g., pericarditis).
   d. giving instructions for home care including dressing changes of patient's temporary hemodialysis catheter at time of discharge.

2. Dialysis specific quality assurance (QA) is performed monthly and may include a review of
   a. patient census, acute dialysis treatments outside of regular hours of operation and nurse/patient ratio.
   b. incidence of access thrombosis and infection rates as well as requirements for access interventions to maintain patency.
   c. issues related to monitoring the dialysis unit's water quality and equipment breakdown.
   d. all of the above.

3. Staffing challenges in the acute care setting include
   a. coping with the demands of an acute care environment that do not always allow for planning.
   b. maintaining the annual competency requirements for equipment that is highly complex.
   c. the need to provide support to both patients and their families in the management of a disease process with limited prognostic certainty.
   d. all of the above.

4. Challenges related to acute care organizations include all of the following except
   a. costs associated with acute care is less now than it has ever been.
   b. the level and nature of demands for acute care are changing rapidly.
   c. advances in technology offer both advantages and challenges to institutions.
   d. maintaining an adequate, but yet not overly staffed workforce is difficult in an acute care environment.

5. Some of the resources that are commonly offered in the acute care setting include
   a. pastoral care.
   b. ethics committee.
   c. both a and b.
   d. all of the above.

6. All of the following are true about Hospital Consumer Assessment of Healthcare Providers and Systems (HCAHPS) except
   a. Inpatient Prospective Payment System (IPPS) annual payment update provisions must collect and submit HCAHPS data in order to receive their full annual payment update.
   b. HCAHPS does not allow valid comparisons to be made across hospitals locally, regionally and nationally.
   c. HCAHPS is the first national, standardized, publicly reported survey of patients' perspectives of hospital care.
   d. HCAHPS performance scores are included in the calculation of the value-based incentive payment in the Hospital Value-Based Purchasing program.

Chapter 2

7. Acute kidney injury affects approximately what percentage of hospitalized patients worldwide?
   a. 10% to 12%.
   b. 7% to 18%.
   c. 5% to 8%.
   d. 23% to 26%.

8. Acute kidney injury in the hospitalized patient is most commonly related to acute tubular necrosis secondary to all of the following except
   a. hydration.
   b. sepsis.
   c. ischemia.
   d. nephrotoxicity.

9. What is the role of biomarkers to predict AKI?
   a. To determine the etiology of AKI in only patients with potential for recovery.
   b. Permit early diagnosis of AKI, primarily to detect tubular injury.
   c. To determine the best treatment options.
   d. To determine renally adjusted drug dosing.

10. Which nursing interventions/collaborative treatment is the most effective in treating patients with AKI?
    a. Identify patients at risk.
    b. KRT.
    c. Provide education and support to patients and their families.
    d. Discuss and institute palliative care as deemed appropriate.

11. Your patient was diagnosed with hepatorenal syndrome and is hemodynamically unstable, and is started on CRRT. Why is CRRT the preferred renal replacement therapy for this patient?
    a. It will provide the most rapid correction of acidosis.
    b. It will lead to a rapid correction of volume overload.
    c. It will cause a rapid correction of hyperphosphatemia and thus preserves calcium and phosphorus homeostasis.
    d. It offers kidney replacement in a manner guided towards preserving hemodynamic stability.

12. Your patient is elderly and has developed AKI. What is unique related to signs and symptoms of AKI?
    a. The elderly may become symptomatic at lower levels of serum BUN and creatinine.
    b. Elderly patients do not develop rapid fluid shifts.
    c. Mortality risks in the elderly patient are the same as risks for any other age group.
    d. Will develop constitutional symptoms of sepsis before experiencing a decrease in urine output.

Chapter 3

13. Isolations precautions in the inpatient setting are used
    a. whenever someone is admitted with a diagnosis of having HIV.
    b. when routes of transmission are not interrupted by use of standard precautions.
    c. as a standard measure for anyone that is unkempt or had poor hygiene.
    d. for anyone that has not received the influenza or pneumonia vaccination.

14. Medications that routinely require dose adjustments for patients with kidney failure that are actively receiving dialysis include:

a. all categories of calcium channel blockers.
b. one class of potassium-sparing diuretics.
c. aminoglycosides.
d. guaifenesin.

15. Fluid that is immediately accessible for ultrafiltration during hemodialysis includes fluid that is found in
    a. brawny edema.
    b. ascitic fluid.
    c. the intravascular compartment.
    d. a pleural effusion.

16. Invasive hemodynamic monitoring provides information about
    a. pulmonary structure and function.
    b. information about cardiac output.
    c. cardiac tissue perfusion.
    d. paradoxical pulses.

17. Factors that may contribute to intradialytic hypotension include
    a. left ventricular ejection fraction of 60%.
    b. autonomic dysfunction with fluid overload.
    c. hemoglobin of 10 to 11 g/dL.
    d. corrected serum calcium 9 to 10 mg/dL.

Chapter 4

18. Which of the following is a symptom of exposure to chlorine during hemodialysis?
    a. Leg cramps.
    b. Hemolysis.
    c. Angioedema.
    d. Polycythemia.

19. Carbon filters are required in water treatment for hemodialysis in order to
    a. reduce the bacteria in the water.
    b. remove chlorine and chloramines.
    c. increase the sodium content of the dialysis fluid.
    d. remove turbidity from the source water.

20. A rejection rate refers to
    a. the number of particles rejected by the RO membrane.
    b. the percentage of particles presented to the RO membrane that are rejected to the drain.
    c. the amount of pressure placed on the RO membrane.
    d. the number of components that fail monitoring testing.

21. The most important component of the water treatment system for acute dialysis is
    a. the carbon tanks.
    b. the RO membrane.
    c. a competent staff.
    d. the endotoxin retentive filter.

22. The allowable level for total chlorine in dialysis treatment water is
    a. less than 0.1 ppm.
    b. equal to or greater than 1.0 ppm.
    c. achieving 2.0 ppm between the first and second carbon tanks.
    d. achieving 3.0 ppm between the first and second carbon tanks.

23. Disinfection of the water treatment system should be done
    a. only when there is evidence of bacterial growth.
    b. on a set schedule sufficient to prevent bacterial proliferation.
    c. only if there is suspicion of contamination.
    d. only if the city water supply is contaminated.

24. Portable water treatment equipment is at more risk of contamination due to
    a. intermittent use requiring more frequent connections.
    b. intermittent use requiring a larger water supply volume.
    c. lack of carbon tank filtration.
    d. lack of a distribution loop.

Chapter 5

25. When providing peritoneal dialysis in an acute care setting, daily patient assessments need to include
    a. the character of the peritoneal effluent
    b the patient's weight at the same time of day and in the same manner of dress.
    c. evaluation for adequate clearance by reviewing routine laboratory parameters.
    d. All of the above.

26. The frequency of peritoneal dialysis exchanges will depend on all of the following except
    a. patient fluid volume status.
    b. intact parathyroid hormone level.
    c. electrolyte abnormalities.
    d. presence of metabolic acidosis.

27. Contraindications for peritoneal dialysis include all of the following except
    a. reduction in visual acuity requiring glasses and living alone.
    b. traumatic injury to abdomen resulting in development of numerous adhesions.
    c. need for urgent dialysis due to hyperkalemia, serum potassium over 7 mg/dL.
    d. patient preference for hemodialysis as their kidney replacement modality.

28. With a standard silicone PD catheter, a 2-liter exchange volume can be expected to infuse in less than _____minutes, and to drain in _____minutes.
    a. 20, 15 to 20.

b. 25, 20 to 25.
c. 10, 15 to 20.
d. 10, 25 to 30.

29. Factors that are more likely to result in development of complications in the provision of acute peritoneal dialysis include all of the following except
    a. using a high concentration dianeal in someone that is volume contracted.
    b. using a low concentration dianeal in someone that is volume expanded.
    c. performing high volume exchanges in someone immediately following catheter placement.
    d. performing low volume exchanges in someone immediately following catheter placement.

30. Issues that have a higher incidence of occurrence following emergent temporary Tenckhoff catheter placement include all of the following except
    a. accidental disconnection of the temporary catheter and/or tubing.
    b. a higher risk for infection, peritonitis.
    c. referred pain to shoulders.
    d. bowel or bladder perforation.

Chapter 6

31. Choose the best definition of heart failure as described by the Heart Failure Society of America.
    a. Progressive heart dysfunction, characterized by ventricular dilation and/or hypertrophy.
    b. Inability of the heart to pump enough blood to maintain adequate perfusion.
    c. Systolic and/or diastolic dysfunction leading to neurohormonal and circulatory problems.
    d. A syndrome resulting in symptoms of fluid overload, shortness of breath and fatigue.

32. A normal left ventricular ejection fraction (EF) is represented by which of the following percentages?
    a. > 35%.
    b. > 45%.
    c. > 25%.
    d. > 55%.

33. What are the four parameters that need to be monitored/documented during hemodialysis?
    a. Speed, flow, pulsatility index, and power.
    b. Battery charge, flow, power, and speed.
    c. Alarms, battery fuel gauge, AC power, and flow.
    d. Power, alarms, flow, and speed.

34. Because the HM II LVAD is a continuous flow pump and a patient's pulse is most often not palpable, the best way to obtain a blood pressure is
    a. using a dynamap machine on the thigh.
    b. using a dynamap blood pressure machine on the arm.
    c. using a manual cuff, sphygmomanometer, and a Doppler probe over the brachial artery.

d. inflating a manual cuff on the patient's arm and obtaining a palpable reading.

35. After LVAD implant, acute kidney failure remains a significant problem most often caused by which of the following?
a. Right ventricular dysfunction, preexisting CKD, older age.
b. Respirator dependent pre-op, severe left ventricular dysfunction, elevated bilirubin.
c. Cachexia, anemia and Intra-aortic balloon pump preoperatively.
d. Elevated BNP, pulmonary hypertension and female gender.

36. Suction events or LV collapse is more likely to occur during hemodialysis when
a. the patient is hypovolemic from excessive ultrafiltration.
b. the patient is volume replete, but has electrolyte abnormalities.
c. the hemodialysis blood pump speed is reduced to what the access can safely deliver.
d. the hemodialysis blood pump speed is set at below what the access can deliver.

37. Choose the most important safety issues in order of priority when caring for LVAD patients:
a. Monitor changes in parameters, avoid MRIs, swimming, and tub baths.
b. Avoid chest compressions and be prepared for emergencies (e.g., power outages).
c. Keep room equipment dry, and avoid any potential to elicit a static electric shock.
d. Transport patient on batteries, and never disconnect both power leads simultaneously.

Chapter 7

38. You are doing your morning rounds on a patient on CRRT in the ICU and notice that the patient has been on the incorrect potassium bath for the last 6 hours. What is the next most appropriate nursing action?
a. Change the dialysate bath to coincide with what was prescribed and document.
b. Change the potassium bath to the correct one and document accordingly Notify the ICU charge nurse.
c. Notify the nephrologist.
d. Collect a stat potassium level and determine what dialysate is appropriate based upon result obtained.

39. Physician writes order for CRRT requesting net UF of zero mL per hour. Pt receiving IV meds; Levophed 10 mL/hr, calcium chloride 5 mL/hr, a PICC with TKOs NS 20 mL/hr and an IJ pig tail TKO NS 20 mL/hr plus Diprivan at 13 mL/hr.

Assigned RN is flushing system with 100 mL q hr. What UF rate should be programmed per hr on the machine?
a. 150 mL/hr.
b. 168 mL/hr.
c. 200 mL/hr.
d. None of the above.

40. The nephrologist orders CRRT with citrate for anticoagulation. What additional orders would you expect?
a. Hemoglobin and hematocrit every 3 to 4 hours.
b. Calcium and Phos protocol as dictated by physician or facility policy.
c. D5W drip @ 30 mL/hr with hourly glucose monitoring.
d. Rotation bed with hourly neuro checks.

41. Why is CRRT the best treatment option for critically ill patients with AKI?
a. Removes fluid and electrolytes quickly in order to avoid congestive heart failure.
b. Removes fluid/solutes slowly to reduce risk for hemodynamic instability.
c. Allows high ultrafiltration goals to be achieved in short period of time.
d. Allows low ultrafiltration goals to be achieved without changing electrolytes.

42. The filtration fraction (FF) should be below 10% because a
a. higher percentage will result in poor clearance.
b. higher percentage will result in supraphysiologic clearance.
c. lower percentage reduces the liklihood for clotting the dialyzer.
d. lower percentage will offset dialysate deliver and fluid replacement.

43. What is the recommended delivered dose of CRRT?
a. 25 mL/kg/hr.
b. 35 mL/kg/hr.
c. 20 mL/kg/hr.
d. 40 mL/kg/hr.

44. Severe hypophosphatemia may result with CRRT causing:
a. prolonged anticoagulation.
b. elevated blood pressures.
c. neurologic dysfunction
d. elevated serum calcium.

Chapter 8

45. List two methods of plasma separation.
a. Centrifugation and osmosis.
b. Filtration and osmosis.
c. Centrifugation and filtration.
d. Centrifugation and absorption.

46. Extracorporeal photopheresis (ECP) uses
    a. a one step process of infusing photoactivated mononuclear cells from a qualified donor.
    b. a two-step process of leukapheresis with photoactivation and reinfusion of treated cells.
    c. red blood cell exchange.
    d. plasma exchange.

47. Transfusion associated graft versus host disease
    a. rarely occurs.
    b. occurs frequently.
    c. occurs at a higher rate with available immunosuppression.
    d. occurs at a higher rate with kidney transplant compared to other solid organs.

48. Which device is an intermittent-flow device?
    a. Spectra Optia.
    b. UVAR-XTS cell separator.
    c. Amicus cell separator.
    d. Com.Tec cell separator.

49. The "buffy coat" layer consists of
    a. primarily red blood cells.
    b. primarily white blood cells.
    c. red blood cells and white blood cells.
    d. red blood cells and platelets.

50. Centrifugal devices separate blood components according to their
    a. size.
    b. solubility.
    c. saturation.
    d. color.

51. Low-density lipoprotein (LDL) apheresis is only FDA approved in the United States for treatment of patients with
    a. sickle cell crisis.
    b. cutaneous T-cell lymphoma.
    c. familial hypercholesterolemia.
    d. acute leukemia.

Answer Key

Chapter 1
1. d
2. d
3. d
4. a
5. d
6. b

Chapter 2
7. b
8. a
9. b
10. a
11. d
12. a

Chapter 3
13. b
14. c
15. c
16. b
17. b

Chapter 4
18. b
19. b
20. b
21. c
22. a
23. b
24. a

Chapter 5
25. d
26. b
27. a
28. c
29. d
30. b

Chapter 6
31. a
32. d
33. a
34. c
35. a
36. a
37. b

Chapter 7
38. c
39. b
40. b
41. b
42. c
43. a
44. c

Chapter 8
45. c
46. b
47. a
48. b
49. b
50. a
51. c

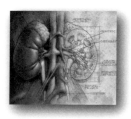

INDEX FOR MODULE 4

Page numbers followed by **f** indicate figures.
Page numbers followed by **t** indicate tables